TOTAL BREAST HEALTH

TOTAL BREAST HEALTH

The Power Food Solution for Protection and Wellness

Robin Keuneke

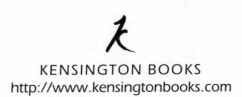

KENSINGTON BOOKS
http://www.kensingtonbooks.com

The guidelines presented in this book can be followed as part of a breast cancer prevention program, and also as an adjunct for women who may be healing breast cancer. Let your doctor or nutritionist know about any herbs or supplements you are taking. The information in this book is not intended as medical advice.

KENSINGTON BOOKS are published by

Kensington Publishing Corp.
850 Third Avenue
New York, NY 10022

Library of Congress Card Catalog Number: 97-074361
ISBN 1-57566-269-8

First Printing: June, 1998
10 9 8 7 6 5 4 3 2 1

Printed in the United States of America

ACKNOWLEDGMENTS

For their help in the making of *Total Breast Health*, I would like to thank the following people: Neenyah Ostrom for her steady hand, counsel, and humor during the long months of hard work; Lee Heiman for believing in this project; Tracy Bernstein for her skillful editing; Vicki Accardi; Udo Erasmus and Donald Yance for their generosity in sharing time and knowledge in contributing to this book; my friend Myrna Baye for her support and her keen eye in editing the recipes, and Susun Weed for her knowledge and creative energies for all women, and for her inspiration.

Thanks also to Lendon Smith, M.D.; Dixie Mills, M.D.; Michael Schacter, M.D.; Jon J. Michnovicz, M.D. (from the Foundation for Preventive Oncology in New York City); Alan Cohen, M.D.; Dimitrios Trichopoulos, M.D. (from the Harvard School of Public Health); and Carlo La Vecchia, M.D. (from the Instituto Di Richerche Farmacologiche Mario Negri in Milan, Italy), for their valuable time and information; and to Michael David Winther (from Efamol Institute); Ann Louise Gittleman for sharing her time and knowledge in the field of women's health; Dr. Blonnie Thompson (from the University of Bridgeport School of Nutrition) for her encouragement and input; Bert Schwitters, Joan Friedrich, Ph.D., and Carolyn Heller-West for their help; and Robert Crayhon.

Thanks to Josephine Mahi and Lyle Hurt from *Total Health* magazine; Jill Dotlo from WEBE and WICC radio in Connecticut for her interest in my work early on; and to Lori Duke and Diane Daddona from *Women's Magazine* in Connecticut.

With loving thanks to the following friends for their help and their recipes, which they have allowed me to include in *Total Breast Health*: Myrna Baye,

Pam Hatfield, and Rachel Luna; and to Ann Katz, Susan Kalev, and Marianne Hickey for their interest and support, and for sharing their stories with me. Gratitude also to my friend Marianne Hickey for contributing the chart on progesterone.

Thanks to Chef Alice Waters for her information and wonderful books; to Deanna Cross and Mindy Green for their help in aromatherapy; to Brigette Mars for her inspiration and knowledge in the field of herbs; and to Kimberly Gordon for supplying information on reflexology.

Thanks to Rosemary Gladstar for her work and inspiration; to herbalist and author Brigette Mars for her help; to Christiane Northrup, M.D., for her inspiration; to Francie King and to Oldways Preservation and Trust for their interest in this book. I particularly appreciate the use of Oldways' food pyramids.

Much appreciation to Paul Schulick for his time and information about ginger; to Anthony J. Cichoke for his work on enzymes; to the Herb Research Foundation; to the New York Academy of Medicine and Anthony Taylor; and to the wonderful Norwalk Public Library and the help of Judith Stark.

Gratitude to Suzanne Diamond for her articles and information; to Julie Baily at Mountain Rose Herbs; and to the following people who have helped in various ways to support this project: Cristina Salas-Porras; Tracy Roberts; Cristin Dicks; Gary Senecal, Trish Lefevre, and Bob Brownson.

Thanks to Caroline MacDougall, Susan Martin, Joan Rioux, Jean Eckrich, Cynthia Tenney, and the many other people who have helped and encouraged me in the creation of this project.

DEDICATION

This book is dedicated with love to the following significant people in my life: Thomas, my beloved husband and partner; my mother, Nancy Grant; my dear stepfather, Richard Grant; and my beloved grandmother, Edith Rottner, the most proficient cook I know. This effort is also for my Aunt Judith Ellison, a remarkable pastry chef; and the following creative women, who happen to be my cousins, and whose encouragement means so much: Nancy Thal, and Susan Kipperman. This dedication would be incomplete without acknowledging Gabriel Lightfriend, who helped to inspire this book; and all the researchers and health professionals who build the foundation of prevention, brick by brick. My profound gratitude to you all.

Finally, *Total Breast Health* is dedicated to my brother, Peter, in loving memory. I wish we could have shared this together.

CONTENTS

PART THREE

PART FOUR

FOREWORD

I want to apologize to the world and all the people who have read my books. I have been remiss because I did not know of the best methods of getting people well and keeping them that way until they are around one hundred years old. Now we have a big answer in *Total Breast Health*. We have all the evidence. We now know what to do.

We were taught in medical school that all we had to do—and that was plenty—was to make a diagnosis and then treat the condition with a drug supplied by the pharmaceutical industry. If that didn't work, try surgery. Then for those who did not fit into that paradigm of treatment, send the patient off to the psychiatrist. Our professors told us they had science on their side. Weren't all these methods tested and approved by the Food and Drug Administration? What more did we need? Anyone who doubted us medical doctors was a quack, or an unscientific know-nothing. I was trained in those methods, and did not question what I was taught until I hit some snags on the march to truth and decency.

What was wrong with our practice methods in the last few decades, if my patients were still getting sick? The parents of my pediatric patients asked me, "Why is he sick all the time? He is getting good foods, and we love him. What more are we supposed to do?" One of my little patients actually lived next door, and he never seemed to be sick. He even played in a mud puddle in the street outside, and never seemed to fall apart with some exotic intestinal calamity. What was going on? I was standing by to treat him when he was invaded by the germs and viruses in which he was swimming—but it never happened. I thought, "Maybe those neighbors are on to something." I began to do a little outside-of-the-mainstream reading, and it became obvious that modern "science" had been fooling us with their promise of a drug for every disease. That was a Band-Aid approach.

The big question for me was, 'Why had all these new diseases been showing up since the turn of the century? Heart attacks, Alzheimer's disease, autism, lupus, and autoimmune diseases have all become rampant in the last several decades.' Although antibiotics were helpful for those nasty diseases we love to treat, like pneumonia, pyuria, meningitis, and osteomyelitis, it appeared that we were saving people so they could get some degenerative disease or cancer. What was our purpose?

It became clear to me that we all must go back to our ancestors' diet: they had raw foods, no sugar, no white flour products, little dairy, and some seeds and whole grains. Lean meat only if one could catch the animal. But how do we get people today to run naked through field and forest, eating natural foods? We would probably be arrested and put in jail with a diet of doughnuts and coffee.

We now have some answers, and they are in this book. Robin Keuneke has researched the diets of people around the world. I would not have believed her work two decades ago, but there is no doubt about the wisdom of the proper diet and optimal cooking of our foods. I had thought that maybe just getting the right vitamins and minerals would solve all these twentieth-century diseases. They help, but we need the next step. Robin Keuneke has provided that step, and makes it easy for us. She supplies the motivation, the research findings, and the practical methods of getting a healthy diet, despite your doctor and the local supermarket. Pay attention! She is trying to save your life.

—Lendon H. Smith

I confess—I'm a foodie. My earliest memory of the feeling of pure joy is watching my mother, my maternal grandmother, and my aunt—all women I love dearly—make their way around my grandmother's kitchen in Connecticut. When I was old enough to cook, I loved the responsibility of helping my mother by making lunch and sometimes dinner. I sure could mess up a kitchen—and still can! Generous Aunt Judy actually encouraged my cousin Karen and me, when we were barely tall enough to reach the counter, to bake all kinds of confections in her kitchen. What a stack of dishes and pots and pans we left her, but our lopsided cakes and other creations tasted just right.

As an adult, I learned to appreciate more fully how food touches so many areas of our lives. Food creates pleasure, delighting and surprising our sense of taste. It also provides beauty. The true, pure colors of fruits and vegetables exemplify the richest palette—nature's. Where does a more beautiful shade of red exist than in a tomato? The presentation of food, a form of expression that reflects the cook's personality, can also provide beauty and surprise. Food is a source of endless enlightenment, linking us to other cultures and lives in all parts of the world. Food can also remind us of times gone by. Consider the unforgettable taste of a summer tomato allowed to ripen on the vine, picked at the peak of flavor, and eaten that same day. When you taste that perfect tomato, doesn't it bring you back to your childhood when your mother or grandmother fed you a summer lunch on the porch, in a tree house, at the beach?

Food is memory. It is nourishment. It is art. It is even existential, providing elements of health—or of illness.

This book was written to inspire. Food is delicious, but it can also help to protect us and the people whom we love. Although more funds for research are needed, especially for prevention, there already exists quite a bit of very specific information about how vegetables, fruits, herbs, and foods such as freshly pressed oils; fresh, fatty-rich fish; and grains can help to protect our health. Certain phytochemicals in vegetables, for example (phytochemicals are the nonnutrient substances in vegetables that we cannot see, taste, or smell), can detoxify potential carcinogens (like pollutants), protect DNA, and block tumor growth. A nutrient-dense, whole foods diet can help to create health in many ways.

In the process of writing this book, it became evident to me that the recipes and information in *Total Breast Health* have implications for preventing many illnesses besides breast cancer. Studies indicate that flax seed and extra virgin olive oils help to protect the prostate and colon from cancer. Also protective for the prostate and colon are cruciferous vegetables, soy foods, and common herbs such as parsley and rosemary. Attention deficit disorder (ADD) in children can be positively affected by the recommendations in this book, as can adult diseases like arthritis, heart disease, and depression. Many studies show, for example, that addressing a deficiency of essential fatty acids by adding healing oils to the diet can help to prevent all of these problems from developing.

Let's go back to that juicy, flavorful tomato—symbol of the sun, of warmth and summer. Take just a few moments to make a simple vinaigrette for that tomato: extra virgin olive oil, lemon juice, shallots, mustard, and a touch of fresh rosemary. Season it with sea salt and freshly ground pepper. What a delicious dressing for that fresh tomato! But did you know that olive oil helps to protect the arteries and keeps dangerous cholesterol from building up, regulates blood sugar, and may help to prevent cancer? Furthermore, the oil acts as a transport system for the antioxidants contained in the tomato and the rosemary, helping the body to metabolize these nutrients. Did you know that in animal studies shallots dramatically block cancer? Shallots are the strongest source of quercitin, a powerful antioxidant known to protect against stomach and other cancers. This type of simple, but healthful, vinaigrette of olive oil, lemon, and herbs is commonplace in the Mediterranean, in France, and in Italy—cultures known for their wonderful food. We *can* combine flavor and health; one does not have to be sacrificed for the other. It is this revelation that inspired *Total Breast Health*.

I love food, and have studied its preparation all over the world. I've eaten herring in Oslo, paprika stews in Budapest, mezas in Jordan and Istanbul. I've enjoyed the wonderful and varied foods of Europe. The people with whom you share an experience can also be a source of nourishment. One of the most memorable refreshments I was ever honored to receive was freshly brewed jasmine tea served to my husband and me by a Bedouin family in Jordan as we all sat on carpets. The memory of drinking tea with this Bedouin family, their donkey tied up outside their tent, will forever be imprinted in my heart, because this warm family offered us the very best they possessed. To help keep the memory alive, we searched for the exact type of tea and glasses the Bedouins had used to bring home with us from Jordan.

Focusing on health, by nourishing ourselves and those we love, goes beyond food. Taking a little extra time to select and prepare healthy foods (as opposed to eating poor-quality, processed foods that are perhaps more convenient) reflects other forms of nourishment. Being loving and forgiving, for example, is another. Exercising on a regular basis is yet another. Caring for oneself, and making healthy choices in all aspects of our lives, is what focusing on health is all about.

Creating Breast Health

It is time to focus attention on the things you can do to lower your risk of developing breast cancer: What and how much you eat, how you move your body and whether you smoke cigarettes. While the importance of such factors is not as firmly established as that for cancer genes and menstrual history, the accumulating data have convinced many experts that behavioral adjustments are more than justified.

—Jane Brody, *New York Times,* May 1997

There is no doubt that women fear breast cancer more than any other illness, or that the media feeds this fear with constant reports that the malady is on the rise.

We are confronted almost every day with potential but unconfirmed new causes for breast cancer that concern prudent women: Are the birth control pills taken years ago contributing factors? What about the estrogen levels associated with early menarche of late menopause? Are the potential benefits of estrogen replacement therapy, like decreasing loss of bone mass, negated by an elevated risk of developing breast cancer? Are environmental factors—such as pesticides, chlorine, or formaldehyde—partly to blame for the explosion in numbers of breast cancer cases? Does sunlight protect against cancer or increase our risk? What is the impact of weight gain?

Although we are limited in how much we can change our environment and heredity (as well as our children's), women's fear and feelings of helplessness can be offset by the knowledge that influencing our health is really in our power. We do have choices! Instead of becoming resigned to the seemingly inexorable advance of breast cancer, we can become informed about our choices, and take steps that protect our health and help to prevent breast cancer. We can also make choices to prevent heart disease and lung cancer, which take more women's lives each year than breast cancer.

An important pathway to preventing or reversing degenerative conditions such as breast cancer is to influence our health positively: We can improve the food we eat, we can exercise, and we can learn to relax more. Researchers are still investigating the role a person's mental state has on well-being; most people, however, understand that there is a direct correlation between what we choose to feed our bodies and how they respond. I also feel that emotions and thoughts have a strong influence on our health. If we put to practical use all that is known about stress reduction and nutrition and their effects on preventing breast cancer (and other illnesses), we will be accomplishing something very significant: focusing on health, not disease.

Men can also benefit from what researchers are learning about using foods to prevent cancer. Foods containing substances that are protective against breast cancer also protect against cancers of the prostate and colon. For example, Jon J. Michnovicz, M.D., director of The Foundation for Preventive Oncology in New York City, and co-author of *How to Reduce Your Risk of Breast Cancer*, has found that indole-3-carbinol (a phytochemical found in cruciferous vegetables like kale and broccoli) is beneficial in preventing all of these cancers.

In addition to what is already known about nutrition and its impact on breast cancer, there is a great deal of exciting research being made public almost daily about specific foods, herbs, and teas with powerful, and often clinically documented, "chemoprotective" effects. Consider, for example, flaxseed.

Flaxseed, in addition to being the richest source of one of the two essential fatty acids, has been found to contain plant lignans that are precursors for the protective estrogens called phytoestrogens. Lignans possess antiviral, antifungal, antibacterial, and anticancer properties. This class of chemical compounds, according to the *Women's Health Advocate Newsletter* (June 1996), "protects against a number of hormone related conditions, ranging from hot flashes and fibroids to breast and ovarian cancer."

Soybeans, too, are phytoestrogen-rich. In 1992, *The Lancet*, a British medical journal, reported a study of Japanese women going through menopause. The study concluded that these women had infrequent hot flashes because of the phytoestrogens consumed in soy sauce, miso, and tofu—all made from soybeans—as well as from eating soybeans themselves. Not surprisingly, Japanese women also have minimal breast cancer, heart disease, and osteoporosis. A study conducted at the University of Alabama in 1996 found that genistein, a soy isoflavone, is able to inhibit the spread of breast cancer cells. Omega-3 fatty acid from diets that include flaxseed oil or fish oil offer significant protection against breast cancer in animal studies.

Breast Cancer Prevention Is Effective Against Many Hormone-Related Problems

A simple but powerful fact is this: What benefits breast health helps the entire body, particularly the endocrine system. The endocrine system is a vast complex, interactive group of glands (including the thyroid, pituitary, and adrenals), nervous system tissues (like the portion of the brain called the hypothalamus), and the hormones they produce (like insulin, estrogen, and cortisone). Imbalance of the endocrine system's hormones can result in conditions as diverse as diabetes, hypoglycemia, goiter, and cancer. Conditions that Western women, especially Americans, take for granted—such as mood swings, menstrual cramps, and symptoms of menopause—result from hormonal imbalances. These conditions are the direct result of the Western diet, which has a profound deficiency of fresh vegetables, fresh organic oils, and soy foods, as well as excesses of sugar, hormone-laced meat and dairy, and junk fats such as margarine and highly refined supermarket oils.

It is no secret that North American women suffer from among the highest rates of cancer, heart disease, and osteoporosis (loss of bone mass)—not to mention symptoms of PMS and menopause—of women anywhere in the world. Sadly, with the spread of American fast food worldwide, we will share our junk food legacy with other cultures, thereby profoundly affecting the health of people everywhere.

Colon cancer is a hormone-sensitive cancer, taking more lives a year than breast cancer. The recommendations in this book will help to prevent colon cancer: eating lots of vegetables and fruit; a nutrient-dense, whole foods diet prepared without the use of heated oils, broiling, or grilling, and lifestyle modifications like daily exercise and reducing or eliminating alcohol.

How I Began My Journey to Natural Foods and Holistic Health

Soon after marrying my husband, Thomas, in San Francisco in 1976, I began to study French cooking. San Francisco was a beautiful place to live as newlyweds, a great place to enjoy gourmet meals in exotic restaurants and food shopping in the many different ethnic markets. My cooking skills, which were already well developed, improved during our time in San Francisco. Food was (and is) a passion.

In 1980, we moved to New York City, and one day, in the basement of our Manhattan apartment building, I found a discarded book on macrobiotics. I remember that, as I leafed through it, I couldn't believe people made a steady diet of such foods as tempeh, natto, and seitan. What were these foods, anyway? More to the point, these foods and their preparation were beyond my experience. Nevertheless, I felt drawn to the message of macrobiotics.

As a result of my serendipitous discovery, Thomas and I embarked upon a journey that would turn my notion of nutrition on its head. Thomas was definitely not as enthusiastic as I was; in fact, he hated to give up dishes such as chicken with apples, Calvados brandy, and cream. Nevertheless, I began incorporating a few of the book's suggestions, such as eliminating sugar and dairy, cutting back on coffee, and adding nutritious foods such as whole grains and dark leafy green vegetables to our regular diet. Soon, we were eating tofu and beginning the process of eliminating meat. The temple that had been our diet of gourmet-quality meals heavily reliant on fat, sugar, and animal products was slowly being deconstructed and rebuilt from the ground up! The trick, as I soon realized, was to make natural foods actually taste good, a detail that Thomas didn't consider minor.

Although I was open to the possibility that food and physical well-being were connected, I was not prepared for the dramatic, almost immediate reversal of health conditions that I had always viewed as lifelong afflictions. The same was true for Thomas, as he hesitantly admitted.

I had battled insomnia for years, but now found the instant, delicious sleep of my childhood and the incredibly precious gift of waking rested and energized. With the disappearance of the insomnia went my reliance on aspirin, as well—no more daily headaches. One month into this new way of eating, I experienced my first pain-free menstrual period—no cramps!

Thomas found that on his trips overseas, jet lag soon ceased to be a problem. His body adjusted with amazing speed to changing time zones, which were sometimes as much as twelve hours apart. His spring-summer allergy, with its debilitating sneezing jags, runny nose, and postnasal drip, never recurred. Talk about positive reinforcement! I have never experienced a clearer or more striking demonstration of cause and effect: Replace empty calories, processed foods, and sugar with fiber-rich, nutrient-dense, natural foods, and the body responds. We were amazed! There was no going back and no thought of it, really. We were facing a lifestyle change, and there was only one thing left for me to do. Go back to school. I couldn't wait.

Focusing on Health: Cooking School

My cooking skills gradually adjusted to this radical method of food preparation as I voraciously absorbed knowledge about creating health through selection and preparation of natural foods. The Macrobiotic Center in New York City reinforced what I was learning, and introduced me to a seemingly endless variety and combination of foods utilizing a wide array of vegetables, whole grains, soy foods, beans, sea vegetables, sugar-free desserts, pickles, noodles, and more. I learned about "healing foods" such as umeboshi, burdock root, and daikon. I was fascinated to learn that the philosophy of yin and yang, the need for balance in all things, applied to the amount, type, and combination of foods we eat. It was pretty esoteric stuff, many times without scientific basis, but with the weight of centuries of practice behind it—a precedent I couldn't resist. It was while studying macrobiotics that I first learned Asian women have lower rates of heart disease, cancer, and osteoporosis than do women in the West—another reinforcement.

One of the most profound aspects of the time I spent at The Macrobiotic

Center was the opportunity to associate with people who were pursuing methods of healing, including the healing of illnesses such as breast cancer. Their stories of survival and gaining a second chance at life through a fundamental change of diet were moving, affirming, and empowering.

Even our beloved bulldog, Gertrude Stein, was co-opted into our nutritional rebirth, and she reaped the benefits of renewed health along with her owners. Bulldogs have a propensity to suffer benign tumors on their paws, as well as chronic eye infections. They also snore a lot, and Gertie was pure bulldog. Surgically removing the tumors is expensive and relatively risky for this breed, and besides, they just pop out again somewhere else. Her eye problem required ever-increasing applications of antibiotic ointment; for the snoring, her owners required ear plugs.

Then, we changed to a holistic vet. Following his advice, we threw out Gertie's commercial chow and the ointment and began feeding her our leftovers. She became quite fond of miso soup, squash (one of her favorites), daikon, broccoli, kale, seaweed (no kidding), tofu, tempeh, and brown rice. Gertie would drool with anticipation as we scooped servings of these foods into her bowl—can you imagine? Almost overnight, her health seemed to respond. The eye infections eventually cleared, and the tumors never reappeared. At the risk of stretching believability, even her snoring subsided—though it never did stop.

After New York, my journey took me to holistic centers throughout Europe, including the East-West Center in London and René Levy's Macrobiotic Center in St. Gaudin, France. The natural food movements in Lisbon, Paris, and Milan, with their many wonderful restaurants and inventive dishes, were exotic and impressive.

But perhaps most revealing for me was the purity and quality of foods in developing countries like Jordan where, out of necessity, everything is locally grown, raised, or produced, and eaten fresh, whole, and unprocessed. Without question, the best-tasting, most nutritious meals I've ever eaten were prepared in these faraway places whose people have never heard the word "macrobiotics." What I knew as the natural foods movement was, to them, simply food preparation as their ancestors had practiced it for generations. But the spirit of what the macrobiotic and other natural foods movements advocate is alive in these cultures, and they have a lot to teach us about creating health.

Leaving Macrobiotics Behind

As I became more knowledgeable about nutrition through my own research and practical experiences, I realized that there is no one way to possess the truth about nutrition, but many paths toward that truth. Macrobiotics is only one such path; however, in my opinion, it is not perfect, and perhaps the single most important area in which it is deficient is fats and oils. Macrobiotics does not offer enough information about these substances or advocate their role in health—a serious oversight. People are more deficient in essential fatty acids than in any other nutrient.

Practitioners of macrobiotics are not alone in this oversight. Until 1994, when the work pioneered by Udo Erasmus—a researcher, lecturer, and author with a Ph.D. in nutrition—became known in this country, little or no thought was given to fats and oils, except for the general belief that they should be avoided.

The indisputable fact is that we need certain of these substances, the "good fats," in as natural a state as possible, unheated and fresh. They provide essential nutrients not available elsewhere. For all there is to rejoice in about the macrobiotic diet, its advocacy of heating oils for cooking (or using soy margarine), or eliminating oil altogether, may not contribute to health.

Learning about fats and oils was a real epiphany for me. Freshness of ingredients had always been important in my food preparation, but became paramount as I came to understand more about its relationship to well-being. This understanding was enhanced by my experience overseas. The Italians, for example, wouldn't plan the menu for a dinner party before going to the market to see what was fresh that day. This is the basis for creating not only flavor, but also health. At my home, garden-fresh, dark, leafy greens are preferable to yesterday's leftovers. The same is true of oils. Why buy highly processed, rancid oils in clear bottles in supermarkets, when what is needed and available are freshly pressed, unprocessed oils in light-protective dark glass, complete with pressing date to ensure freshness? Why roast seeds and nuts if heat destroys the nutrients?

The Truth About Fats and Oils

Research groups from around the world have identified the cancer-protective effect of Omega 3 oils.
—Jeffrey S. Bland, Ph.D., *Delicious!*, September 1997

The truth is, as Udo Erasmus has articulated, fats and oils can create health or destroy it. That's a powerful statement about substances that most people take for granted, yet are widely misunderstood. Although this subject will be explained in greater detail in later chapters, it's important to possess a fundamental understanding of why certain oils are essential to good health, while others can harm or even destroy it.

In 1994, the year Erasmus introduced me and other Americans to proper oil usage, Harvard published a study acknowledging that margarines doubled the risk of heart disease. What people in the natural foods movement had suspected for years was finally validated by one of the most respected medical institutions in the land: Margarine is, indeed, not a healthy choice. In 1997, a study from the University of North Carolina offered further confirmation, correlating the consumption of trans-fats found in processed margarines, vegetable oils, and other foods with an increase in breast cancer.

There is evidence that consuming saturated fat increases the risk of breast cancer in women, as well as evidence that consuming olive oil may prevent it. While some studies associate breast cancer risk with margarine consumption, margarine was always examined within a general group of fatty foods, so its specific risk has been hard to evaluate. In 1975, researchers found a correlation between consumption of fried foods such as French fries and an increased risk of breast cancer—another finding that needs further evaluation. There is clearly a need for researchers to focus on the specifics of this puzzle.

Nevertheless, much exciting information has been generated during the last several years about the protective qualities of flaxseed and olive oils and fatty-rich fish, particularly in relationship to breast cancer.

The fats and oils we consume function in our bodies as precursors for powerful, hormone-like substances called prostaglandins. We are constantly making prostaglandins, of which there are many types. The various types frequently have opposing actions. Some increase inflammation, for example, while others reduce inflammation. Researchers have discovered that, by altering the type of dietary fats we eat, we can change the balance of these various prostaglandins. By replacing our intake of harmful fats such as transfats, margarines, shortening, hydrogenated oils, and saturated fats with fresh, unprocessed oils, we can protect against cancer, lower triglycerides and cholesterol, reduce platelet aggregation (which can reduce heart attack risk), and reduce inflammation.

Essential fatty acids are so vital to our health that they used to be called "vitamin F." These substances in unprocessed, fresh oils are absolutely necessary for health and are as important as the other essential vitamins, minerals, and amino acids. Because there is a general unavailability of healthy oils, and because of mass commercialization of highly processed oils, most women (and men) are deficient in essential fatty acids. Omega-3 and omega-6 (the two essential fatty acids) are needed for proper immune and organ function, healthy cell membranes, proper kidney and hormone function, and oxygen transport. Adding fresh, unheated oils in small amounts to the diet is a great way to consume them, since many vitamins and nutrients in our food are oil soluble.

Consider flaxseed oil, the richest source of omega-3. Studies show that consumption of flaxseed oil (and flaxseed) can result in reducing tumor size by more than 50 percent. Consuming both flaxseed and flaxseed oil may be important for breast health.

The journey I began years ago in the basement of my apartment building not only taught me to recognize such misconceptions, but provided the inspiration to help others discover the correct ways to use health-giving oils in food preparation, for both disease prevention and healing.

Food Offers Protection Against Pollution

Many women I meet, intimidated by the pervasiveness of problems with our air, water, and food supplies, seem resigned to the inevitability of the statistical advance of breast cancer. Why bother to take care of ourselves when air pollution may get us anyway?

The amazing thing is that some foods available to us can actually help to protect us against pollution. Glutathione, for example, a nutrient found in parsley and raw spinach, can help to eliminate pollutants. If my journey of discovery convinced me of anything, it is that food can be a powerful ally in creating health and preventing disease. As long as we have this potential arsenal at our disposal, we should use it.

For instance, the person whose livelihood depends on logging innumerable hours in front of a computer screen, knowing the risks involved, need not feel helpless. Studies show that sea vegetables, particularly wakame and kombu, help to remove radiation from the body. There is also no reason to fear that cancer is inevitable when there are foods and other natural substances that can help prevent its development. For instance, according to research done in Japan, Russia, and India, green tea has powerful anticancer properties and the ability to suppress solid tumor formation completely. While health is neither destroyed nor restored overnight, we can make choices as informed individuals to safeguard our health and remove some of the anxiety of living in a dangerous world. It is comforting and empowering to have these choices. It's also important to acknowledge that cancer and other illnesses are more easily prevented than treated.

A New Paradigm for Ourselves, and Our Daughters

Will my generation, the Baby Boomers, be the first to stop the epidemic of breast and other cancers? We certainly are the first generation to think in terms of prevention. The health food movement began, was nurtured, and flourished on our watch. The magazine ads of the 1940s and 1950s, pitching the health advantages of margarine and even cigarettes, are now long gone. We were the first generation in America to question much of the status quo our parents had accepted. Baby Boomers were the first generation to question conventional medicine, with its emphasis on treating disease, and to begin looking to holistic practitioners who advocate prevention and the importance of nurturing well-being. That is our rich legacy to future generations: the knowledge necessary to create and maintain health naturally, through nutrition, diet, exercise, and relaxation.

Women in my generation created a new paradigm for health. We coined the term PMS, bringing menstruation "out of the closet." Some of us even breastfed in public. Twenty-five million Americans will enter menopause by the end of this century, more than at any other time in history. Pharmaceutical companies, armed with sophisticated market research, have targeted our generation for "new and safer treatments for menopause" (as was advertised in 1995 in the *New York Times*), realizing that we ask far more questions than our mothers did. Women today are less likely consumers of artificial hormones to treat symptoms of menopause. How can we ignore the alarming results of the 1995 Harvard nurses study of 122,000 women, which showed that estrogen, even when combined with progestin (an artificially produced progesterone formerly thought to be protective against estrogen's cancer-promoting qualities), was found to increase breast cancer risk by 30 to 40 percent? Another study, published in the *New England Journal of Medicine* in 1997, indicated that long-term use of postmenopausal hormones is implicated in increased mortality from breast cancer.

Our mothers were, and quite possibly still are, avid consumers of artificial estrogen and progestin. They were the ones who made Dr. Robert Wilson's now out-of-print 1968 book *Feminine Forever* a bestseller. In it, he spoke degradingly of menopausal women as "sexless creatures, caricatures of their former selves," who "would become the equivalent of a Eunuch." We can laugh at Dr. Wilson's book today. What is not so funny, however, is that Wilson's advocacy of artificial hormones has resulted in questionable consequences for millions of women. While Wilson's language now seems dated, drug companies continue to exploit the confusion surrounding the issue of hormone replacement therapy to tap into the multibillion-dollar market that it still is. Drug companies continue to foster fear in women through a relentless and well-funded advertising campaign that claims postmenopausal life without these drugs is one of high risk for heart disease and osteoporosis. I find this misleading. There are women living elsewhere in the world—in the Mediterranean, for example, as well as in China and Japan—who do not take hormones and do not develop heart disease or osteoporosis. Shouldn't researchers begin studying groups of women who have never taken hormone replacement therapy and do not have heart disease or osteoporosis? Isn't it time to begin studying health and prevention more aggressively?

I don't think my generation and those to follow can be manipulated by messages of fear. We know how to protect our bodies by selecting healthy foods, engaging in physical exercise (studies show light weight training protects bones from osteoporosis), and utilizing nutrition to maintain health. In other words, *we are a generation ready to focus on health, instead of disease.*

None of these conditions—osteoporosis, post-menopausal heart disease, or breast cancer—is the inevitable result of aging. Are artificial hormones required to prevent them? I am convinced that the foundation for preventing breast cancer, in particular, lies in strengthening the immune system and other vital bodily processes by changing our diets to include more nutrient-dense foods. There is much we can do to safeguard our health and actually prevent breast and other cancers.

More people than ever before are turning to natural medicine and nutrition to improve their personal well-being. Moreover, much exciting research is showing that certain foods contain powerful phytochemicals that help to prevent illnesses such as breast cancer. Researchers are supporting the need for better food selection, including consuming a wider variety of vegetables. Studies are showing that whole foods (such as vegetables, grains, and herbs) are the best source for vitamins. A 1994 study conducted at the Dartmouth Medical School found that vegetables, because of their antioxidant properties, are better than vitamin supplements for lowering the risk of colon cancer, for example.

In an interview, Jon J. Michnovicz, M.D., shared with me the following statement: "Preventing breast cancer is do-able. It is not out of reach. It is easier to prevent breast cancer than people realize. My best advice for women is to begin now. Begin by eating five servings of different fruits and vegetables each day. This is the most important aspect of breast cancer prevention." Foods and their phytochemical compounds figure prominently in alternative anticancer agents because they are not cytotoxic (damaging to all cells, not just cancer cells). There are already enough toxic cancer treatments, including chemotherapy and radiation.

Sir David Weatherall, Oxford University's Regius Professor of Medicine, has written that much of this century's scientific focus has been researching "the major killers of western society, particularly cancer." He added that, "Although we have learned more and more about the minutiae of how these diseases make patients sick, we have made little headway in determining why they arise in the first place." The focus of research has been on sickness, not prevention.

Total Breast Health offers women a guide to foods that are rich in breast-protective phytochemicals, as well as the most recent research exploring those phytochemicals and how they *specifically* contribute to breast cancer prevention. An exciting collection of recipes, featuring a broad spectrum of vegetables and herbs as well as protective oils, utilizes these power foods and describes the healthiest ways of preparing them.

Many people are confused by the mixed messages they're receiving about using fats and oils in their diets, in part because this area of nutritional research is relatively new. For example, some cookbooks recommend frying, broiling, or sautéing with flaxseed oil. Heating flaxseed oil is *not* a healthful practice. In fact, studies show that light and heat are damaging to flaxseed oil; special care must be used in pressing and bottling this important, immune-enhancing, cancer-preventing nutrient. Special care, too, must be taken to use flaxseed oil *unheated*. Heat may also alter potentially protective effects of olive oil. Trans-fats and other unidentified, harmful substances are created when oil is heated, and there is evidence that these substances promote breast cancer. Other recent studies have shown that people who eat roasted meat—which is cooked at a much lower temperature than fried or grilled meat—have no increased risk of stomach cancer; frying and grilling of meat, however, is linked to increased risk of stomach cancer. It is important to know what foods provide in terms of protective properties and nutrients, and to understand how to prepare those foods.

Lifestyle is also important in creating breast health, and Chapter 20, "Personal Care Guide," contains important information on natural medicine, exercise, body care tips, aromatherapy, and other information designed to encourage a strong immune system.

I have collected the recipes and other information in *Total Breast Health* during many years of counseling women about their diets. I've witnessed all kinds of wonderful improvements in health as women incorporate these power foods into their diets, and some of these women are interviewed in *Total Breast Health*. It is evident to me that a healthy diet, rich in vegetables and protective oils, is of primary importance in restoring health. I have seen conditions such as breast cancer, depression, chronic yeast infections, arthritis, heart disease, and other chronic ailments ameliorated when a nutrient-dense diet is consumed. Witnessing so many women restore their health by changing their food selections and preparation techniques inspired me to make the information presented here as specific and complete as possible.

In May 1997, the *Townsend News Letter for Doctors and Patients* noted that, "The most successful way women have beaten breast cancer is with diets high in phytochemicals." *Total Breast Health* grew out of a wish to inspire women to make healthier choices in their lives each and every day, choices that current research indicates can protect against breast cancer.

The research areas of food chemistry, nutrition, hormones and cancer (breast, colon, and prostate), and cardiovascular disease have all contributed tantalizing hints about the relationship of fats and oils to health. For example, *Supplement to Nutrition* published a study in 1996 indicating that dietary omega-3, from flaxseed oil and fatty-rich fish, is important in preventing breast cancer. As with omega-3, it is extremely important to consume omega-6 (linoleic acid) from *unprocessed* sources only, such as sunflower seed oil or sesame seed oil, and to strictly avoid *processed* sources, including margarine, to obtain this benefit. *Cancer Research* published a study in December 1994 showing that mammary tumors grow faster in animals fed a diet containing more linoleic acid. Specifically, it was noted that linoleic acid encouraged metastases (secondary tumors that spread). The linoleic acid in commercial feeds is highly processed.

Important pieces of the nutrition-cancer puzzle are being identified more rapidly than ever before, especially with respect to oil consumption. Studies of the protective effects that extra virgin olive oil can provide in preventing breast cancer have been reported by Dimitrios Trichopoulos, M.D., at the Harvard School of Public Health. Carlo La Vecchia, M.D., from the Instituto di Ricerche Farmacologiche Mario Negri in Milano, Italy, has also studied the beneficial effects of extra virgin olive oil in preventing breast, pancreatic, and colorectal cancer. Increased vegetable consumption, and the use of olive oil in dressings (instead of heating it in cooking), also seemed to be factors in lowering the risk of lung cancer, a recent Italian study revealed.

My hope is that one day very soon there will be cancer research centers which can evaluate the validity of specific information about nutrition and cancer prevention. More research is crucial—not just laboratory research, but also clinical studies. There is a pressing need to fund research into disease prevention; however, there is also a need for more coordination, and the sharing of ideas and findings, between researchers in different scientific disciplines in order to identify the missing pieces of the puzzle of nutrition and breast health.

PART ONE

CHAPTER 1

The Effects of Fats and Oils on Breast Cancer

I will devote more time to a discussion of fat than to any other aspect of diet, because I believe the implications of research on how fat affects the body are vitally important.

—Andrew Weil, M.D., *Spontaneous Healing*

Despite the disturbing increase in breast cancer cases over the last fifty years, little progress has been made by conventional medicine in developing prevention strategies. Knowledge gained in the field of nutrition and the natural foods movement, however, has resulted in practical, alternative approaches to preventing breast cancer, and it is now generally accepted that diet can work in conjunction with medicine to heal breast cancer. Most doctors now agree, for example, that a diet high in fiber and low in saturated fat can help protect against breast cancer.

Recent research has shown, however, that specific fats and oils, when properly selected and used, complemented by a plant-based diet, can actually be powerful allies in strengthening the immune system and preventing breast cancer.

Certain fats and oils are not only beneficial to good health, they are essential for good health. These oils contain one or both of the two essential fatty acids, alpha-linolenic acid or omega-3, and linoleic acid or omega-6. Most people are more deficient in essential fatty acids than any other nutrient.

Healing Benefits of Fresh Oils

A variety of freshly pressed, unprocessed, organic oils contain essential fatty acids, or EFAs. Available only from plant sources, they are called essential because like forty-three other nutrients (minerals, vitamins, and essential amino acids), they cannot be manufactured by the human body.

While the modern Western diet provides a sufficient amount of omega-6, it is profoundly deficient in omega-3. In fact, consumption of omega-3 has declined to one-sixth its level in the mid-1800s. As much as 95 percent of today's population may be deficient in this essential nutrient.

Since the mid-1800s, cancer has increased dramatically. Is this increase in cancer due in part to an omega-3 deficiency? While that direct connection has not been proved, it is known that omega-3 essential fatty acids inhibit tissue inflammation and reduce tumors.

Even if breast cancer develops, omega-3 EFAs appear to be able to inhibit the cancer's spread; conversely, breast cancer tissue that metastasizes has decreased levels of this essential nutrient. In one study of 121 patients, the amount of omega-3 was found to be lowest in the breast cancer tissue that metastasized.

> Many nutrients that are breast protective, such as carotenes, vitamin E, and lycopene, are oil soluble. Fresh, unheated, and unprocessed organic oils act as a transport system for many of the nutrients in the foods we eat. Adding small amounts of flax or extra virgin olive oil to food helps these nutrients to be utilized by the cells.

Flaxseed oil is by far the best source of cancer-protective omega-3 essential fatty acids. Moreover, flaxseeds (from which flaxseed oil is pressed) contain important plant-derived nutrients called lignans, a phytochemical possessing antiviral, antifungal, antibacterial, and anticancer properties. Lignans were at the heart of a $20.5 million study by the National Cancer Institute into the prevention of cancer. (Unfortunately, this study was canceled before it was completed.) Flaxseeds, which contain approximately 100 times the amount of lignans found in other plant foods, were among the first foods included in the study.

Lignans have been shown to be protective against breast cancer. Lignans from flaxseed help to prevent breast cancer in several ways. For information on flaxseed, see Chapter 6, "Flaxseed and Flaxseed Oil: Nature's Super Foods for Breast Health."

> "Perhaps the most significant action of the lignans is their anti-cancer effect. A substantial amount of research has shown that flaxseed lignans are changed by bacteria in the human intestine to compounds that are extremely protective against cancer, particularly breast cancer."—Julian Whitaker, M.D., *Dr. Whitaker's Guide to Natural Healing.*

The richest source of protective lignans is freshly ground flaxseed; only 2% of the lignan content of flaxseed ends up in flaxseed oil; the other 98%—plus nutritionally beneficial fiber, mucilage, and other nutrients—remains in the seed meal.

However, both flaxseeds and flaxseed oil have been found to be instrumental in the dissolution of existing tumors. When animals with mammary or colon cancer are given flaxseed, they demonstrate a greater than 50 percent reduction in tumor number and size in one to two months.

> TIP: How much flaxseed oil should you consume? If you are actively healing breast cancer, ask your physician or nutritionist for an individualized program. Nutritionists generally recommend one tablespoon of flaxseed oil daily.

Cold water fish such as salmon, rainbow trout, tuna, sardines, cod, and herring are also excellent sources for the omega-3 derivatives EPA (short for "eicosapentaenoic acid") and DHA (short for "docosahexaenoic acid"); they offer powerful protection against degenerative diseases such as cancer. For instance, among the Inuits of Canada and fishermen in Japan on traditional diets—people who get more than half of their diet from the fatty flesh of whales, seals, and salmon—both heart disease and cancer are rare.

The effects of omega-3 fatty acids on breast cancer are being studied by John Glaspy, M.D., at the UCLA Medical Center. Dr. Glaspy has discovered that breast cells respond more radically to dietary changes than do any other cells in the body. After only one month of increased consumption of omega-3 oils, Dr. Glaspy found that breast cells not only have higher omega-3 fatty acid levels, they also have a decreased amount of omega-6 fatty acids. Additional research has shown that omega-3 fats appear to protect against the development of tumors. Much more research is needed on the topic of fats, oils, and cancer. It is also important to study the effects of all *unprocessed,* fresh organic oils.

The role of extra virgin olive oil in preventing several kinds of cancers has become an area of intense research. While its possible role in reducing the risk of breast cancer has been investigated for several years, in July 1995, a group of Italian researchers reported in the *Journal of the National Cancer Institute* that *unheated* olive oil also protects against lung and colon cancers. A lowered risk of these cancers was linked to using unheated olive oil as a dressing on salads and vegetables. No protective effects were seen with the regular use of olive oil for cooking. Researchers explained this observation by noting that the protective polyphenols in olive oil are destroyed during the cooking process; therefore, olive oil was cancer protective only when used in salad dressings. Fresh herbs were also found to offer protection against lung cancer, including common herbs popular in the Mediterranean diet, such as rosemary, parsley, and basil. Because natural antioxidants present in the olive oil (and fresh herbs) encourage the repair of potentially carcinogenic oxidative damage from free radicals, researchers theorize that the loss of polyphenols during cooking lowers the natural resistance of olive oil to oxidation. This new information was gathered in a hospital-based, case-control study conducted in Rome. One of the tables in the published article provided specific information illustrating that the type of olive oil used (dressing versus cooking) was a significant part of the research. It is clear that the potentially protective role of unheated, unprocessed oils on human health warrants further investigation.

Prostaglandins and Breast Cancer

Prostaglandins are hormone-like substances that regulate virtually every organ system and process in the body: the nervous system, immune system, reproductive system, digestive system, and cardiovascular system, as well as inflammation, healing, and many other processes. There are more than thirty kinds of prostaglandins, which are very short-lived—meaning we have to make them every single day. Prostaglandins are created by very specific, enzyme-controlled metabolism of the essential fatty acids. Omega-3 and omega-6 nutrients are metabolized into different classes of prostaglandins that have very different functions—which is why it is important to eat a diet containing the correct balance of omega-3 and omega-6 EFAs. If too much omega-6 fatty acid is consumed, and not enough omega-3 fatty acid, prostaglandin production can become unbalanced.

There are three families, or series, of prostaglandins (abbreviated "PG"). Series 1 and 2 are metabolized from omega-6 nutrients; series 3 prostaglandins are made from omega-3 nutrients.

Not all prostaglandins are beneficial. One of the harmful prostaglandins in the series 2 group, PGE2, causes the kidneys to retain salt (which can lead to high blood pressure), and also causes inflammation. Inflammation, in turn, can lead to the development of immune system malfunctions; overproduction of PGE2 hampers the immune system in its ability to kill cancer cells. Women with breast cancer, for instance, make an excess of PGE2.

The food source of the dangerous prostaglandin PGE2, linked to breast cancer, inflammation, and rheumatoid arthritis, is animal fats. PGE2 is also made from omega-6 under stress.

The series 3 prostaglandins are metabolized from omega-3 nutrients. The intermediary substance produced when omega-3 EFAs are metabolized, called EPA (eicosapentaenoic acid), is more important to health than any of the series 3 prostaglandins: EPA inhibits the production of the harmful PGE2.

Foods that result in the production of the protective EPA, which blocks the production of PGE2 and guards against breast cancer, are:

- Flaxseed
- Fresh, organic, unrefined flaxseed oil
- Cold water fish
- Dark, leafy greens

The Dangers of Processed Fats: Refined Oils, Hydrogenation, and Trans-Fatty Acids

Traditional—that is, unprocessed—foods, including fats, have nourished people throughout the ages. According to experts, it is the increased consumption of *processed* fats during this century that is a key factor in the proliferation of degenerative diseases.

"Breast cancer risk seems to be associated with dietary fat. But this is only part of the problem," says Christiane Northrup, M.D., member of the Women to Women clinic in Yarmouth, Maine. "We did not see the great increase in breast cancer (or heart disease, or all kinds of cancer) until hydrogenated fats were added to the diet in huge amounts, starting in the 1930s, when the process was developed to blow hydrogenation into the fat at very high temperatures, creating artificial fats with a shelf life higher then your life's expectancy. Don't eat them! Unfortunately, they are in everything. They are in Wheat Thins, baked goods, everything. Avoid them at all costs. This kind of fat is a transfatty acid that increases free radical damage in your tissue, and this is the beginning of cellular damage."

There are a number of processed fats that are unhealthy to consume, including refined oils, fried or deep fried oils, hydrogenated fats, and foods resulting from partial hydrogenation.

Refined oils are heated to high temperatures, and treated with chemicals such as deodorizers, bleach, and solvents. This process destroys the oils' cancer-fighting antioxidants—substances that prevent cell damage—and creates dangerous free radicals that can damage cells. "Expeller-pressed" oils—a label you may have seen in the health food store—are usually the equivalent of refined oils; they may be heated, deodorized, and/or bleached. Look for labels that say "unrefined" when purchasing oils, and most importantly, avoid clear oils. Unrefined oils are golden to amber in hue. Many supermarket oils contain trans-fats, but do not indicate that on the label.

Hydrogenation and Trans-fatty Acids: Hydrogenation was developed not to increase products' nutritional value, but to extend their shelf life, and to make them less expensive. Hydrogenated fats, for instance, were developed

to provide consumers with a cheap version of butter (margarine). Hydrogenated tropical oils (made from coconut or palm) are utilized in products like
chocolate, keeping it hard enough not to melt in the store. (Makes you think
twice about chocolate, doesn't it?)

> Did you know that margarine melts above body temperature? Think
> about what it does to cells, tissues, and arteries as it accumulates
> within the body.

During industrial hydrogenation, liquid oils are artificially saturated with
hydrogen gas at very high temperatures. Hydrogenation also generally employs
nickel and aluminum as catalysts. As nutritionist Udo Erasmus points out in
Fats That Heal, Fats That Kill, "Remnants of both metals remain in products
containing hydrogenated or partially hydrogenated oils, and are eaten by
people. . . . Aluminum is particularly worrisome, because it is associated with
Alzheimer's, osteoporosis, and may facilitate the development of cancer." He
goes on to say, "Hydrogenation . . . destroys Omega 3 [essential fatty acids]
very rapidly, and Omega 6 [essential fatty acids] only slightly more slowly. It
is impossible to control the chemical outcome of the process. We cannot
predict the quantities of each different kind of altered substance that will be
produced."

The altered substances may contribute to various health problems. Of these,
trans-fatty acids have received most of the attention of researchers because
they make up the largest part of the altered substance. However, numerous
other, still uncharacterized and largely unstudied, chemicals are produced
during hydrogenation. Professor G. J. Brisson at Laval University in Quebec
has pointed out (in Erasmus's *Fats That Heal, Fats That Kill*), "It would be
practically impossible to predict with accuracy either the nature, or the content, of these new molecules [produced in the process of hydrogenation]
between the parent vegetable oil, sometimes labeled 'pure,' and the partially
hydrogenated product. . . . There is a world of chemistry that alters profoundly
the composition and physiochemical properties of natural oils."

Herbert Dutton, a respected oil chemist working with Professor Brisson,
has commented (in *Fats That Heal, Fats That Kill*), "If the hydrogenation
process were discovered today, it probably would not be adopted by the [food]
oil industry. . . . The basis for such comment lies in the recent awareness of
our prior ignorance concerning the complexity of isomers formed during
hydrogenation and their metabolic and physiological fate."

Trans-Fatty Acids and Breast Cancer

Trans-fatty acids have been linked to breast cancer. American women's intake of trans-fats is twice that of European women. In a 1997 study conducted by researchers at the University of North Carolina at Chapel Hill, trans-fats were found to have several detrimental effects on women's health. The fatty acid content of women with breast cancer was measured in body fat—fat taken from the buttocks reflects the dietary intake of various fats—instead of determining how much fat the women consumed by asking about their diets. It was found that body fat with a high level of trans-fats indicated a higher risk for breast cancer. These researchers, led by Dr. Lenore Kohlmeier, also noted:

- Trans-fats have an adverse effect on protective enzymes in the body that potentially have an antiinflammatory effect.
- Trans-fats are associated with chromosome breakage.

The effect of a given increase in trans-fats may depend upon the level of polyunsaturated fat competing with it for binding sites. Women with the lowest levels of polyunsaturated fat had a 3.6-fold greater amount of trans-fats. In other words, trans-fats *displace* other, healthier fatty acids.

Trans-fatty acids are produced by the high temperatures (120-210° C; 248-410° F) and hydrogenation that turn cheap, liquid, refined oils into creamy fats like margarines, shortening, and other oils that are often then used as ingredients in convenience foods. During this process, essential nutrients are destroyed and trans-fatty acids are produced in huge quantities; they make up from 9 to 50 percent of most hydrogenated products.

Trans-fatty acids have much the same chemical form as healthful fatty acids, which allows them to usurp the place of fatty acids inside cells. However, trans-fatty acids do not contribute to cell growth or metabolism; their presence actually blocks the essential fatty acids from functioning properly.

The Center for Science in the Public Interest (CSPI) is urging manufacturers to include trans-fat content on nutritional labels, and the Food and Drug Administration (FDA) is considering a proposal to require listing their presence on food labels. Many vegetable oils contain trans-fats, but do not list them on the label.

Trans-fatty acids also have detrimental effects on cardiovascular function, by increasing "bad" LDL cholesterol and decreasing "good" HDL cholesterol. They make platelets stickier, thereby doubling the risk of heart attack. It's estimated that 15,000 women die each year from heart attacks resulting from consuming trans-fats. In November 1997, Jane E. Brody reported in the *New York Times* that women's heart risk is linked to the type of fat consumed, not the total amount of fat, as researchers previously believed. In a fourteen year study of 80,000 women, it was found that the consumption of trans-fats was the most serious coronary risk factor, ahead even of smoking. Trans-fatty acids have a negative impact on cell membranes, certain aspects of the immune system, essential fatty acid function, insulin response and function, pregnancy (including increasing the possibility of having a low-birthweight baby), and breast milk quality. Trans-fatty acids have also been linked to diabetes.

Currently, the federal government knows enough about the harmful effects of trans-fatty acids not to allow them in baby foods. Let's hope they publicize the dangers these substances pose for us all.

"I believe that trans-fatty acids in the diet damage the regulatory machinery of the body, significantly compromising the healing system," says author Andrew Weil, M.D. "Remember that TFAs are rarely found in nature, only in fats that have been subjected to unusual chemical and physical treatment."

Health Destructive Effects of Frying

We have already seen from the 1995 *Journal of the National Cancer Institute* report that unheated olive oil offers protection against lung cancer but that protective effects were not seen with the use of heated oil for cooking. Nearly all nutritionists now agree that highly saturated animal fat and margarine are bad for us. Nevertheless, a trend toward avoidance of fried foods has developed among many progressive physicians and nutritionists. But there is still no consensus about the health risks of heating vegetable oils (despite some compelling evidence), or about which varieties are the least harmful to heat. Amazingly, even the argument over butter use has come full circle, and a growing number of nutritionists now advocate using butter instead of margarine.

> When oil turns to smoke, and/or food is browned, destructive processes occur, including the process that turns protein into the carcinogenic substance acrolein. Also, protective polyphenols, offering antioxidant benefits, are lost during the cooking process. These same polyphenols offer healing benefits, when unprocessed oils are consumed unheated in dressings poured over vegetables and salads.

While cooking obviously involves heating food, we don't generally think about the chemical changes that occur in foods when they are heated. Although heat affects some fats and oils more than others, all undergo profound biochemical change when heated. Beyond a certain temperature, the healthful antioxidant properties of fats and oils disappear and destructive free radicals form. Eventually, the molecular structure of the heated fat or oil is modified and dangerous molecules are created. Frying is particularly destructive of the healthful properties of fats and oils.

Is there evidence that being exposed to smoking oil and fat on a daily basis contributes to the formation of cancer? There is at least a strong correlation. In 1995, the *Wall Street Journal* reported that a study conducted by the National Cancer Institute found that North American cooks have higher rates of lung cancer than cooks in countries where little or no food is prepared by frying.

Frying and deep frying present a profound danger to health because of the rapid oxidation and other chemical changes that take place when oils are heated at high temperatures in the presence of light and oxygen. (Proper production of fresh, unprocessed oils is performed in darkened rooms at low temperatures. Donald Rudin, M.D., and Clara Felix, authors of *Omega 3 Oils* [Avery, 1996] recommend that oils be bottled in dark brown glass. Proper bottling utilizes opaque glass bottles to further protect the oil from light.)

> Infrequent use of butter for sauteing produces fewer health problems than the use of fried oils. Be sure to sauté at gentle, low temperatures.

The protective fats are protective primarily because of their chemical structure. The oxidation that occurs when a fat is heated to a high temperature destroys the chemical structure that makes the healthful fat good for us. The antioxidants and vitamin E that nature puts into oils to protect from oxidation and rancidity are destroyed by frying. Additionally, free radicals—substances that are highly reactive, and generally harmful—are produced and can start harmful chain reactions in oil molecules.

> In restaurant frying, the same batch of oil is sometimes re-used for days, and heated to very high temperatures. Many altered substances known to be very damaging to health are present in these oils.

An epidemiological study done in 1975 found that fried foods and French fries were the foods consumed most frequently by Seventh Day Adventists with breast cancer. These foods were listed as two of the five most frequently consumed foods by all women with breast cancer.

There also appears to be an increased risk of pancreatic cancer among people who consume large amounts of fried potatoes and other fried foods, according to six studies published during the last two decades.

Breast Cancer and Fried Foods

- Destruction of breast-protective antioxidants (polyphenols) in oil.
- Production of free radicals, which are potentially carcinogenic.
- Creation of many unnatural breakdown products, such as polymers, with unknown effects on health.
- Destructive factors are cumulative. After ten, twenty, or thirty years of fried foods, eventually our health is affected at a cellular level.

Frying may also produce some trans-fatty acids. In addition to the unhealthy effects already described, trans-fats impair the protective (lipid, or fat) barrier around our cells, as well as interfering with the production of prostaglandins (hormone-like substances made from the essential fatty acids). Trans-fats change the efficiency of protective essential fatty acids, reducing or eliminating their potential benefits. They are broken down more slowly than healthy fats by our enzymes. Since enzymes are naturally depleted by age, our bodies are less likely to be able to break down these harmful transfats as we get older. Even when not impaired by age, the body's ability to break down trans-fats is limited. When our absorption of trans-fats exceeds our ability to metabolize them, degenerative diseases can begin.

> TIP: Since it's best not to fry at all, try using a couple of tablespoons of water, soup stock or diluted miso, instead of oil. Even onions can "sauté" nice and golden, with no oil at all.

Many other products of oxidation even more dangerous than trans-fats are produced by frying, including a spectrum of unnatural breakdown products that have unknown effects on health. As Erasmus points out in *Fats That Heal, Fats That Kill,* "Frying once or twice won't kill us, but after ten, twenty, or thirty years of eating fried foods, our cells accumulate altered and toxic products for which they have not evolved efficient detoxifying mechanisms."

Fried foods or heated fats and oils cannot be recommended for health, and should be avoided by anyone trying to heal cancer or prevent its recurrence, particularly if there is a family history of breast (or other) cancer(s).

For some people, it will be hard to abandon heating oil, even when cancer may exist in the family. It is helpful to know some practices are safer than others.

For sautéing use in this order of preference:

- *Butter,* a natural substance, remains relatively stable in the presence of heat, light, and oxygen.
- *Untoasted sesame oil and olive oil.* While unsaturated oils are less stable

than saturated fats, some may be heated more safely than others. Relatively speaking, the most stable unsaturated oils are untoasted sesame oil and olive oil. When heating either oil, do so over low temperatures, and use sulfur-rich onions and garlic to protect against free radical damage. In addition, put a small amount of water in the pan first. Just 1-2 tablespoons of water before you add a touch of oil (1-2 teaspoons) keeps the temperature at the nondestructive level of 100° C, or 212° F, the point at which water boils.

I do not recommend using heated oil of any kind while trying to heal breast cancer.

It is becoming increasingly popular to use safflower, corn, and canola oil for frying foods. All three, particularly canola oil, are relatively unstable when heated.

Moreover, much *safflower oil* has been genetically engineered from regular safflower seeds and may contain some irritating properties.

Corn oil has been linked to tumor formation and harmful prostaglandins. Much of the corn oil available commercially is highly processed, heated in production, treated with chemicals, and sits around in huge containers for months—or even years. For these reasons, never use it.

Canola oil also tends to be highly processed, and may be linked to heart problems. Also, because of its omega-3 content, much canola oil commercially available is rancid. Canola oil is derived from processed rapeseed oil. The rape plant is a source of highly toxic erucic acid; this acid is known to cause cancer and heart disease. Although the Canadian government (which markets canola oil) claims to have found a way to eliminate the erucic acid from the oil, there is a concern that canola oil may still contain some erucic acid.

The rape plant, part of the mustard family, contains a seed low in saturated fat, high in unsaturated fatty acids, and a highly toxic fatty acid, erucic acid. Furthermore, supermarket canola oil has been processed. The fatty acids have been altered, and because rape is heavily treated with pesticides, it is likely that some of these substances end up in the oil.

By far the biggest problem facing those of us concerned with this issue is letting people know that it's not a healthy choice to cook with garden-variety supermarket oils. These oils are chemically treated with sodium hydroxide and phosphoric acid, and are bleached, deodorized, and heated at high temperatures.

For Occasional Gentle Sautéing

Always use a little water in the pan first, to act as a buffer between the heat and oil. This helps to protect the oil from the damaging effects of the heat. Use a very small amount of either butter, unroasted sesame oil, or olive oil. Be sure to keep the flame low, and gently sauté. Never, ever fry. Frying employs a high temperature, which is not desirable for health. Better still, use a few teaspoons of water to sauté vegetables over medium to high heat.

TIP: Flaxseed oil is an unstable oil that oxidizes very quickly. This simply means it goes rancid easily. That is why flaxseed oil is protected from both light and heat during pressing, and (hopefully) packaging. This is also why it needs to be refrigerated, and why bottles should have a pressing date.

Try using several tablespoons of water in your pan, without adding any oil. I have been "water-sautéing" for years, which allows me to avoid heating oil or butter. Instead, I drizzle a small amount of fresh oils on food after cooking. Extra virgin olive oil, flaxseed oil, and others can be added to food right before eating, for both flavor and health. The Mediterraneans drizzle fresh, extra virgin olive oil on their food before serving and, in general, don't use a lot of heated oil. Food prepared this way tastes great! In Greece, fresh olive oil is drizzled on salads and grape leaves, and in the Middle East, olive oil is drizzled on humus, salads, and other foods. In Southern France, people eat a lot of salads and vegetables. They poach, braise, and lightly cook much of their food. In southern Italy, olive oil is drizzled on food after cooking.

Extra virgin olive oil also offers healing benefits. Studies conducted by researchers from the Harvard School of Public Health and the University of Athens in Greece found that women who consume olive oil at more than one meal a day have a much lower risk of breast cancer than those who used olive oil less frequently. And women in Crete have been found to have very low rates of breast cancer, even though they consume approximately half of their calories from fat (in the form of olive oil). The significance of this breast cancer statistic lies not only in the fact that women in Crete consume so much fat from olive oil, but in *how* they consume the oil—freshly pressed and unheated, much of it consumed with vegetables. All the studies showing lower rates of breast cancer among women following the Mediterranean diet highlight consumption of extra virgin olive oil—not light olive oil.

"Minor ingredients" in extra virgin olive oil (beta-carotene, vitamin E, chlorophyll, squaline, and phytosterols) improve liver and gall bladder function; increase bile flow; improve digestion; benefit heart and arteries. Light olive oil is lower in minor ingredients. Avoid light olive oil.

Olive oil may have a favorable impact on the risk of pancreatic cancer. This new role for olive oil was suggested in a study conducted in Italy between 1983 and 1995 on 362 people with pancreatic cancer.

Information about the potential for olive oil to help prevent breast cancer has been accumulating rapidly over the last decade. While Dr. Antonia Trichopoulou of the Harvard School of Public Health is not ready to state unequivocally that consuming olive oil will prevent breast cancer, she wrote an editorial in the June 1995 issue of the journal *Cancer Causes and Control* noting that, since mid-1994, four important studies—one from Greece, one from Italy, and two from Spain—were published that show a beneficial effect of olive oil consumption on breast cancer risk. Dr. Trichopoulou also notes that olive oil is frequently consumed with vegetables in these countries, and points out that consuming large amounts of vegetables also plays a role in reducing cancer risk. "Nevertheless, the necessary caution should not overshadow the fact that the existing evidence converges in support of a protective role of olive oil against breast cancer," Dr. Trichopoulou concludes. She also urges increased research into the effect of olive oil on preventing breast cancer.

Cookbooks that recommend flaxseed oil for frying or sautéing are incorrect. Remember, because flaxseed oil is rich in omega-3 EFA, consume this oil in as fresh a state as possible. Heating flaxseed oil creates a toxic oil instead of a healing one. Julian Whitaker, M.D., author of *Dr. Whitaker's Guide to Natural Healing,* points out, "Because flax oil is a highly polyunsaturated oil, it is extremely susceptible to damage by heat, light, and oxygen. Once damaged, the oil is a rich source of toxic molecules known as lipid peroxides. These molecules can actually do the body harm and should not be ingested."

Tips for Eliminating Harmful Fats and Oils

1. Purchase only organic, freshly pressed, unrefined oils in dark glass bottles, labeled with pressing date to ensure freshness. Use within two to three months to avoid rancidity, and always refrigerate. Erasmus advises people to freeze oil that is not going to be consumed within four to eight weeks. Freshly pressed oils should be treated as perishables: "They require a lot of care," Erasmus says. "They are a reminder that health requires care."

> TIP: The term "cold-pressed" can be misleading—and so is the term "expeller-pressed." The higher the heat, and the greater the pressure in pressing, the greater the yield. Temperatures can go as high as 200° F. Oils produced in this way can still be described as "cold-pressed."

2. Purchase only organic seeds and nuts, *unroasted*. Even tahini should be unroasted.

3. Water sautéing, blanching, steaming, poaching, slow roasting, and cooking in parchment offer an exciting choice of food preparation. Add a drizzle of fresh, unheated oil after cooking.

4. Barbecuing, broiling, frying, or sautéing fatty-rich fish such as salmon, cod, or sardines destroys their valuable oils. Cooking these fish at high temperatures actually creates carcinogens.

5. High heat is also damaging to meat such as beef or lamb, which becomes three times more carcinogenic when cooked at high temperatures. ("Heterocyclic amines" are the cancer-causing chemicals that are formed when animal protein is heated at high temperatures.) When oil turns to smoke, and/or food is browned, destructive processes occur. During cooking, animal protein breaks down into creatinine, an excess of which can be unhealthy. Animal protein can also degenerate into acrolein, a carcinogen. In the most authoritative study, how the meat was cooked made a more important contribution to higher rates of cancer than the amount eaten, or how often.

6. If you eat dairy, consider purchasing organic butter, yogurt, and other dairy foods to limit exposure to harmful hormones and antibiotics. Many women notice a drastic decrease in painful breast lumps after switching to organic dairy, suggesting that our breasts are sensitive to the artificial hormones in nonorganic dairy foods.

Truly Light Cooking: Sixteen Ways To Prepare Foods Without Heating Oil
(Avoidance of Frying and Charcoal Grilling Protects Breast Cells)

• **Sautéing in water, diluted miso, chicken or vegetable broth.** This is a flavorful way of preparing vegetables without using added fat or oil. Water sautéing has been used for many years by macrobiotic cooks in healing cancer, but we can enjoy this wonderful cooking technique for prevention as well. Simply use 1-2 tablespoons water or broth for each 2 cups of chopped or sliced vegetables. Begin by cooking over low to medium heat, while stirring. (You may want to use a lid for 5 minutes or so for larger, more fibrous pieces.) Keep a little extra water in a small cup right by the stove. Saute for 5-20 minutes, depending upon how finely the vegetables have been sliced. Cook until the vegetables are just slightly tender and still retain their bright colors. Suggested vegetables for this cooking method: broccoli, cabbage, corn, cauliflower, leeks, spinach, onions, collard greens, kale, sugar snap peas, yellow squash, green beans, daikon radish, carrots, turnips, rutabagas, and other root vegetables. For variety, employ different cutting techniques, such as julienne strips for carrots, turnips, and daikon radish.

Very delicate, light vegetables such as spinach or scallions may require just 2-3 minutes of water sautéing.

> TIP: Bok choy sautéed in low-fat chicken stock is light and delicious.

• **Poaching.** Simmer foods in very hot water or vegetable broth until just tender. Salmon or sea bass are excellent choices for poaching.

• **Steaming.** Place vegetables, tofu, or fish in a steamer basket over boiling water. Steaming several different kinds of vegetables together in a steamer basket is an easy way to add more variety.

• **Pressure cooking.** This is an ideal way to cook brown rice. It's also convenient for quick-cooking beans and is used a lot in macrobiotics. Pressure is built up in a specially designed pot with a tight-fitting lid. (*See* Chapter 18, "Secrets of a Healthy Kitchen," for information on pressure cooking.) One of my favorite winter foods is pressure-cooked brown and wild rice, chewy and fragrant with chestnuts.

• **Stewing.** Cooking chunks of lamb, chicken, seafood, onions, garlic, assorted vegetables, and herbs in simmering liquid until done is a popular method of food preparation in all cultures. An example of delicious stewed food is a popular San Francisco seafood dish called Cioppino. Chunks of fish and shell fish are cooked in a tomato broth with garlic and herbs until just tender. A "ragout," simply another form of stewing in which foods and flavor meld together quickly, is composed of foods that have been lightly cooked separately—such as a combination of water-sautéed onions; lightly steamed shrimp; lightly blanched snow peas; slow-roasted shiitake mushrooms and garlic—cooked together in a little hot vegetable broth with herbs for about five minutes until the flavors have blended. A "navarin" is a light stew, traditionally made with lamb and early spring vegetables. Adding drizzled oil and freshly chopped herbs to stews and ragouts before eating complements them beautifully. *Many cultures, relying on traditional foods, reduce saturated fat consumption by combining only a small amount of meat with vegetables and chickpeas, lentils, or soybeans in stews.*

• **Bolito Misto, Pot Au Feu, Mongolian Hot Pot.** Cultures all over the world have traditionally boiled lean meat, vegetables, herbs, and aromatics (onions, shallots, leeks, and garlic) for appealing cold-weather meals.

• **Blanching.** Several quarts of salted water are brought to a boil, and vegetables such as bright yellow summer squash (1 pound of vegetables to 3 quarts of water) are added to the boiling water. Vegetables cook for 3-5 minutes, so that they are still a little firm when pierced with a knife. A delicious way to "finish" blanched vegetables is to dress them with sea salt, ground black pepper, freshly chopped chervil, basil, or parsley, with a drizzle of your favorite vinaigrette while the vegetables are still warm. Many vegetable dishes in France and Italy are prepared this way, and I urge you to use this wonderful method of preparing vegetables frequently.

• **Braising.** In the French Mediterranean, braising is often employed when fennel is cooked, especially if cooking large fennel bulbs. Braising is simply the use of boiling water in a large pot with a lid (adding fresh or dried herbs, such as a "bouquet garni"). Braising uses less water than stewing. Simmering in liquid over a low flame, as is done in making Yosenabe (a Japanese stew; see page 301), is another form of braising.

• **Slow roasting.** This method is simply slow cooking in an oven at moderate temperature, such as 250-375 degrees, until food is cooked. Some of the foods I slow roast include portabello mushrooms, onions, potatoes, and seafood. Sometimes I slow-roast an organic chicken with slivers of garlic and rosemary or tarragon under the skin.

TIP: Chicken with the skin attached has 47 grams of fat per serving; with the skin removed, only 10 grams of fat.

• **Clay pot cookery.** This cooking method dates back thousands of years. Clay pot cooking is easy, healthy, and delicious; it retains natural juices, eliminates the need for heated oil, and allows the flavors to intermingle. I first became aware of the gourmet quality of clay pot cooking when I discovered a wonderful dish of rice, "tree ear" mushrooms, spices, onions, and shrimp (with a tangy peanut sauce) at a Vietnamese restaurant. The dish was cooked and served in a clay pot. (For information on clay pot cookery, *see* the Resource Guide. Look for Romertopf unglazed clay pots; glazes contain chemicals.)

TIP: Look for Beyond Gourmet unbleached parchment paper imported from Sweden (available in most health food stores).

• **Cooking in parchment.** I like this method because it employs slow roasting, prevents browning, and is really very easy. Most of all, I find it a terrific way to intensify the flavors of foods, as in lamb chops roasted with garlic and sage (*see* page 323.) Parchment roasting also works for fish. Be sure to select chemical-free parchment paper from your local health food store.

TIP: Increasing raw vegetables provides an important source of healing enzymes, a major factor in breast health.

• **Salads.** Don't underestimate the benefits of eating raw vegetables. Consuming a variety of vegetables and changing the vegetables you select to include in your salads provide many breast-protective benefits. These benefits include phytochemicals, phytonutrients, and a very important breast ally, enzymes. (Refer to Chapter 5 for details on enzymes.) Research has shown that the greater the variety of vegetables we eat, the greater the breast (and other cancer) protection. Cultures that have low rates of breast cancer consume much smaller amounts of meat than people in Northern America and Europe, and larger servings of vegetables. In the Mediterranean, where rates of breast and other cancers are low, salads are emphasized and meat consumption is minimized. Salads often include a variety of alliums—such as purple, white, or green onions, as well as minced garlic in the vinaigrette—which offers even greater breast protection. Turkey, lamb, or lean beef paillards, over salad, makes a delicious lunch or dinner.

The American Institute for Cancer Research recommends eliminating commercially pickled foods. Natural pickles avoid the use of excessive salt, chemicals, and vinegars found in commercial, bottled pickles.

• **Natural pickles.** Commercially bottled pickles are not recommended for health. Natural pickles that you can make yourself, however, contain valuable enzymes and friendly bacteria. **Light pickling:** Pickling, using a little sea salt, shoyu or tamari sauce or umeboshi plum vinegar (*see* the Resource Guide), is an important part of healthful Asian cuisine. Many cultures with low rates of breast and other cancers eat lightly pickled foods every day. Light pickling begins the digestive process by adding naturally occuring, friendly bacteria to the foods for complete digestion and assimilation of minerals and other nutrients. Light pickling can be done conveniently, as well (as opposed to longer pickling, which can require lengthy storage, boiling of jars, and so on). Here's an example of how easy it is to lightly pickle food: Simply cut into thin julienne pieces your favorite vegetable (or combine two or three). Spread out on a dish. Add several pinches of sea salt, and allow to pickle for 10 minutes to 1 hour, until the vegetables are slightly wilted and liquid begins to accumulate in the dish. Suggested combinations: onions, radishes, and carrots.

TIP: For a quick version of Korean "kim chee pickle," which is renowned for its health benefits and spicy flavor, consider the following: Cut daikon radish and savory cabbage into thin strips. Add a few pinches of sea salt and minced garlic. Allow to marinate for 1 hour. Add some cayenne pepper (full of breast-protective antioxidants) and enjoy.

• **Natural pickling.** If you are healing breast cancer, it's worth the extra effort to make pickles. In macrobiotics, pickles are a part of every diet. When miso is used in the pickling process, women healing breast cancer receive the added benefits of the protective isoflavones found in soy. Additionally, when miso is used, the mineral content is increased and its potent, anticancer enzymes work more efficiently. Traditionally, vegetables pickled in miso have been part of the Japanese diet for centuries. Many beneficial, immune-enhancing enzymes are created during the pickling process. Both the burdock and the garlic recipes I've chosen to illustrate how easy it is to pickle foods are powerhouses of breast-healing nutrients. Use either brown rice miso or country barley organic miso from the health food store.

Burdock pickles. Scrub burdock with natural bristle brush. Cut into thin strips, like matchsticks. There is no need to peel, just scrub well (mineral content is high in the skin of the vegetable, so don't discard). Use equal parts miso and burdock, and mix well. Put in a small glass bowl or jar and cover with a bamboo mat for 1 week to 1 month. Wipe miso off with a clean dish towel, and the pickles are ready to enjoy. Try burdock pickles with tofu and vegetables, and a little brown rice.

Garlic pickles. Garlic, used more in Korea than Japan, is delicious for pickling. Simply follow the same recipe as for Burdock pickles, substituting garlic. Begin by peeling and slicing the garlic. Uncooked garlic contains the most cancer-preventative phytochemicals and enzymes, so this delicious recipe contains many benefits. I especially enjoy garlic pickles with fish.

• **Crushing or gently crushing foods.** Herbs, garlic, citrus juices, vinegars or oils can release a great deal of flavor when crushed together and then mixed with salads to marinate. Suribachi grinding is the optimum way to puree miso. **Suribachi grinding:** Grinding miso and broth (for gentle pureeing)and blending raw garlic, fresh herbs, lemon, and fresh oils for dressings is best done by hand. Traditional cultures have always used a mortar and pestle to grind spices. The gentle blending obtained with a wooden pestle helps to release protective enzymes from foods like garlic or miso. In fact, macrobiotic cooks use a suribachi, a ceramic bowl with a raised geometric pattern on the inside bottom, to grind foods. The bumpy interior of the bowl helps to purée the food gently, especially when a wooden pestle is used.

• **Grinding.** Some dishes can be prepared in large, cone-shaped bowls, which help to combine and crush ingredients together when making salads. Juices and flavors are thereby released, which is a definite advantage in food preparation. Asian markets carry these bowls; their use is quite common in Thai cuisine, for example. Some salads in Asian cuisine are simply lemon grass, herbs, and citrus juice combined with raw vegetables. The herbs are ground together with citrus juice and spices, and the vegetables added to marinate.

• **Chiffonade.** The addition of julienne strips of raw, carotene-rich, leafy greens provides color and texture to food. The refreshing flavor and crisp texture of a chiffonade of uncooked greens makes an attractive bed for steamed or poached fish, or as garnish for pasta, rice, etc. It is so important to include greens each day; a chiffonade is extremely convenient because it eliminates the need to prepare another green vegetable. To make a chiffonade, simply select one of the following: Napa cabbage, spinach, chard, basil, bok choy (only the leafy part), mustard greens, or dandelion greens. Wash and dry eight leaves. Fold the leaves in half, right along their stems. Using a sharp knife, cut across the stems every ⅛th of an inch. If the green does not have a stem in the middle, like napa cabbage, you can cut the leaf in half, fold over, and use the same cutting technique to create julienne strips.

• **Pressed salads.** In macrobiotics, it is said that pressing vegetables helps to break down the fibers of the raw foods so that they are easier to digest. I love pressed salads; the pressing creates another texture for the salad, and melds the tangy condiments with some of the liquid from the vegetables. Pressing is very easy. Cleaned, sliced vegetables are arranged on a plate, lightly sprinkled with your favorite condiments, and covered with a second plate and weighted down. A book or a sack of cornmeal can be used to weigh down the top plate. Here's an example of a pressed vegetable dish:

Pressed Vegetables with Dill

2-3 thinly sliced radishes
1 small cucumber, thinly sliced
1 small onion
1 tsp finely minced dill (or any fresh herb)
⅓-½ tsp. sea salt to taste
¾ tsp umeboshi vinegar
touch of lemon juice (freshly squeezed)
ginger root
1 tbsp flaxseed oil

Place the cleaned, sliced vegetables on a plate. Add the minced herb. Sprinkle salt and vinegar on the vegetables. Put a second plate on the vegetables with an 8-10 pound weight on top. Leave for 10-20 minutes. Gently squeeze juice from vegetables. Drizzle pressed vegetables with lemon juice, or grate some fresh ginger root and squeeze out the juice. Add a drizzle of oil and enjoy.

TIP: If there is no liquid from the pressed vegetables, simply add a little more salt, or try again with a heavier weight.

Breast Health Plan: Adding Fresh, Organic Oils to Food

The following food combinations illustrate ways to use freshly pressed, unheated, organic oils on food. Once you begin using delicious, fresh oils on food, I'm sure you will be inspired to come up with some favorites of your own.

- Fall squash soup (use either Kabocha, buttercup, or butternut squash), drizzled with pumpkin seed oil.
- Asian rice salad, with bits of shrimp, lemon grass, scallions, and cilantro, lightly drizzled with fragrant sesame seed oil.
- Poached Chilean sea bass with fennel and plum tomatoes, perfumed lightly with extra virgin olive oil.
- Angel hair pasta primavera with delicate spring vegetables and a trio of fresh herbs such as marjoram, basil, and parsley. Complete with a touch of fragrant sunflower seed oil.
- Beet salad with chives, walnut oil, and a touch of balsamic vinegar.
- Sugar snap peas, ground Szechwan pepper corns, minced scallions, red wine vinegar, and a touch of sesame oil.
- Wild rice, a crisp apple (cubed), and chopped hazelnuts, drizzled lightly with hazelnut oil.

• Black bean salad with minced jalapeño pepper, purple onion, and red pepper, garnished with cilantro and a light drizzle of extra virgin olive oil.

Trans-Fats and Heart Health
Centers for Disease Control and Prevention
Leading Causes of Death 1990-1994
(Death rate per 100,000 women in the US)
Number 1 killer: Heart disease.
Number 79 on the list: Breast cancer.

Trans-Fats Trigger Problems Related to Heart Disease As Well As Breast Cancer

Walter Willett, M.D., chair of the nutrition department at the Harvard School of Public Health in Boston, said, "Fifteen thousand women die prematurely every year because of heart disease resulting from a high trans fat intake." In a study of 85,000 nurses in the late 1980s, Willett found that those with the highest intake of trans-fats had double the risk of heart disease.

Trans-fatty Acids Have Been Found in Studies to Have the Following Adverse Effects on Heart Health:

Increase bad cholesterol (LDL)
Decrease good cholesterol (HDL)
Make platelets stickier

The "It's About Time" Award: In 1997, the Federal Trade Commission and the Food and Drug Administration banished the "Get Heart Smart" slogan from Promise Margarine packaging and advertising because of hidden trans-fats.

Harmful Fats at a Glance

• Commercially produced, clear, refined vegetable oils (may contain trans-fats).
• Hydrogenated and partially hydrogenated oils (trans-fatty acids made from these substances).
• Fried oils.
• Excessive consumption of saturated fat.
• Trans-fats (found in candy, chips and junk foods).

CHAPTER 2

An Interview with Udo Erasmus, Author of *Fats That Heal, Fats That Kill:* The Importance of Fats to Women's Health

After Udo Erasmus was poisoned by pesticides, he turned his attention to the field of nutrition to begin a personal odyssey back to health. Since the publication of his landmark book *Fats and Oils* in 1986 (which earned him a Ph.D. in nutrition and is now available as *Fats That Heal, Fats That Kill*), he has become an internationally recognized authority and sought-after lecturer on the subject of fats, oils, cholesterol, and human health.

In *Fats That Heal, Fats That Kill*, Erasmus explains that there are good fats and bad fats. Some fats promote cancer, but other inhibit it. Some fats make stroke or heart attack more likely, and others make them less likely. Some fats block insulin function while others are necessary for insulin function. Bad fats damage cells, tissues, and organs, but other fats protect them.

Healing fats are required to prevent and reverse so-called incurable degenerative diseases, such as heart disease, cancer, and Type II diabetes. Healing fats also help reverse arthritis, obesity, PMS, allergies, asthma, skin conditions, fatigue, yeast and fungal infection, addictions, certain types of mental illness, and many other conditions.

The most dangerous fats are the result of processing. *Fats That Heal, Fats That Kill* exposes the manufacturing practices that turn healing fats into killing fats, explains the effects of those damaged fats on human health, and discloses the information that enables you to choose health-promoting oils.

In addition to his Ph.D., Erasmus's education includes a B.Sc. degree in honors zoology with a major in psychology from the University of British Columbia, followed by post-graduate studies in genetics and biochemistry. In addition, he earned an M.A. in counseling psychology from the Alfred Adler School of Professional Psychology in Chicago.

Could you give us background on how your expertise evolved?

I was poisoned by pesticides. I used them carelessly in my work. The one I used most was 2,4-D, which is the more toxic part of Agent Orange. It has dioxins in it, which are highly carcinogenic, but 2,4-D is carcinogenic even without dioxins. Medicine had nothing to offer for pesticide poisoning, so I turned to nutrition, the most likely self-help option for dealing with my problem. I specialized in fats and oils because the information I needed was not easily available. I had cancer to look forward to and knew that cancer often involves fats, but didn't know how, so I buried my head in the journals for three years full-time and three years part-time to find the information I needed. Drawing on seven years of university studies in science and life sciences, with biochemistry and genetics as my special disciplines, I had a good background to be able to research the information I needed to solve my own problem.

How is the information that you uncovered about the omega-3 oils linked to preventing cancer?

The omega-3 essential fatty acid inhibits tumor growth. The omega-6 essential fatty acid does not. There are derivatives of both the omega-3 and the omega-6 essential fatty acids that also inhibit tumor growth.

In general, what are the effects of low-fat or no-fat diets on health?

A no-fat diet will kill you eventually, because it deprives you of essential fatty acids, two substances from fats that you have to obtain in order to live and be health, that the body cannot make from anything else you eat, and that therefore have to come from food. A no-fat diet deprives you of these vital nutrients, and leads you to deteriorate until you die. You won't die overnight, but you will die if you don't bring them back into the diet.

On a low-fat diet, you just become sick. People on a no-fat or low-fat diet commonly experience symptoms such as low energy and dry skin. Sometimes people lose their hair. Low-fat diets stunt the growth of children. They also interfere with muscle development in athletes. Testosterone cannot be made without essential fatty acids.

It's especially detrimental for women to be deprived of essential fatty acids. Don't glands throughout the body depend on the nourishment of the essential fatty acids?

One of the functions of the essential fatty acids, especially the omega-3, is energy production. They increase oxygen metabolism. They give every gland and every organ more energy to do its job. They are helpful in cancer. Cancer hates oxygen, and essential fatty acids increase oxygen metabolism, which inhibits cancer. You can use essential fatty acids to sweat oil-soluble toxins out of the body; many oil-soluble toxins are carcinogenic, such as pesticides,

PCBs, and other chlorinated hydrocarbons. Essential fatty acids are also required for developing tumor necrosis factor (a substance created by the body that helps destroy tumors).

Can you briefly describe omega-6 and omega-3?

Our bodies cannot make the omega-6 and omega-3 essential fatty acids, but every cell requires them to be able to function normally, and therefore has to get them from the diet. Our bodies make from those two essential fatty acids several essential fatty acid derivatives that have functions in our cells and our cell membranes. From three of those derivatives, our bodies make hormone-like regulating substances called prostaglandins, that have vital, hormone-like regulating functions in all of our cells. The two essential fatty acids, the derivatives, and the prostaglandins are all part of the story of the omega-6 and omega-3 essential fatty acids.

Prior to the midpoint of the century when the cancer rate began its slow but steady climb, was the American diet richer in omega-3 essential fatty acids?

It was. We have decreased our omega-3 intake to one-sixth of the amount that was being eaten in 1850. We've also increased pesticides and pollution. We've also decreased our intake of other nutrients that are required for immune function and cancer inhibition. All of these factors play a role in increasing cancer.

Most supermarket vegetables are high in omega-6 essential fatty acid. Do you think the dramatic increase of omega-6 essential fatty acid is linked to higher rates of cancer as some studies have suggested?

We have doubled our omega-6 increase in the last hundred years. But is that the reason for the higher rates of cancer? Only in part. More likely, what has led to higher rate of cancer has to do with *processing*.

You see, it doesn't make sense that the omega-6 essential fatty acid, which every cell in our body requires to function, would at the same time give you cancer. On the one hand, it's required for health. On the other hand, it kills you. Doesn't make sense. Processing changes essential fatty acid molecules chemically; that's what we need to look at to explain why increased polyunsaturates have been associated with increased cancer. For instance, when we fry them, they are known to increase cancer. When they're in their natural state like we find them in seeds, or in carefully pressed oils bottled in brown glass bottles, refrigerated in health food stores, they have been processed in a way that is not destructive to the molecules. There is increasing research evidence that when you press omega-6 oils with care, they do not promote tumor growth.

What are some of the more popular omega-6 rich oils?
My favorite omega-6 oils are in sunflower and sesame seeds. Besides omega-6, they contain substances known as "minor" ingredients which have health benefits. Sesame is particularly stable because it contains powerful antioxidants, and sunflower has antioxidants and vitamin E in it as well. But oils must be fresh. Supermarket oils have had most of these beneficial "minor" ingredients removed.

The source material should be organic if possible?
You bet. We don't like our oils with pesticides in them.

Can you describe the harmful ingredients found in supermarket oils and explain how they are produced? Could this also be a factor contributing to tumor development?
In the processing of supermarket oils, the natural antioxidants—vitamin E and carotene—are removed from the oil. Then a cheap synthetic antioxidant, BHT, is added. Some research suggests that there are toxic side effects from BHT, because it doesn't quite fit into the body's very precise molecule architecture.

Most of the harmful ingredients found in supermarket oils result from processing. To make supermarket oils, fresh oils are treated first with Drano (a very corrosive base called sodium hydroxide), then with window washing (phosphoric) acid, then they're bleached (causing rancid taste and odor), and then they're heated to above frying temperature (deodorized). In the course of those processes, molecules are altered: double bonds shift; molecules get fragmented; molecules are cyclized; molecules are cross-linked within a triglyceride, or cross-linked with other triglyceride molecules; a few trans-fatty acids are formed—many chemical changes can take place in the essential fatty acid molecules as a result of this very harsh processing. Some of these altered molecules are toxic, and a connection to cancer is likely.

More research on this topic is surely coming out soon.
There's already quite a bit of research information available on the toxicity: effects on liver function, on detoxification, effects on the platelets, on cardiovascular function, on insulin function, on pregnancy. Studies have clearly shown the toxicity of some of the substances produced by processing oils.

Why did you develop Udo's Choice Perfected Oil Blend?
We need to balance our intake of omega-3 and omega-6 essential fatty acids. If we get too much omega-6, we become deficient in omega-3; if we get too much omega-3, we become deficient in omega-6. Omega-3 and -6 must be balanced properly, because they share enzyme systems and compete with each other. We take great care to balance the Omega 3's and 6's. We

make the blend omega-3-richer because they are missing from standard North American diets, and are therefore more "therapeutic." The blend has all of the ingredients from fats that we need, contains no fats that we should avoid, and is packaged in a dark glass bottle, within a dark box to protect it from light. What we recommend to the consumer is to use it right. The blend can be used in all foods, but should not be fried because frying destroys very quickly the health benefits of the blend. It can be used on steamed dishes and on cold dishes. It goes with every type of food: fruit, vegetables, grains, pastas, starches, and proteins.

Some people may ask, "Aren't we getting enough omega-6 in the average American diet? Why do we need an oil with omega-6?"

There are two answers to that. First, the omega-6s we get in the normal North America diet have been somewhat altered and are not the same as omega-6s that are simply pressed from seeds and not further processed. Second, although we do get some omega-6 (one reason why we make the blend omega-3 richer), if you get too much omega-3—and this can happen, for instance, if someone uses flaxseed oil exclusively—then you can l become omega-6 deficient. We put enough omega-6s in the blend so that someone using it exclusively can't hurt their health.

Please address concerns of vitamin B6 deficiency with omega-3 supplementation.

Vitamin B6 is required in essential fatty acid metabolism, along with about twenty other minerals and vitamins. It is important not to think that essential fatty acids are magic bullets that act alone. You need all forty-five essential nutrients in optimum quantities in order to get optimum cell function, which translates into optimum health. You do need to make sure that your body's getting the vitamin B6 it needs.

Through supplementation?

By whatever way ensures adequacy. Flaxseed and flaxseed oil require B6 to be metabolized properly. Vitamin B6, which is important for the immune system, is also required for protein metabolism. A product I developed, called Udo's Choice Beyond Greens, supplies adequate B6 through other ingredients it contains. People do not need to take a B6 supplement if they are using Udo's Choice Beyond Greens, which was developed to compensate for the downside of consuming flax by itself, which may create deficiencies in the following nutrients: iodine, sulfur, zinc, B6, and omega-6. Udo's Choice Beyond Greens addresses all these concerns. Additionally, Udo's Choice Beyond Greens is immunosupportive, and contains flaxseed lignans and good fiber. The government's RDA (recommended daily allowance) for B6 is 1.6 milligrams a day. You should be sure to take at least 1.6-10 milligrams of B6 to ensure that there's no deficiency while taking flaxseed. As much as 25-50 milligrams of B6, and even up to 200 milligrams per day, is safe. Use more than that only under the supervision of a health professional.

Women with breast cancer, PMS, menopausal symptoms endometriosis, and fibroids generally have improperly functioning livers, and the liver is where the important work of detoxifying potentially dangerous forms of estrogen takes place. Aren't the medium chain triglycerides in your blended oil protective to the liver?

They're helpful because the liver metabolizes them easily. They put less of a burden on the liver, because the liver has to process all fat. Medium chain triglycerides go directly to the liver, through the portal system, and are metabolized there as fuel. They bypass the lymphatic system, which transports all other fats. But essential fatty acids are also protective of liver function, as are many other nuts, oils, and herbs.

The lymphatic system is a factor in breast cancer. What supplements prevent breast cancer? For women interested in maintaining health, what is a general nutritional program that you recommend?

The number one food is lots of greens, meaning vegetables. Number two is good protein and good oils. Third are carbohydrates, but use only as much as you actually need for energy. Fourth is a high-dose, multimineral, multivitamin containing 200 micrograms of selenium. Selenium is a very strong anticancer mineral. Also B6. There are about fifteen different vitamins and mineral deficiencies which impair the immune function enough to allow cancer to proliferate. So those need to be there, but the best way is to use a good, solid, high-dose, multimineral, multivitamin. I get them in capsules because there are fewer fillers and they're absorbed better. I usually add chromium and selenium, extra zinc sometimes, and extra vitamin C.

Please share with us your favorite supplement program for women wanting to recover from breast cancer. There are some "designer supplements" that you may have some recent information on. I'd like to ask you about NAC, CoQ10, alpha-lipoic acid, vitamin E, beta-carotene, Vitamin C, and lycopene.

You also want to include the phytoestrogens that come from soybeans and flax, because they protect estrogen receptors. In terms of cancer, the following nutrients are critical: vitamin A, B3, iodine, magnesium, D, zinc, and essential fatty acids as well as NAC, CoQ10, alph-lipoic acid, vitamin E, beta-carotene, vitamin C, and lycopene. CoQ10, vitamin E, betacarotene, and lycopene are oil-soluble antioxidants. Alpha-lipoic acid is water-soluble, as is vitamin C. You need antioxidants, both in the water system and the oil system in your body, because both are subject to free radical and oxidative damage to tissues, which these antioxidants prevent. Tissue damage ties up the immune system in repair functions, and makes it less able to go after cancer cells.

Can you explain the role enzymes play in cancer?

Every organism in nature eats all its food raw. Raw foods contain enzymes that are part of its own repair mechanism. They digest dead cells back into the basic building materials for making new cells. Enzymes also repair damaged cells. When we eat raw foods, the enzymes they contain do part of the digestion. When we cook food, the enzymes they contain are destroyed. That means our digestive system, which was made for raw food, carries a heavier load. If it can't carry that load, then the immune system gets involved in digestion. The immune system then becomes less able to do other important work in the body—destroy viruses, fungi, bacteria, and cancer cells.

We recommend replacing the enzymes that were destroyed by food preparation. They ease the load of the digestive system, which in turn eases the load of the immune system. Enzymes are also helpful in allergies, which can be forerunners of cancer. We're simply helping the immune system do its job in the bloodstream rather than tying it up in the digestive system.

Further, we know that proteins can be absorbed intact into the body. That's what happens in allergies. There is clinical evidence that enzymes might be absorbed intact into the body through the immune cells that line the intestinal tract. There is evidence of clinical benefits in the treatment of cancer from taking enzymes between meals on a continuous basis.

How many enzymes would you recommend for women with breast cancer?

Digestive problems vary in severity. In order to improve digestion—gas and bloating are the most common symptons—take enough enzymes with meals, preferably mixed through the food, for the symptoms to disappear. Enzymes in capsules can be opened and their contents spread through the food. The food should be warm, not hot, because heat will destroy enzymes. The symptoms stop with anywhere from one to five or six capsules per meal for people with seriously impaired digestion.

For a woman with breast cancer, ten enzyme capsules mixed into the water bottle and sipped all day may be helpful. Continual delivery of enzymes throughout the day is an optimum way to supplement with enzymes.

And the quality of the enzyme supplementation is extraordinarily important.

The best enzymes are rich in protein-digesting proteases, because most of the immune problems caused by foods result from poorly digested proteins. A key factor is therefore that the enzymes be high in protease, to ensure complete digestion of proteins.

The full spectrum, plant-based enzymes supplement that you developed would be good for women to know about.

I've noticed improved circulation from taking the enzyme blend, which is important in healing cancer. Digestive problems improve; many allergy symptons like inflammation are alleviated. They help prevent colds, used in the same way as they're used in cancer. Just sip them in water. If I mix ten to twenty capsules in water in a day, I can get rid of a cold in a day or two.

It really is interesting. I think we've found the cure for the common cold.

I'd like to talk about using fats and oils in food preparation. A recent study at the University of North Carolina at Chapel Hill discovered women with breast cancer stored a lot more trans-fats than women without breast cancer. The theory that trans-fats may trigger breast cancer and other cancers is not new to you. What are trans-fats and which foods contain them?

Trans-fatty acids are what I call the "twisted sisters" of essential fatty acids. They are heat-twisted molecules with double bonds—monounsaturated or polyunsaturated fatty acid molecules whose shapes have been changed. Their shape changed, they no longer fit into the molecular architecture of the body, and interfere with the functions of the essential fatty acids. You find trans-fatty acids in margarines, shortenings, shortening oils, and in partially hydrogenated vegetable oils, which are really widespread in our food supply. They are found in breads, cakes, cookies, candies; in dried soup mixes and frozen foods; in most crackers in some salad dressings; in chocolate; in granola bars. Even the croutons we use for our healthy Caesar salad contain trans-fatty acids.

Trans-fatty acids interfere with liver detoxification and that's very important. When toxins back up in the body, cancer can proliferate. Whatever interferes with liver function cannot be good for cancer patients and will take you closer to cancer. Trans-fatty acids also interfere with essential fatty acid functions and the antitumor effects of omega-3's. Trans-fatty acids make platelets stickier and thereby interfere with circulation, which decreases oxygenation of cells—another factor in producing cancer. Otto Warburg showed in 1927 that one can induce cancer experimentally by oxygen deprivation. Trans-fatty acids may also have adverse effects on estrogen metabolism, which may play a role in producing cancers.

Aren't freshness and quality more important than terms such as monounsaturated and polyunsaturated when it comes to understanding oils?

One of the key points that I make when I talk about the fats that heal and fats that kill is that the health problems usually blamed on fats are actually the result of the processing to which the fats have been subjected, because processing damages oils. To make colorless, odorless, tasteless supermarket oils—some of which you also find, unrefrigerated, on shelves in health food stores—requires treatment with Drano; with window washing acid; with bleach, which produces rancidity; and then with overheating to above frying temperature (in a process called deodorization to get rid of the bad odor of rancidity). These four processes change and damage oils.

To make health-supporting oils (essential fatty acids are very sensitive to destruction by light, by oxygen, and by high temperature), we need to treat them with a lot of care—in production, in storage, and in food use in the home.

In 1987, we pioneered ways to make oils with human health in mind. We had to modify the machinery that's used to make oils and we had to develop new packaging systems. We use dark glass, we put a shelf date on the oil, we keep it in the refrigerator. In fact, for best storage, we tell people to freeze oils solid. Buy oil by the case, get your discount, freeze it (oil shrinks when it freezes, so the brown glass bottles will not break!), and keep the bottle you're using in the fridge. Use the oil within four to eight weeks of opening if it's an oil rich in essential fatty acids.

Good oils need to be treated like perishable groceries, because they can spoil (unlike minerals and vitamins, which can be dried and powered and stuck on a shelf for three years with little deterioration). Good oils require a lot of care. They are a reminder that health is not a convenience, but requires care.

How long can flaxseed oil and Udo's Choice Oil be frozen?

If you freeze oils solid so the molecules don't move, their shelf life is three to five years. The only way to get that long shelf life is by freezing oils solid. Vitamin E, vitamin C, and carotene (antioxidants) extend the shelf life maybe by sixty percent if you're lucky. Refrigerated, flaxseed oil has a three-month shelf life. Antioxidants might take it up to five months, but you have to freeze the oil to get three years. That's how delicate the essential fatty acids are.

A recent article on fats and oils stated that monounsaturates and polyunsaturates are not harmful and, in fact, are probably beneficial. Frank Sacks, a researcher with the Harvard School of Public Health, was quoted as saying this. The article also stated that research has not borne out the connection between polyunsaturated fats and human cancer. The article concluded with a recommendation to use corn, canola, olive and safflower oils. What are your thoughts on this?

I referred to this before: If the omega-6s are not damaged in processing, they do not produce cancer. I do not agree with the recommendation that we should stock up on corn, canola, olive, and safflower oils because the corn, canola, and the safflower oils have been heated to above frying temperature before they go into your kitchen. Harvard's recommendation doesn't tell you not to fry with these oils, but they should have! There is a correlation between fried oils and cancer.

Extra virgin olive oil has not been overheated—it's the only oil in the supermarket that hasn't been treated with Drano, window washing acid, bleach, and overheating. But extra virgin olive oil should not be used for frying either, because frying damages all oils.

We tell people to fry only with water. Add good oils to the food on their plates to prevent oils from being damaged in food preparation. Poaching, boiling, steaming, and pressure-cooking food is really only a small change. In all food preparation—toasting, roasting, baking, broiling, and barbecuing, only the outside of the food dries out and burns. From the point of view of health, or if we have breast cancer, we should remove the browned, charred outside part of foods.

When we steam, poach, boil, or pressure-cook, we save ourselves the work of having to remove the burned portion. The only noticeable change to the food is that the burned taste is lost. Easy to get used to.

If people do not have breast cancer and they feel they want to use an oil once in a while, do you recommend untoasted organic sesame seed oil, bottled in dark glass, used with water in the pan first, sautéed at low temperatures?

Always put water or vegetables in the pan first, and add the oil afterwards. When you put oil in the frying pan by itself, it overheats and is damaged long before it turns into smoke. Water in the pan keeps the temperature down and then you don't burn the oil.

Do overheated fats and oils block the protective effects of flaxseed oil and fatty-rich fish?

They compete for enzyme sites and thereby block out the essential fatty acids. The body has to make more enzymes and clean up the mess. They interfere with the functions of the essential fatty acids, both omega-6 and omega-3. But overheated oils cause other toxic effects as well.

Could you comment on canola oil?

One hundred fifty million dollars were spent on marketing canola oil. That's why it's getting a lot of attention. But canola oil is processed like all the other oils: with Drano, window washing acid, bleach, and then overheated. It shares the processing problems with all the other oils. Then it's recommended for frying and further damage is done to it.

Does it contain omega-3?

It has about ten percent omega-3, 25 percent omega-6, and about sixty percent monounsaturated.

So it wouldn't be a choice for heating because it does contain some omega-3s?

Omega-3s and omega-6s become more toxic when they're overheated than do monounsaturates and saturates. The more omega-3 an oil contains, the worse off you're going to be if you overheat it.

There's been some controversy over canola oil not really being heart healthy.

It's heart healthy, in theory. If you consumed the oil the way it exists in the seed or in an oil that is simply squeezed out of the seed at low temperature and protected from light and oxygen, it does have heart healthy omega-3s in it. But you do better on oils that have been made with more care and that also contain more omega-3s such as the blend we talked about and flaxseed oil. Because of the processing, I put canola oil low on the list of healthy oils.

Federal standards don't permit the use of trans-fatty acids—margarines, shortening, or partially hydrogenated vegetable oils—in baby foods. Is this important for adults to be aware of as well?

The metabolism of babies and adults is similar. Babies are more sensitive, but the metabolism is the same. Trans-fatty acids interfere with a baby's liver detox, but they also interfere with adult liver detox. I don't understand why the government decided that after we're two years old, they don't care anymore. Maybe they're trying to kill the voters, so they can impose their ideas on babies. I'm joking, of course, but the care is not there. Poison for children is poison for adults.

The oil and margarine industry is a strong lobby in Washington.

That's true. Huge lobby with financial interests to protect.

Please comment on the use of soy margarine. Is this simply another hydrogenated product? How about the so-called nonhydrogenated spreads— good or bad?

Soy margarine, if it says "partially hydrogenated" or "hydrogenated vegetable oil" (if the "H" word is on the label), has trans-fatty acids in it. And yes, then it's simply another hydrogenated product. Whether you find it in a grocery store or a health food store, the biochemical problem is the same.

In manufacturing non-hydrogenated spreads including some margarines, processed oils that have been treated with Drano, window washing acid, bleach, and overheating are used. Because people don't know the processing that has taken place, they assume that, if it's not hydrogenated, it's good. From the research I have read, I have to disagree. The spreads have been processed and changed too much from their natural state. From a health point of view, you want to eat things the way nature makes them, not the way they've been chemically changed by high-tech processes.

Could you tell us the difference between partial hydrogenation and complete hydrogenation?

Partial hydrogenation produces trans-fatty acids. Completely hydrogenation produces a saturated fat with no trans-fatty acids in it.

Partial hydrogenation creates a softer product, and complete hydrogenation creates a harder product?

That's true. If you completely hydrogenate canola or another oil, it becomes so hard that you need a chisel to chip it out of its container. It melts at about 160 degrees Fahrenheit (body temperature is 98). Manufacturers make some margarines by combining completely hydrogenated oil and liquid oil. But both ingredients are highly processed. The "minor" ingredients are gone. Toxic molecules that are the result of the oil having been refined, bleached, and deodorized even before it was hydrogenated are present. Not a natural product. Health is about living in line with nature.

Can you comment on the use of cottonseed oil and peanut oil, both prevalent in packaged foods?

Peanut oil contains only small amounts of omega-6 and no omega-3 essential fatty acids, is high in saturated fats, and includes a twenty-carbon saturated arachidic acid, a very hard fat. Peanut oil is treated with the four processes; the same is true for cottonseed.

Cottonseeds are garbage from the cotton industry. The oil must be put through all those processes—to get rid of toxic pesticides and natural toxins present in the cottonseed. Both oils have been overheated. Both oils only contain omega-6s and are not sources of omega-3s.

Please comment on the use of grapeseed oil for cooking.

Grapeseed oil is another omega-6 oil. It is made from the seeds, material that used to be thrown away, a cheap starting material. The oil from grapeseeds is similar to corn oil; it has some healthful minor ingredients when it's unrefined. Those are removed to some extent when the oil is refined. Using it for "cooking" causes the same damage that frying does to other oils, and it's already been overheated in the process of being made. Although it's getting a lot of marketing attention, I am not impressed with grapeseed oil.

Oils from organically grown seeds, made with care, packaged in brown glass, refrigerated in health food stores, not used for frying, are the kinds of oils I recommend for health.

I've noticed that some cookbooks recommend the use of safflower oil for heating, and I've also heard you mention in your lectures that safflower oil contains some irritating properties. Can you explain?

The irritating properties of safflower oil come from its "minor" ingredients. What are "minor" ingredients? "Minor" ingredients in extra virgin olive oil improve liver, gall bladder, digestive, and cardiovascular function. They have antioxidant functions that prevent random damage from free radicals in the body. "Minor" ingredients can have very powerful healing effects. In fact, in extra virgin olive oil, the "minor" ingredients that make up only two percent of the oil (hence the "minor") are the most important aspect of the oil. [Author's note: Light olive oil contains no "minor" ingredients.] But "minor" ingredients can also make an oil unpalatable or even toxic. According to Ayuervedic tradition, some minor ingredients present in safflower oil have irritating properties.

Safflower is like corn oil for heating, but safflower has even more omega-6. Heating damages the Omega-6 essential fatty acids. Safflower has no Omega-3s. Heavy consumption of processed safflower oil (and other omega-3-deficient oil) promotes cancer in animals. Hardening of the arteries, and probably inflammation, are also associated with such oils.

That's important information because so many natural foods cookbooks recommend safflower oil. On another subject, what is olestra and how will this phony fat affect the immune system?

We call olestra the "anal leakage" fat, because it's not absorbed. The body doesn't take it apart, because it has no enzymes to do so. Olestra is a synthetic product that never existed in nature, so the body has never had to make something to break it down.

The olestra concept is based on the mistaken notion that all fats are bad and that you should be on a low-fat diet. But to get the mouth feel and flavor enhancement that fatty substances bring to foods (and olestra will do that), you add something that isn't fat to foods. Because olestra is not digested, it ends up in your stool and then it's hard to hold your stool. Hence, anal leakage.

Olestra, because it's not absorbed, will dissolve oil-soluble nutrients in foods, which include vitamin A, carotene, vitamin E, vitamin D, vitamin K, and many of the oil-soluble phytonutrients including anticancer lycopene found in tomatoes, and many others that have benefits. The Harvard School of Public Health told the FDA that if olestra becomes widespread in the diet, we will be looking at increased cancer, increased cardiovascular disease, increased diabetes, and increased other degenerative conditions. They asked the FDA not to okay it. The FDA decided that since occasional diarrhea is not life-threatening, they would allow it in foods.

This is outrageous, because antioxidant nutrients are so important for women who want to prevent breast cancer.

Extremely important, because if you don't have antioxidants, you get random tissue damage, and tie up the immune system in something other than cancer prevention and healing from cancer.

Why is butter better than most oils for heating?

Butter fries at a lower temperature, around 300 degrees Fahrenheit, as opposed to oils which fry between 360 and 420 degrees Fahrenheit.

Tell us about the origin of ghee.

Ghee was invented in India, in a hot climate without refrigeration. Butter goes rancid quicker because it has debris from the milk cells in it. Indians take the cell debris out. You end up with just a purer oil, which is more resistant to bacterial growth and to rancidity.

Is soybean oil a source of protective isoflavones? Isoflavones are important for women with breast cancer. Also, is it a recommended oil for cooking or for salad dressings?

That's an interesting question. Most of the isoflavones, because they're water-soluble, are found in the bean, not in the oil. You might get a little bit in the oil, but I think you're better off to eat tofu for isoflavones. Eat the soybeans. Soybean of from the supermarket has all the problems that all the processed oils have.

Even some oils sold in health food stores may not be fresh and unprocessed.

There are colorless, odorless, tasteless oils in health food stores that come from the same suppliers as the oils sold in supermarkets. There's a mistaken perception in the health food trade that these oils are better, but most of them are exactly the same.

I have begun to notice recipes calling for "high oleic" safflower or sunflower oil for frying. Could you comment?

High oleic safflower and sunflower oils are a product of genetic engineering; scientists have destroyed a gene that makes an enzyme that turns oleic acid into linoleic acid. So they have less omega-6s in them. Neither of them contain omega-3s and they can be heated to a higher temperature, but that means there is more molecular damage and that means there's more damage to health. Again, frying is not a healthful practice. And those oils are usually fully refined, treated with the four—Drano, window washing acid, bleach, and overheating—before you get them. The "minor" ingredients have been taken out. These are highly processed oils.

In Spain, sunflower oil is often used instead of olive oil; Spanish cooks say sunflower oil is less heavy. What do you think?

Sunflower is less heavy than olive oil. Oils richer in essential fatty acids are lighter. Sometimes we mix extra virgin olive oil with my blend and make humus that way. The dish is lighter. Sunflower oil is less heavy than olive oil, but neither should be fried.

Most of us don't think about the fact that many peanut butters are partially hydrogenated.

You have to look for the "H" word. We say if you see the "H" word on the label, get the "H" out of there. If there's oil on top of your peanut butter, it's not hydrogenated. The reason they hydrogenate it is so that the oil can be mixed into the peanut butter and will stay mixed. If your peanut butter has no oil on top of it, it's likely to be hydrogenated. You will see that listed on the label as "partially hydrogenated."

We already established that eating cold-water fish is breast protective. I'd like to ask you to define EPA and DHA.

Eicosapentaenoic acid (EPA) and docosahexaenoic acid (DHA) are derivatives of the omega-3 essential fatty acid. Both are found in high-fat, cold-water fish. Most people's bodies make them from alpha-linolenic, the omega-3 essential fatty acid. They have benefits: EPA is the parent from which the prostaglandin 3s are made. They have protective functions against the damage that the prostaglandin 2s can do. EPA has anticancer as well as heart-protective properties.

People may not realize that farm-raised salmon is low in EPA and DHA. Susun Weed pointed out that she recommends that people eat tuna, which provides more EPA and DHA, because it is a wild fish. Do you think that's a better choice?

The farm-raised salmon is lower in EPA and DHA than the open-ocean fish. I prefer open-ocean fish to farm-raised salmon. Because the omega 3s are perishable, commercial feeds contain less of it because of the rancidity problem. In nature, fish eat living foods that contain the omega-3s, including the EPA and DHA. I recommend high-fat, cold-wrater fish from *natural* sources: trout, salmon, albacore tuna (white tuna—the red tuna is a low-fat fish), mackerel, and sardines.

Commercial foods have to have shelf life. When we change foods for better shelf life, we especially alter essential fatty acids, because they are easily altered or destroyed. It takes care to make foods well. The pet food industry also never gets the fats right. The essential fatty acids should come from living foods or from foods made with a lot of care and handled with a lot of care.

So breast-protective omega-3s are in the fatty albacore tuna?
Yes. The belly of the tuna, around the fins and behind the gills, are the fat-richest part. Canned tuna contains only the low-fat part of the fish: the back part that contains the backbone. About one-third of the oil is lost in the canning process.

How do you feel about broiling or grilling fatty-rich fish?
The essential fatty acids in the burnt part of the fish are changed and become toxic. It's better for health to poach fish.

Poached or steamed salmon is delicious. What do you think about charcoal grilling in general?
Grilling has a strong association with cancer. When charcoal burns, it produces toxic substances. Burnt food is also toxic.

So, it's the charcoal that's the issue. Traditional people used to cook elk and venison and wild game over a wood fire.
You're going to get toxins from smoke, too. The high heat causes damage and the smoke adds cancer-causing chemicals. That's been known for a long time.

Oil freshness is of paramount importance. That's why I've learned to look for refrigerated oils in small, amber glass bottles, complete with a pressing date. Are rancid fats and oils detrimental to our endocrine system? How do we know if an oil is rancid?
Rancid oil has a painty smell. If an unprocessed oil is two percent rancid, it is completely unpalatable. With a processed supermarket oil, it's harder to tell because most of the flavor is removed, but there may be a painty or fishy smell. Fresh fish doesn't smell fishy—that's deterioration. The "fishy" smell is nature warning your body against rancid oils.

What do rancid oils do to our health?
Rancid oils interfere with the functions that essential fatty acids are required for. They are changed molecules, and they cause inflammation in the digestive tract.

Should nuts and seeds be refrigerated as well?
It's not necessary, but okay. Most nuts and seeds have a protective skin around them that protects them both from light and from oxygen; then the temperature is not as critical. Broken nuts and seeds are best refrigerated.

A lot of unroasted or untoasted almonds or Brazil nuts that don't have shells are available in stores.

If they're broken, certainly for walnuts, I would recommend refrigeration, because they're broken and they do go rancid. Almonds are fairly stable. Sunflower seeds I would probably refrigerate as well. Peanuts are stable. Brazil nuts are mostly monounsaturated, but they do go rancid—you can taste the rancidity—so I would probably refrigerate those. I wouldn't use Brazils much, because they're poor sources of essential fatty acids.

I'd like to talk about food selection and breast cancer. What type of diet should women follow to facilitate the process of maintaining and restoring breast health?

Lots of green veggies. Good fats, whole foods, and organic foods.

Raw foods?

Raw foods are great, although you have to convert to eating raw foods gradually. Otherwise, you may get uproar in your digestive system if you're not used to them. Freshly made raw vegetable juices are easier to digest. Specific supplements that are helpful, besides the essential fatty acids, include iodine, niacin, magnesium, and nuneral ascorbates. Some healers use very high closes of vitamin A in cancer treatment for a time, doses that are considered toxic by RDA standards, like two million IU [international units] a day.

So, people should go to a naturopath or a nutritionist for a plan that is individualized when they are healing breast cancer?

Yes, I would work with the healing professional competent in nutrition. Dosages of vitamins will vary for different people. They depend on the kind of cancer, the stage of advancement, and the rest of the woman's lifestyle. It also depends on her metabolic rate, which is in part genetically determined. Many factors need to be taken into account. Programs need to be individually tailored.

Is it necessary to follow a strict vegetarian diet to heal cancer and other degenerative diseases?

If you've been on a high-meat diet, going strictly vegetarian (vegan) may be helpful for a while, but I would not go on it life-long. I would not take it beyond three years. There's no traditional vegan diet anywhere in the world. That's probably because all the people who followed it died out. There are some substances from animal proteins that we seem to need. Even the vegetarian chimpanzees will eat a baboon every once in a while. If you have been vegan or fruitarian for a long time, meat may be helpful to healing cancer.

I didn't know that!

A little bit of animal product seems to be better for health than being strictly vegetarian. [Author's note: Studies are now being conducted on benefits of amino acids and other nutrients in meat for cancer. Meat is a source of breast-protective and cancer-fighting lipoic acid.]

Also, there's the movement towards increasing protein because people have been consuming so many carbohydrates.

You want to malce sure you get fresh green vegetables. This is the green planet; green vegetables are the number one food. Get good proteins and good fats and eat only as much carbohydrates as you actually burn. The carbohydrates you eat in excess of what your body burns in activity turn into and are stored as fat. Those fats interfere with essential fatty acid functions, so they have a moderate correlation to increased cancer. So does sugar.

I think when people add adequate protein they have fewer sugar cravings.

Also, adequate essential fatty acid-rich oils decrease cravings. By the way, there's a lot of sugar in sweet fruit, and excess fruit consumption causes the same problems as sugar. An apple a day keeps the doctor away, but the second apple brings him back.

Are you at all concerned that a life of strict vegetarianism may lead to the body's inability to naturally convert omega-3 essential fatty acids to their important derivatives?

No, not really, except for those who have a genetic problem converting. In the general population, probably less than one percent of people can't convert omega-3 to EPA and DHA. On a strict vegetanan diet, you are likely to get better conversion of omega-3s because your diet is less likely to have a lot of interfering substances in it. Now, that's not entirely true, because sugar and fried oils can be part of a vegan diet. Even margarine and shortening can be present in a vegan diet, and these do interfere with omega-3 conversion. Vegans have to be extremely knowledgeable in their food selections if they want to be healthy.

I think that dietary choices are determined by health, age, climate, and constantly changing factors in our lives. There have been a lot of dietary recommendations suggesting a new trend, eating according to blood type. Could you give us your guidelines on putting it all together?

Anybody who tells us, "This is the diet for everybody," is wrong. People are different and must experiment with their food choices (even though Mother told us not to play with our food). They must figure out individually what works best for themselves. It's different for different people.

If a cave man had a Big Mac attack, he didn't say: Let me chip a rock, turn it into a spear, and go after a deer. He looked around to see what was available to eat. It was usually something green, roots of something green, or fruits, seeds, berries, and nuts of something green. That was the number one food available everywhere. And number two was good protein and good oil. The oil came from the seeds and nuts, mostly. The good protein came from a rock they'd throw at a rat, or a rabbit, or a bird, occasionally. Cave men were greater braggers then hunters. They came home meatless a lot. The women fed the tribe with vegetable foods.

I'm not surprised.

Blood type may play a role in dietary requirements. It remains to be determined how strong a role. Fads often precede (or evade) knowledge.

As I mentioned before, you only need enough carbohydrates to burn for energy. Athletes may need sixty percent of their calories as carbs, but somebody who is mostly sedentary may only need forty percent. When I work out more, I crave carbohydrates and protein, because I need more carbs for energy and more protein for muscle building. If you become quiet enough inside to notice what your body is telling you and then observe what you're doing and how that manifests in terms of energy levels and how you feel, you can work your food needs out for yourself, given the nutrition guidelines.

Could you tell us about prostaglandins, how they are formed, what are they for? Can prostaglandins protect a woman's hormonal system, or can they harm it? How can we facilitate the production of beneficial prostaglandins?

The prostaglandins are hormone-like, regulating substances that are made from three derivatives of essential fatty acids. Prostaglandin-1s come from dihomo-gamma-linolenic acid or DGLA. Prostaglandin-2s come from arachidonic acid. Prostaglandin-3s come from eicosapentaenoic acid. So prostaglandin-1 and -2 are made from omega-6 derivatives and prostaglandin-3s are made from omega-3 derivatives. Generally speaking, in our way of life, prostaglandin-1 and 3s have beneficial functions, prostaglandin 2s have a mixture of beneficial and detrimental functions. The latter (detrimental) had survival value in the jungle, but work against us in the modern sedentary situation in which we live, where we can't indulge in fight-or-flight behavior. We are exposed to stress that induces us to fight or flee, but when we're not allowed to fight or flee (in social situations), the prostaglandin-2s become detrimental.

Prostaglandins-3, made from omega-3 essential fatty acids, prevent the production of detrimental prostaglandins 2s. Prostaglandins have many regulatory functions in all of our cells. These include platelet stickiness, inflammatory mechanisms, blood pressure regulation, and water metabolism by the kidney. Prostaglandins are also involved in water regulation in our tissues, along with histamines. Uterine contraction is prostaglandin-based. Many female conditions, including endometriosis, result from prostaglandin imbalance.

Menstrual cramps and premenstrual syndrome also involve prostaglandin imbalances. Some breast conditions are also prostaglandin-related.

Can prostaglandins protect a woman's hormonal system or harm it? They can do both, depending on the balance of prostaglandins. Prostaglandins are in fact a part of the hormonal system of women (as well as men).

How do we facilitate production of beneficial prostaglandins? EPA, the omega-3 essential fatty acid derivative, blocks the production of prostaglandin-2s with proinflammatory, blood pressure-increasing, water-retaining, and platelet-stickying functions. Because most omega-3s have been removed from our diet, we enrich people's diets with omega-3s, which is why the oil blend I developed is twice as rich in omega-3s as it is in omega-6s. It helps to block prostaglandin-2 production.

Adrenal glands, significant in hormone production, are nourished by essential fatty acids. Again, we're back to the problems with fat-free, which can actually create adrenal problems that can turn into PMS or symptoms of menopause.

Fat-free diets don't just create adrenal problems, they create problems in every cell, tissue, gland, and organ in the body, because they deprive us of essential fatty acids. Fat-free diets are lethal if sustained long enough. One of the symptoms of essential fatty acid deficiency is that glands dry up, not just adrenals, but also thyroid, pancreas, male and female reproductive glands, kidneys, liver, and brain—and we consistently get improvements when people get the fats right. One of the reasons why the essential fatty acids are important in gland functions is that they increase energy production and, therefore, gland performance.

The Western diet is rich in omega-6 and deficient in omega-3. Most persons with cancer are found to benefit by increasing consumption of omega-3 essential fatty acids, found abundantly in flaxseeds. There are exciting studies which substantiate the use of flaxseed in the treatment of breast and other hormone-sensitive cancers. This is something you have known about for quite some time and there's a lot of research showing flaxseed modulates estrogen. Could you comment on the way flaxseeds and oil have the ability to shrink tumors?

There are several issues here. First of all, many women with cancer improve with flax or flaxseed oil or a combination of the two. (There are some people who need oils from fish to make the conversion from omega-3 to EPA and DHA. Eating fatty-rich fish provides the EPA and DHA.) The omega-3s, are antitumor. Phytoestrogens called lignans found in flax are antitumor. The fiber in flax improves colon function and detoxifies, and has antitumor properties in that regard. So there are at least three antitumor components in flax. The fiber and most of the lignans don't end up in the oil, but the omega-3s obviously are concentrated in the oil. The best source of lignans and fiber are flaxseeds.

Please comment about flax and colon bacteria.

The fiber, besides being wonderful for bowel regularity and taking toxins out of the body, is also very good food for the friendly microorganisms in our intestines. It is important to remember, though, that flaxseed and flaxseed oil also have a downside. The downside for the seed is that omega-3-rich but omega-6-poor. Flaxseeds increase our requirement for zinc, iodine, sulfur, and B6. But obviously flax has a strong upside in the omega-3s, the lignans, and the fiber.

Evening primrose, black currant, and borage oil all contain gamma-linolenic acid, or GLA, an omega-6 fatty acid derivative used to alleviate symptoms of **PMS. GLA is also a precursor to some favorable prostaglandins.** *In fact, most sources of GLA are far richer in linoleic acid than GLA (as you have written in Fats that Heal; Fats That Kill).* **Evening primrose oil, for instance, contains seventy-two percent linoleic acid, but only nine percent GLA. Is this the reason that practitioners knowledgeable about nutrition only recommend short-term use of GLA supplements? Comment also on the increased tissue levels of arachidonic acid, which can produce prostaglandins that cause problems.**

Evening primrose and borage oils contain no omega-3s. Most of the GLA studies were done on the omega-3-deficient population. If Omega-3s are provided in optimum quantities, GLA will lose some of its appeal. We have consistently switched people from GLA supplements to oils rich in alpha-linolenic acid, and have achieved similar results. There are overlapping effects between GLA and alpha-linolenic acid, because both are similar in their structure. Both have eighteen carbons, three double bonds, and a similar kind of chemical reactivity.

When you use GLA-containing oil, I recommend using Efamol evening primrose oil. It's the only one that is unrefined—hasn't been treated with Drano, window washing acid, bleach, and then overheated. That makes a difference, because the "minor" ingredients in evening primrose oil appear to be part of why it is more effective than other GLA-containing oils. Also, most of the research on GLA was done using this specific brand of oil.

Stress produces "stress hormones" that increase production of arachidonic acid, from which the body makes prostaglandins that increase platelet stickiness, blood pressure, water retention and inflammation. These are protective in the jungle for fight or flight. For us, it is better to reduce stress to decrease prostaglandin-2 production. Stress reduction is an important healing factor in (breast) cancer.

Do you think most people would be better off using flaxseed oil over the more expensive GLA supplements in terms of economics as well as health?

GLA supplements provide about six grams of oil, mostly omega-6. We recommend about one to three tablespoons and sometimes up to five or more per day, because essential fatty acids are major nutrients. That's about fourteen to seventy or more grams of oil. You would be better off using flaxseed oil or the omega-3-rich, better-balanced blend I developed, both in brown glass. Oils play many roles in health: in the structure of cell membranes, in protection of DNA against damage, in the functions of glands and organs—much more than the role of just GLA by itself. I do not recommend oil in plastics, because there are too many unanswered health and environment questions. Oils and plastics are similar materials. When I learned about estrogen mimickers that leach out of some kinds of plastic, I changed my view on plastic. I began to wonder what other problems with plastic are we going to find in about five or ten or fifteen years that we haven't thought about? Just like we never thought about the estrogen mimickers until they were widespread in the biosphere and affected sexual behavior and reproductive ability in many species of animals, and probably also in people.

Another important area of discussion is lymphatic vitality, which is key to detoxifying the body and preventing breast cancer. Please talk about how fried foods, and poor quality fats and oils, adversely effect lymphatic health.

The fats—both fried and poor-guality fats and oils, as well as food fats—are absorbed from our intestine into the lymph. From there, they go to the blood, then to the liver, from the liver to all cells, then back to the liver, into the intestine, and then into the toilet. The lymphatic system is involved in cancer; it's also involved in toxin movement and fat transport. The more garbage fats you load into your lymphatic system, the more problems you are going to create in your lymphatic system. Since the lymphatic system is extremely important in oil metabolism, it is obvious that the oils that we dump into our lymph system ought to be oils that promote health rather than oils that cause disease. Food choices are extremely important.

What suggestions to you have for improving lymphatic health?

The single best recommendation for improving lymphatic health, other than getting clean foods; good, fresh oils; and detoxifying fiber (through water-soluble fiber-rich products, like The Missing Link), is rebound (mini-trampoline) exercise and sweating, which removes toxins from your body through your skin, and spares the liver and kidneys from damage done by toxins.

Rebounding is great for detoxifying the lymph. [For information about rebounding, please refer to the section on the lymph system and the Resource Guide.] How does flaxseed oil nourish the lymphatic system?

Flaxseed oil provides the omega-3s, as long as it's fresh and properly made. Of course, the lymphatic system also needs the omega-6s. The lymphatic system is made of cells, all of which need both essential fatty acids to have the energy to do their jobs.

Obesity is linked to a high rate of breast cancer. Let's focus on weight loss for a moment. Why should people not be afraid of flaxseed oil, if they are on a diet?

The essential fatty acids, especially the omega-3s, increase metabolic rate. You can measure the increase in oxygen metabolism, increased rate of oxidation, called the VO_2 max. Body builders use flaxseed oil for six to eight weeks before a competition in order to lose the fat under their skin so that their muscle fibers shows (look "shredded"). That's really important in body building. We tell people when they count calories they should not count the essential fatty acids as calories because that's not how the body uses them. And for every gram of omega-3s in their diets, they should subtract two or three calories from their total count, because these are actually anticalorie fats—they increase the metabolic rate and you burn more calories. They also make you feel like you have energy so you are likely to be more active. And they also make you calmer and elevate mood or lift depression, so you are less likely to overeat because of depression. They help reduce cravings for junk foods, junk fats, and sugars. They make your skin nice. When your skin is nice, your mood is up, and your energy is high, you are more likely to feel like you're worth taking care of.

What oils put weight on?

Fats don't make you fat. In fact, if you go on a high-protein, high-fat diet, you will lose weight, because fats form ketones that suppress appetite. Of course, you want to use the right kind of fat. What makes you fat is excess sugar and carbohydrates, because if you eat more of those than your body is actually burning, they turn into fat. Fats stored in your body can also store fat-soluble carcinogenic toxins.

Does flaxseed oil help to maintain stable blood sugar levels, preventing "binging"?

Any oil will help to some extent, because oils slow down stomach emptying time, slowing down digestion. Much better results for maintaining stable blood glucose levels come from water-soluble, mucilage fiber found in flax and in The Missing Link. We give the latter to diabetics and hypoglycemics, six to ten tablespoons a day, and we get consistent, remarkable blood glucose stabilizing, effects. Great for anyone with blood sugar fluctuation problems. Fiber is superior to oil in that regard.

What happens when a woman tries to diet but doesn't have any omega-3 oil?
One of the reasons why women gain even more weight when they come off a weight-loss diet is because they get depleted of omega-3s, which results in lowered metabolic rate.

That's an important point. I'd like to talk about Udo's Choice Beyond Greens.
Udo's Choice Beyond Greens is made of twenty-five whole foods and food concentrates. It has been carefully put together to provide balanced omega-3s and -6s. The increased zinc, iodine, sulfur, and vitamin B6 requirements caused by flaxseed have been dealt with. Udo's Choice Beyond Greens provides dozens of immune-enhancing phytonutrients. These come from vegetables and herbs publicized by the National Cancer Institute as containing immune-supporting, immune-enhancing, and cancer-inhibiting phytonutrients.

This is an important product for women who want to prevent breast cancer. How many tablespoons of this product would you recommend women consume for this purpose?
We suggest one tablespoon per 33 pounds of body weight per day. A 100-pound woman would take three tablespoons per day; a 200-pound man would take six. I take five because I weigh 170 pounds. I put my five tablespoons of Udo's Choice Beyond Greens in a glass in the morning, mix in a couple of capsules of digestive enzymes, then I mix in two tablespoons of my oil blend. The oil sticks to the granular material Udo's Choice Beyond Greens is made of. Then I add tomato juice (which contains cancer-inhibiting lycopene) or water or another juice, and stir it, and that's my breakfast. A two-ounce breakfast. Tastes good. My breakfast lasts me from eight A.M. to one or two P.M. Udo's Choice Beyond Greens can also be put in shakes or mixed in yogurt or put on salads—you can eat it lots of different ways.

It has a nice nutty kind of a slightly wholesome, sweet taste to it.
The sweet taste comes from licorice root, which is immune-enhancing. We don't use sugar, because cancer cells like sugar.

Please comment on the Mediterranean diet, and why you think people who naturally eat the diet have such low rates of cancer and heart disease.
By using oil on their steamed or boiled vegetables, Mediterraneans get improved absorption of fat-soluble phytonutrients with health benefits, like

lycopene in tomatoes. There are lots of oil-soluble phytonutrients in all fresh vegetables.

Italians don't fry olive oil. Extra virgin olive oil's "minor" ingredients have many health benefits. Italians eat more fresh, fewer processed foods, no trans-fatty acids. They're big on the relaxed lifestyle. They express themselves. They're lovers. People in their fifties and sixties in Italy walk hand-in-hand, still in love, down the promenade. They drink red wine with the protective red antioxidant pigments. There are lots of reasons why they have better health than we do.

The Lyon Diet Heart Study compared the American Heart Association diet to the Mediterranean diet. The AHA diet places no emphasis on monounsaturated fat (like olive oil) and limits fat to thirty percent of calories. The Mediterranean diet consisted of high monounsaturated fat (which is in olive oil), together with vegetables, fruit, fresh herbs, beans, fish, small portions of meat, no butter or cream. It was found during a careful followup period lasting over two years that those who consumed foods outlined in the Mediterranean plan reflected a seventy-six percent reduction in heart attacks compared to those participants who followed the AHA diet. Both groups got about thirty percent of their calories from fat. The researchers speculated that because monounsaturated fats are more stable and resist oxidation, the Meditenanean diet helps to reduce heart disease and breast cancer. The researchers theorized that plant omega-3 fatty acids provided additional protection by reducing blood clotting and arrhythmia, which often precede heart attacks. I'm confused, though. Isn't olive oil a poor source of both omega-3 and omega-6 essential fatty acids? Please comment on both areas of monounsaturated fat, and the fatty acid profile of olive oil.

The thirty percent fats in the Mediterranean diet is mostly unrefined, unprocessed extra virgin olive oil, with protective "minor" ingredients. The AHA diet pays no attention to the quality of the fat, or the omega-3.

Monounsaturates in olive oil are not very stable because olive oil also contains chlorophyll, which speeds oil breakdown. Olive oil is a poor source of omega-3, less than one percent, and it contains about ten percent omega-6, but the "minor" ingredients in extra virgin olive oil improve liver function, so they should be helpful in cancer. They also improve cardiovascular function, improve gall bladder function and digestion.

Some books on cancer prevention and cooking mistakenly recommend the use of light olive oil. What is so protective about olive oil in the context of the Mediterranean diet? Isn't there more here than meets, the eye?

The extra virgin olive oil in the Mediterranean diet is being compared to a diet in North America which consists almost solely of oils that have had their "minor" ingredients removed, that have been processed with Drano, window washing acid, bleach and then overheated. It's important to recognize that most of the health problems blamed on fats are actually caused by destructive processing. "Light" and "100%" olive oil have lost their "minor" ingredients, and are processed the same way as the other supermarket oils.

Italians don't have artificial ingredients or preservatives in their foods, nor do they consume as much sugar as we do. And they eat a lot more fresh fish. I noticed that their salmon is from Norway, which is not farm raised, so they probably have a salmon richer in fish oils. And tuna migrates to the coast of Italy. So, isn't it important to look at the entire picture when discussing their lower rates of breast cancer?

You bet. Scientists tend to have tunnel vision, because they only look at one aspect of something and you just can't get the whole story that way. Examine the entire diet and lifestyle. You can't just isolate one factor and say, "Well, here's proof. This is the reason." You have to look at the whole picture.

Please comment on the use of brown or amber glass containers in Europe for oils, homeopathics, medicines, elixirs, and so on.

Europeans tend to be more health conscious than North Americans because Europe is more crowded and pollution is more of an issue. Europeans prefer dark glass to plastic for packaging material. In North America, we have a Disneyland fantasy way of living. We don't want to acknowledge the consequences of our behavior. We have a Statue of Liberty, but no statue of responsibility.

To a large extent, we live in a fantasy about health, as well. Europeans are up to speed about plastics. Much of the research that raises red flags about plastics, including the pollution that manufacturing plants cause to waterways and environment, come from European studies.

Ancel Keys, who is now ninety-three, created the field of research on diet and heart disease based on the Mediterranean diet. Walter Willett, an epidemiologist with the Harvard School of Public Health, has the utmost respect for Keys, acknowledging that "Much of the research we do was inspired by studies Keys did thirty and forty years ago." Marion Nestle, head of the Department of Nutrition and Food Studies at NYU, says, "Keys has made five or six lasting contributions in as many different fields. He is a giant." Keys, living in Southern Italy, is currently focusing on the differences among various fatty acids. He points out, for example, that not all saturated fatty acids have the same effect on cholesterol in the blood.

That's true. Some of them actually lower cholesterol. Some of them raise it, and some don't affect it at all.

He also acknowledges that more information is needed about the differences between fatty acids and their effect on health, as you've been saying for a long time. These are topics that you've been talking about and have written about, for a very long time. How does it feel to be a pioneer?

I am pioneering the *application* of their research. I use their work, and I follow a lot of case histories. I evaluate the damaging effects of processed fats and oils from what their research and that of others shows. I can say more than some researchers, because I don't depend on grants. I'm pleased to have been able to do what I do without government help and without grants—I am free to say what needs to be said. I use the research of Ancel Keys and David Horrobin and many other researchers. That I've done is to translate the technical information in the journals into something that the public understands, so that it does not remain hidden in research journals or become misrepresented in newspaper accounts, which happens a lot. I've used their work, but I also look at the rest of nutrition, because I'm not just a fat expert. I look at the whole picture. And most importantly, I've changed the way oils are made, stored, and used, with human health in mind.

The topic of how processing affects oils and health is very, very important. Many, studies printed in the journals ought to be repeated with oils made the way we make them. The results of those studies would be different. Researchers into the effects of oils on health and disease have often ignored the processing issue as though it were of no importance.

> The processing of oils is key to understanding how they help (or hurt) our health. Many studies on fats and oils and health should be repeated using unprocessed, fresh, organic oils. Results of those studies would be different.

Let's discuss general health and beauty. How does a fat-free or low-fat diet impact on physical appearance?

You get dry skin, low energy levels, hair loss, brittle nails. You can get eczema-like skin problems, thin, papery skin. You can become susceptible to infections, and wounds won't heal. You can get arthritis-like symptoms. All of these will affect appearance, but the utmost obvious ones are dry skin, brittle nails, low energy levels, and hair loss. And in kids, growth will be stunted—you get growth retardation on the low-fat or fat-free diet.

I've been using Udo's Choice Ultimate Oil Blend since it first came out in 1994. My hair, skin, and nails have shown remarkable improvements. I think that I'm metabolizing Udo's Choice Oil very efficiently. Could you comment on this observation?

Udo's Choice contains flaxseed oil, but it contains eight other ingredients as well. It has a better balance of omega-3s and omega-6s from combining flax with sunflower and sesame, tastes better, and is absorbed better, because of the way we put it together. It contains lecithin. It's stabilized with vitamin E, so it keeps better. It contains the "minor" ingredients of rice germ, wheat germ, and oat germ oils, and medium chain triglycerides, which are easy for the liver to metabolize as an energy source, so there are several reasons why it might be easier to metabolize than other oils. We get feedback like yours on a regular basis. Tastes better, keeps better, and works better, simply because it's a better-balanced oil. It addresses all of the health and processing issues in oils that need to be considered.

A lot of women who suffer from osteoporosis could benefit from estrogen replacement therapy or so say their physicians, but avoid it out of concern for a family history of breast cancer. Since the omega-3 essential fatty acid is supposed to prevent calcium excretion, isn't this just one more reason to include more flaxseed oil and fatty-rich fish in the diet?

Omega-3s and other fatty acids are used in mineral transport and metabolism in the body. The essential fatty acids are important for the metabolism of calcium, a mineral. Yes, that's another good reason to provide omega-3-rich, but also omega-6-rich oils in the diet. Also, phytoestrogens present naturally in Udo's Choice Beyond Greens and in flaxseed reduce the need for estrogen replacement.

Are you familiar with the disturbing practice of boiling down and making feed meal from animals, and if so, what do you think about it? This practice may be profitable, but seems unhealthy. Do you think this rendered material could affect our health? Do you think these commercial products—which include foods, soap, and cosmetics—can be carriers of undesirable substances from these rendered animals to us?

It depends on how they're made. Usually those oils are refined and over-heated. That kills the unfriendly disease organisms. But fried and deep-fried oils are also recycled into feed. The deep-fried and fried oils that go into feeds end up in the animals' bodies, then in animal products that we eat. More health problems are likely to be caused by chemical changes in oil that become part of the food supply than problems caused by organisms. When you deodorize oils, the disease-causing organisms are roasted.

Do you have brief advice for people who are undergoing chemotherapy and may want to prevent weight loss, as far as recommending oils? And maybe whole foods. A new book recommending low carbohydrates, adequate protein, and certain fats for weight loss warns against more than one tablespoon of flaxseed oil a day. This book also recommends EPA over flaxseed oil for weight loss. Please comment, because I find that I can still lose weight

while taking two to three tablespoons of Udo's Choice Perfected Oil Blend
or flaxseed oil. It doesn't stop me from losing weight, if I watch what I eat.

Flaxseed oil and omega-3-rich blends work well for weight loss. Some of
the big body builders use seven or eight tablespoons a day, and lose the fat
under their skin. More typically, people consume two to four tablespoons.
Take antioxidants (vitamins E and C) because the omega-3s create a good
fire, but the fire also throws sparks and you need spark control. Antioxidants
provide the spark control.

Fish oils are usually too processed and may contain contaminants, and in
practice, usually too little fish oil is used to get significant weight loss.

Can you explain how sugar and sweet fruit turn to fat in the liver?

That's really easy. Sugar, a fully digested food, is absorbed very quickly,
because it doesn't need to be digested. It floods the bloodstream (that's called
hyperglycemia), which is one of the problems diabetics have. High blood
sugar is a very toxic condition. Insulin drives sugar into the cells, where the
sugar goes through the cells' furnace (called the Krebs cycle), which turns
sugar into energy. If the energy isn't needed, the body turns the sugar into
hard fats, because hard fats are less toxic than high sugar. The hope is that
at some future famine the body can live off its fat for a while. Absent a famine,
you get fatter and fatter from sweets.

Can you give us some information about artificially sweetened foods and
how they can actually slow weight loss? And what do you think about the
new pharmaceutical fat blockers?

The fat blockers are based on the wrong concept about fats—that all fats
are bad and that we should be on a low-fat or no-fat diet. We do better if we
replace bad fats with good fats. Fat blockers encourage you to keep eating
junk foods, and fat blockers unsuccessfully attempt to prevent you from negative health consequences of junk foods. The concept is wrong, because they
ignore the fats that heal, which fat blockers will also block. If we bring in
the fats that heal and replace the fats that kill with them, the problem is
solved.

The fats that heal help with weight loss, good health, the taste of foods,
skin and brain function, and energy levels; they improve digestion, cardiovascular and immune function; they make our glands, organs, and tissues work
better. To improve health, we have to replace the fats that kill with the fats
that heal. Fat blockers are just ways to make money on fat phobia without
solving the problem.

It seems like the Europeans know this intuitively. They really have a
respect for whole foods, vegetables, and fresh foods. I think that the Mediter-
ranean people do not have a need for flaxseed oil because they eat the fatty-

rich fish in their everyday diet, as well as whole foods. They weren't getting the omega-6 oils or rancid oils or as much hydrogenated fats and oils. They don't have the same imbalances that Americans have.

On the traditional diet, that's true. But flaxseed is used in some of these countries also, and has been for centuries.

There's some confusion about the lignan of the flaxseed; one definition I've read says that the lignan is actually the matrix of the seed. Another definition is that lignan is the hull of the seed.

Lignans are found throughout the seed. Whether they're more concentrated in one part of the seed or another, I don't know. But they are neither matrix nor hull.

I'd like to talk about depression, and how to maintain a positive outlook, which is so helpful for people trying to reverse degenerative diseases. How can a fat-free diet be linked to depression and how does flaxseed oil help to alleviate it?

The essential fatty acids elevate mood and lift depression. They also produce a feeling of calmness. They help improve mental processing. They raise intelligence (IQ) by several points.

We're fatheads; the brain is the fat-richest organ. Its dry weight is half essential fatty acids, omega-3 and omega-6, in a ratio of one to one. The brain is also richest in cholesterol.

How do essential fatty acids elevate mood and lift depression and bring calmness? They're part of the structure of the brain itself. If the brain isn't made right, then behavior is going to be off. Other behaviors, like hyperactivity, criminal behavior, and mental illness also improve by getting the essential fatty acids right.

You've done work with meditation and creating a path for yourself in life. Has meditation benefited your own outlook? Do you think meditation can help people who are trying to strengthen their immunity and prevent breast cancer?

There's no question about it. We live in a stressful world. But the whole time we live in the stressful world, there is something in us that is never affected by that stress. I call it the "quiet place." It makes sense to me to cultivate a way to live from the quiet place that allows us to leave the stresses outside. That allows us to deal more effectively with whatever we have do deal with, without bothering ourselves about things that we cannot change.

Getting unhooked from the stress that we take on is good—stress produces biochemical changes, many of which have negative effects on health. By staying in the quiet place, we're going to have a lot more energy that can be used for healing.

Do you have any suggestions for people who may want to begin a program of meditation?

There are two options. One is to try to find the quiet place by yourself. If you can't find it, find somebody who knows how to show you.

Authors note: For more information on fats and oils, I encourage readers to purchase Udo Erasmus's book, *Fats That Heal, Fats That Kill* (Alive Books). *See* the Resource Guide.

PART TWO

CHAPTER 3

The New Millennium: Challenging the Myth of the Low-Fat Diet

We lament the plethora of fat-free products high in sugar and the avoidance of foods such as nuts and oil-based salad dressings that provide n-3 [Omega-3] fatty acids. However, the failure to distinguish among types of fat and the emphasis on total fat reduction are the very causes of these problems. Lower consumption of saturated and trans fats is desirable, but nonspecific recommendations to reduce total fat consumption have no strong scientific basis and could be harmful if unsaturated fats are avoided.

—*Martijn B. Katan, Ph.D.; Scott M. Grundy, M.D., Ph.D.; Walter C. Willett, M.D. Ph.D.;* "Clinical Debate: Should a Low-Fat, High Carbohydrate Diet Be Recommended for Everyone?" in the *New England Journal of Medicine,* August 1997.

Americans have been getting fatter. Back in 1977, we were advised by the Senate Select Committee on Nutrition and Human Needs to reduce overall fat consumption. In 1979, the U.S. Surgeon General's report, *Healthy People: The Surgeon General's Report on Health Promotion and Disease Prevention,* supported the original advice of the Select Committee, including the general admonishment to "reduce fat." In 1982, the National Academy of Sciences report *Diet, Nutrition, and Cancer* noted (among other observations) that a diet high in fat was linked to an increase in breast cancer.

By April 1996, however, *American Health* magazine reported that Harvard University researchers found "even extremely low fat diets (less than 20 percent of calories from fat) failed to reduce breast cancer risk."

Don't Generalize About Fat Consumption in Breast Health

The kind of fat you eat is key. Studies show that caloric restriction is more significant than reducing fat in preventing breast cancer. People currently eat more simple carbohydrates, often in the form of low-fat or nonfat foods, because they are hesitant to consume any fat. Simply put, people are eating more. The scale shows it. We are becoming a nation of heavier people, despite the craze over the past decade for nonfat foods.

"Then there is the issue of weight gain," Jane Brody warned in her May 1997 *New York Times* article, "Personal Health: Preventing Breast Cancer." Brody explained, "A weight gain of ten pounds after the age of 30 was linked to a 23 percent increase in breast cancer later in life, and a gain of 20 pounds was associated with a 52 percent increase." Brody also pointed to a National Cancer Institute study of 15,000 Asian-American women that demonstrated weight gain, after moving to the United States, was a strong factor in increased breast cancer risk.

When you reduce or eliminate fat, you feel hungrier. What do people turn to? Fat-free snacks are available everywhere—bagels, corn chips (and salsa), cookies, muffins, and pasta—foods which are high in simple, as opposed to complex, carbohydrates. These high-carbohydrate foods tend to make us want to eat more. Eating a high-carbohydrate–low-fat diet is known to raise triglycerides. *I have noticed that people report strong sugar cravings when consuming a diet high in processed, carbohydrate, fat-free foods.*

When the right type of fat is consumed—like extra virgin olive or flaxseed oil, tuna, salmon, or unroasted nuts (along with adequate protein)—the desire for carbohydrates diminishes. Replacing the simple carbohydrates in these empty-calorie junk foods with the complex carbohydrates found in vegetables and fruits and *adding protective, delicious fats* in the form of fresh, unprocessed, vegetable oils, nuts, avocados, and fatty-rich fish helps to prevent the tendency to overeat because it creates a feeling of satiety. There are adequate vitamins, minerals, and essential fatty acids to satisfy hunger when you choose real foods over processed foods like the artificially sweetened "soy bars," bagels, or pasta. Furthermore, flaxseed oil helps to rejuvenate tired metabolisms, helping to increase energy. Many nutritionists recommend flaxseed oil for people on exercise programs.

A starchy diet may contribute to the risk of breast cancer, as Italian researchers reported in *The Lancet* in May 1996. In a study of 2,569 women, it was found that the risk of breast cancer increased with consumption of such carbohydrates as pasta, white bread, rice, crackers, and cookies, whereas a high intake of unsaturated and polyunsaturated fats are associated with a decreased risk of cancer.

Reduce Carbohydrates for Heart Health
Another strong reason to add healthy, unprocessed, unsaturated sources of fat and reduce simple carbohydrates is heart health. Heart disease is the number one cause of death for American women. Simple carbohydrates consistently lower protective HDL cholesterol. "The more HDL you have, the lower your risk of heart disease,"

Nutritionist Robert Crayhon advised in *Total Health* magazine. The 1997 study in the *American Journal of Clinical Nutrition* cited by Crayhon concluded that "substantial evidence indicates that a low-fat, high carbohydrate diet leads to changes in glucose, insulin, and lipoprotein metabolism that will increase the risk of ischemic heart disease."

Women in Greece have a substantially lower rate of breast cancer than women in the United States, despite the fact that they consume almost 50 percent of their calories in fat in the form of olive oil. Women in the United States consume approximately 35 percent of their calories from fat, but not in the form of olive oil. These facts underscore the danger of generalizing when discussing fat.

"In Spain and Greece, women with breast cancer were shown to consume less olive oil than did healthy women," Brody wrote in her February 14, 1996, *New York Times* "Personal Health: Fat and Health" column. "But until recently, monounsaturated oils were not common-place in American diets and may not have been well enough represented in the Harvard study to show up as protective."

Certain fats are health protective, such as fats from vegetable and plant foods like avocados, nuts, olives, and flaxseed. Fatty-rich fish also contains protective fats. Andrew Weil, M.D. (author of *Spontaneous Healing)*, favors eating fish over taking fish oil capsules. In 1991, the *American Journal of Clinical Nutrition* reported that eating fish is more effective than fish oil capsules in controlling cholesterol.

Do You Lead a Sedentary Lifestyle? Don't Just Eat More Fats!

People in the Mediterranean who consume a diet rich in olive oil are more active than we are in North America. Many people in Greece and Spain walk or ride bicycles to work and school. They also consume a plant-based diet, which is lower in saturated fats than the diet consumed in North America.

Fats Can Protect

Udo Erasmus has been educating people about the dangers of a nonfat or low-fat diet for many years. Early symptoms resulting from a fat-free diet are scaly skin, brittle nails, and dry hair. Symptoms that may later develop include arthritis, cardiovascular disease, cancer, depression, and diabetes. There are well-meaning parents who start their babies off on a fat-free or low-fat diet. Researchers at the University of California at Davis have studied these babies and concluded that they have a "failure to thrive" syndrome, which can be fatal. Researchers in Great Britain found that low-fat diets lead to slower mental functioning.

Oil consumption, of course, is one factor among the many that contribute to the multitude of benefits obtained from the Mediterranean diet. Oldways Preservation and Trust in Cambridge, Massachusetts, is an organization dedicated to the preservation of traditional diets, including the Asian and Mediterranean diets. Oldways reminds us that Mediterranean people make vegetables, grains, beans, nuts, olive oil, and other whole foods the main focus of their meals, with small servings of meat or fish. Locally grown produce and unprocessed foods are important components of the protective Mediterranean diet. As a result, Mediterranean people in Greece and Southern Italy have "some of the lowest rates of chronic disease. In addition, they had one of the highest life expectancy rates in the world, according to nutrition research," Jennifer C. Davis reported in *Delicious!* magazine's Annual Guide. Davis also noted that "Mediterraneans consumed fat ranging from 25-35 percent of their overall caloric intake" and "limited saturated fat to no more than 8 percent of their total diets." *Limiting saturated fat is breast protective*. Recently, the *Journal of Clinical Nutrition* reported that "women who ate the skin on their poultry had a 70 percent increase in breast cancer" and that women who did not consume lean or extra lean ground beef had a more than double risk of developing breast cancer.

"Non-specific recommendations to reduce total fat consumption have no strong scientific basis, and could be harmful if unsaturated fats are avoided," Katan, Grundy, and Willett wrote in the August 1997 *New England Journal of Medicine* "Clinical Debate" over low-fat diets.

Certain types of fatty-rich fish have been found to be beneficial in preventing breast and other cancers. In July 1997, an article in the *New York Times*, "Benefits Found in Asian Fish Diet," reported the outcome of a study conducted at the Jonsson Cancer Center (at the University of California at Los Angeles) in which twenty-five American women were put on a diet that mimicked foods—including fish oil—eaten by Asian women, who have a much lower rate of breast cancer than Americans. The head of the study, Dr. John Glaspy, told the *New York Times*, "Asian women typically eat more fish, which is high in a fatty acid called Omega 3." According to these researchers, the experimental diet "caused tissue changes that may lower the risk of breast cancer, although it was noted that much more extensive study" would be needed.

Studies successfully correlating fish consumption to lower rates of breast cancer were first completed as long ego as the late 1970s. One examined the rate of breast cancer in Greenland, and the other in Japan. It has taken nearly twenty years for the protective benefits of fatty-rich fish to begin to gain acceptance in the West. Perhaps Dr. Glaspy's work at UCLA has contributed to Harvard's recent advice to "distinguish among types of fat" instead of focusing on "total fat reduction." The new guidelines from Harvard will, hopefully, encourage people to add good-quality fats and oils to their diets, eliminate trans-fats (in margarines and shortenings), and reduce carbohydrates. Finally science is confirming that it is the quality, not quantity, of fat consumed that is most important.

For Optimum Health, Replace Harmful Fats with Protective Fats

Replace trans-fats, margarine, saturated fats, "phony" fats, and fried foods containing heated fats with life-giving, protective fats like unheated flaxseed and olive oils (and other unprocessed, unrefined oils recommended in *Total Breast Health*), in judicious amounts, along with nuts and seeds, avocado, and fatty-rich fish such as salmon and tuna.

Be sure your total fat intake is around 15–20 percent of your daily calories, and that you are consuming a plant-based diet. Include some form of daily exercise.

CHAPTER 4

The Importance of Organic Food

Distinguished scientists tell us that there is no longer serious argument about what happens to our good earth with overuse of fertilizers, pesticides, and herbicides. It turns sterile. In the old days, before these chemicals were devised and marketed, the earth remained fertile. Sterility and fertility are not unimportant concerns for our planetary health.
—K. Dun Gifford, Oldways Preservation and Exchange Trust

Alice Waters is chef at Chez Panisse restaurant in Berkeley, California. The author of five cookbooks (her newest is *Chez Panisse Vegetables*, HarperCollins, 1996), Waters has been serving only organic fruits and vegetables at the restaurant for the last ten years. Waters says that the decision to support organic farming was a "deliberate decision made to honor the planet and support future generations." She also insists on serving meat from animals that are antibiotic and hormone-free.

"We've been supporting small farms and farmers for fifteen or twenty years at Chez Panisse. I want to know who grew my food, and become friends with them," Waters explained to me.

Waters is committed to organic food for its flavor, as well as for environmental reasons. There has been a dynamic movement by top chefs all over the country toward the exclusive use of organic foods because of the flavor factor. Waters explains, "When food is picked when ripe, it tastes better, and is more nutritious." The flavor of vegetables is enhanced by being able to select, for instance, lettuce "right from the garden," Waters said. "Aliveness is important to me," she emphasized. Commercial growers, for economic reasons, seldom allow produce to reach this state before it is harvested and shipped to market.

"Farmers' markets are great because they bring people together with the farmers," Waters added. This way, consumers not only can feel and taste produce only hours from when it was picked, but also can hear firsthand by what methods it was grown. Waters believes that respect for the earth and preserving the quality of our food supply should be encouraged in young people. Waters wishes that "a food-based curriculum could be available in all schools, where children learn how to grow their own food, cook it, and eat it together." She is doing a lot to foster that in her own Berkeley community by creating the Edible School Yard program at Martin Luther King, Junior, Middle School.

Chefs like Alice Waters, who are enthusiastic members of the organic foods movement, contribute a great deal to the new spirit of cooking. Waters and other chefs like her have helped to dissolve the division between healthy food and *haute cuisine*. These chefs influence hundreds of thousands of people yearly in a very healing way.

There is reason to be alarmed, as Waters is, about the state of the earth. Soil depletion reports show a regression to the very depleted state found thirty or forty years ago.

The World Bank's *World Development Report* (1992) expressed concern about the environment with respect to policy making. "The value of the environment has been underestimated for too long, resulting in damage to human health, reduced productivity, and the undermining of future development prospects," the report stated. It recommended environmental conditions be improved, which will require a "major policy program, and institutional shifts." The World Bank report concluded with the statement, "Governments have to enforce regulations that ban or limit the use of pesticides, which pose large risks to human health and the environment."

Certainly, human health depends on the health of the planet. Pesticides are not good for the earth. Chemicals upset the ecological balance of the earth, the sea, and the air. Environmental agents can negatively affect human health. It is estimated that 80–90 percent of all cancers are caused by agents in the environment. The National Toxicology Council has identified thirty chemicals that are classified as xenoestrogenic. (For more on xenoestrogens, *see* Chapter 11, "Food, Hormones, and Breast Cancer: What's the Connection?")

Minimizing exposure to free radical-promoting substances encourages breast health. Smog, chemicals from machinery, and organochlorines in pesticides all upset the balance of the endocrine system. Limiting further exposure to chemicals by selecting organic food whenever possible limits further exposure to even more free radicals.

Toxic fertilizers may be another threat to our food supply. Investigators in Washington State discovered that impure, potentially hazardous substances— products from municipal waste and the incineration of medical waste, and other undesirable substances, including recycled products from cement-making and wood product manufacturing—are added to some fertilizers. The government actually sanctions this practice to conserve space in hazardous waste landfills. As a result, consumers may end up with cadmium, lead, arsenic and even radioactive materials and dioxins in their fruits and vegetables. Because investigators, led by the Mayor of Quincy, Washington, were concerned about crops and cattle that seemed unhealthy, they discovered that wastes are added to fertilizers without being listed on the label. Legislation is being introduced in Seattle to put a stop to this unhealthy practice.

Many women are buying organic dairy and other animal products because of reports that milk from cows injected with recombinant bovine growth hormone (rBGH) increases risks of breast and colon cancers in humans. Recombinant BGH increases levels of insulin-like growth factor (IGF-1) in milk, according to a January 1996 report in the *International Journal of Health Services.* IGF-1 stimulates and regulates cell growth and division in humans and cows, and appears to be cancer-promoting in breast cells, as well as the cells that line the colon.

Is Organic Food Important?

There are several important reasons to purchase organic produce:

- Commercially fertilized crops yield foods lower in minerals.
- Organic food is lower in other harmful substances such as mercury, lead, and cadmium.
- Several studies link breast cancer to diets low in selenium. Organic produce is significantly higher in selenium.
- Organic food is also rich in potassium, another important mineral.

Phytochemicals from Vegetables and Fruits Help to Protect Us from Pesticides

If you are unable to purchase organic produce, be sure you consume five to ten different vegetables and fruits daily to ensure phytochemical intake. *Phytochemicals help to protect cells and DNA from potentially harmful substances such as pesticides.*

While it is true that you will be exposed to fewer environmental estrogens if you purchase organic produce, it is not always possible to do so. Just be sure you are eating a variety of fresh produce every day.

Research has shown that an increased selenium level leads to an increased number of white blood cells, which are essential in fighting pathogens.

Additionally, it's suspected that selenium's antioxidant properties may contribute to lowered cancer risk. Soil from Utah, for instance, has higher-than-average amounts of selenium. Dr. Gethard Schrauzer from the University of Califomia at San Diego believes this may be an important factor in Utah's distinction of being the state with the lowest rate of cancer in the country.

Dr. Schrauzer's comprehensive research into the possible link between selenium and cancer has led him to state that, if our soil contained adequate selenium, cancer would be reduced by 75 percent.

The greatest concentration of minerals is found in the skin of produce. If you buy organic produce, you can leave the skin on. Just scrub with a natural bristle vegetable brush, available in health food stores.

Our water supply is contaminated with pesticides, fungicides, and herbicides. Thirty-eight states have contaminated ground water supplies, according to the Environmental Protection Agency (EPA). Many farmers experience pesticide-related illnesses, another reason to buy organic produce. Peaches, strawberries, honeydew, apricots, and sweet peppers from the United States and Mexico; cantaloupe, nectarines, and cherries from the United States; and celery and grapes from Chile tested highest for pesticides by the Environmental Working Group (in conjunction with the EPA and Food and Drug Administration).

Many researchers are concerned about the potential problems associated with combining several different pesticides, and their long-term effects on health. There is also concern that exposure to pesticides and other chemicals may pose a significant threat during childhood and the teenage years.

Purchase organic baby food. Children may receive up to 35 percent of their entire lifetime doses of some carcinogenic pesticides by the age of five. Sixteen pesticides, in trace amounts, were found in products from three of the most well-known baby food manufacturers. Furthermore, environmental groups point out that lifetime exposure to pesticides and other chemicals may be cumulative, posing even an greater threat over time. Some researchers are particularly concerned about the effects that pesticides and other chemicals may have on breast tissues during early adolescence, noting that DNA may be at even greater risk at that time.

Websites of Interest

www.organicfood.com   The Organic Trading and Information Center provides answers to questions, and a link to other websites

www.ccof.org   California Certified Organic Farmers

www.openair.org   International website information for farmer's markets throughout the world

www.starchefs.com   Farmer's markets throughout the U.S.

www.ewg.org   The Environmental Working Group's website regarding safe water and food

CHAPTER 5

Raw Foods and Juices Provide Protective Enzymes

Enzymes, found abundantly in raw fruits and vegetables, aid in digestion. They also aid in the metabolism of omega-3 essential fatty acids. If the proportion of cooked food to raw food is too high, levels of health-giving digestive enzymes are diminished. The digestive system then becomes overworked, as it struggles to produce more enzymes.

Cancer cells are constantly being created, in every person. A healthy person makes enough enzymes to fight off cancer cells. When we're exposed to carcinogenic substances (like smoke and environmental pollutants), however, our bodies form free radicals that interfere with enzyme production. The absence of certain enzymes is one reason cancer can take root and grow.

Enzymes are proteins that participate in numerous chemical reactions throughout the body, without being broken down or otherwise changed chemically themselves. In *Fats That Heal, Fats That Kill*, Udo Erasmus defines an enzyme as "a protein produced by the body to catalyze (facilitate) a particular chemical reaction. The enzyme that catalyzes the reaction is not itself changed thereby." Anthony J. Cichoke, D.C., offers this definition in *Enzymes and Enzyme Therapy—How to Jump Start Your Way to Lifelong Good Health*: "Enzyme, from Greek, meaning 'in yeast.' An organic compound which accelerates or produces a catalytic action."

Every plant and animal has enzymes. There are approximately 3,000 different enzymes in the human body that help to build new cells, tissues, and organs. Enzymes are greatly influenced by their environment—temperature, acidity, alkalinity, and other proteins can affect their ability to act. Each type of enzyme has a specific function, such as breaking down fats so they can be digested. Other enzymes are used in the process of breathing, to control respiration, and in other crucial bodily functions.

> TIP: Strive to consume raw vegetables in each meal. Eat salads first, before cooked foods, to start production of digestive enzymes. When we consume a meal made up entirely of cooked foods—like concentrated starches, animal protein, and a minimal amount of vegetables—neither the salivary enzymes nor the upper-stomach enzymes are capable of completing digestion. Foods can then putrify in the digestive system, and dangerous, health-threatening residues are released into the bloodstream. Under these circumstances, the liver, pancreas, and intestines are constantly overworked.

Enzyme-Depleting Substances

- Smog
- Nicotine
- Poor eating habits (processed foods)
- Pharmaceuticals and over-the-counter medications

Juicing Prevents Disease and Provides Stamina

The Gerson Cancer Clinic, renowned worldwide for effective cancer treatment, uses raw juices, consumed throughout the day, as a form of therapy. Some of my favorite juice combinations are:

1	2	3
Cucumber	Beet	Carrot
Kale	Carrot	Spinach
Celery	Parsley	Parsley
Carrot	Spinach	Cucumber
Ginger	Daikon	Chlorella
	1 clove garlic	

> TIP: Chew food well, until each mouthful is liquid. According to practitioners of macrobiotics, chewing aids in enzyme production.

European Enzyme Research

According to Dr. Cichoke, researchers at the Janker Radiation Clinic in Bonn, Germany, noted that up to 90 percent of breast lumps and other painful breast problems disappeared when young women were treated with enzymes.

Dr. Karl Ransberger, director of Medical Enzyme Research Institute in Munich, Germany, has spent more than forty years researching the benefits of enzymes, working with doctors in Europe and America. In an interview in *Total Health* magazine, Dr. Ransberger reported that, "In recent years, over 90 research studies have been completed regarding the beneficial effects of enzymes. Most of the research has been conducted by universities and academic institutions throughout the world. There are presently 125 research protocols in progress. . . . Studies are currently underway to evaluate the benefit of enzymes in the prevention of metastasis of cancer." Details of these studies are available on the Internet at http://www.mucos.de.

Additional studies from Germany show that, when enzymes are used after breast cancer surgery, the following clinical improvements are observed:

- Reduction of recurrence
- Prevention of metastasis (spreading) after surgery
- Reduction of pain
- Reduction of hemorrhaging
- Improvement of morale
- Improvement of appetite and digestion

Research in the 1950s showed that eating cooked food (even 50 percent cooked food, when cooked portion is eaten first) causes an irritation in the stomach and intestines similar to that found around tumors, which involves an accumulation of white blood cells.

Rita Romano's informative book, *Dining in the Raw, Cooking with "The Buff,"* is helpful for anyone interested in learning more about high-enzyme foods and their powers of rejuvenation.

TIP: If you are experiencing indigestion, gas, and/or bloating, con-sider taking a full-spectrum, plant-based enzyme supplement.

The absence of certain enzymes allows some types of cancer cells to grow. Dr. Cichoke explains that enzymes strip cancer cells of fibrin, a sticky substance that coats the inside of blood vessels, protecting them from damage and smoothing any rough areas that impede the blood flow. Cancer cells use this "glue," fibrin, to attach themselves to internal tissues. Once the outside surfaces of the cancer cells are coated with fibrin, their antigens—the surface proteins that allow the immune system to recognize cancer cells as dangerous—are hidden. By destroying the fibrin surrounding cancer cells, enzymes not only remove the "glue" holding them in place, they expose the cancer cells to attack by immune system cells.

A deficiency in enzymes, therefore, can allow cancer cells to grow; the more cancer cells that are present in the body, the more enzymes are required.

Nicolas Gonzalez, M.D., explained in a 1995 lecture in New York City that the combination of excessive estrogen and insufficient pancreatic enzymes contributes to the growth of breast cancer. The pancreas is instrumental in the digestion of essential fatty acids and other nutrients (such as proteins, starches, cholesterol, and triglycerides), and helps to supply the small intestines with fat-digesting enzymes. Enzyme deficiency is indicated by indigestion, gas, and bloating. A Scottish embryologist, Dr. John Beard, has also found the pancreatic enzymes to have inhibiting effects on the growth of cancer.

Juicing

It's easy to experiment with different juice formulas. After you have made two or three juice combinations, you will see how easy it is. Many people experience some wonderful results from consuming fresh juices daily, including increased energy, relief from digestive problems, clearer skin and eyes, and even pain relief. Remember, the nutrients and enzymes in raw vegetables and fruits are important in creating a strong immune system. Refer to the Resource Guide for my favorite juicer, Champion.

Increasing Enzymes in Your Diet

Both animal and plant foods are sources of active enzymes; cooking these foods destroys the enzymes they contain. Many people question the safety of consuming raw meat; however, sushi (raw fish) is a healthy and delicious choice. (I have seen far more reports of *E. coli* and other bacterial contaminants in hamburger than of parasites in sushi.) Tuna, salmon, mackerel and eel are sources of breast-protective fish oils and enzymes when eaten as sushi. Find the very best sushi bar in your area where the turnover is high (meaning the fish is fresh) and the sushi chef is knowledgeable.

TIP: Ginger has antiparasitic properties, so be sure to consume plenty of ginger when eating sushi.

Raw vegetables and fruits are rich sources of enzymes for vegetarians and nonvegetarians alike. If you find that salads are hard to digest, try the pressed salads in *Total Breast Health*. The enzymes are still present but the vegetable fibers are broken down and so are easier to digest.

Enzyme-Rich Foods and Ways to Include Them in Your Diet

- Raw vegetable salads
- Fresh vegetable juices
- Alfalfa, mung bean, and broccoli sprouts in salads
- Raw spinach
- Minced and crushed raw garlic in vinaigrette
- Watermelon
- Papaya
- Lightly cooked asparagus
- Bits of fresh (not canned) pineapple, combined with cous-cous and red pepper
- Sushi with ginger

Be aware that canned foods contain no live enzymes, because the process of canning involves heating the food to very high temperatures. Fresh is best. Freezing, drying, and canning foods strips them of their enzymes.

Broccoli Sprouts Contain Concentrated Amounts of the Phytochemicals "Isothiocyanates," Potent Stimulators of Natural Detoxifying Enzymes

Isothiocyanates from sprouts greatly reduced the size, amount, and incidence of mammary tumors in animals. Broccoli sprouts contain 30–50 times more protective phytochemicals than those found in mature broccoli. Sulforaphane, a compound isolated from isothiocyanate, helps the body to eliminate potentially harmful compounds before they can damage cells.

A Method for Sprouting Broccoli Seeds

All you need are broccoli seeds, a large mason jar, gauze or cheese cloth, and a baking dish or pan large enough to hold the mason jar, which will be placed on its side.

Place seeds in jar; use enough to cover the side of the jar. Cover the jar with a piece of cheesecloth and secure with a rubber band. Cover seeds with just enough water to soak, filtering it through the gauze. Let the seeds soak in the water for 24 hours. Pour out the water and add fresh water (to cover). Lay jar, with cheese cloth cover, on its side in the pan on a sunny windowsill. Drain water and add fresh water 2–3 times a day. In about ten days, you will have crunchy broccoli sprouts, rich with protective sulforaphane.

CHAPTER 6

Flaxseed and Flaxseed Oil: Nature's Superfoods for Breast Health

W hen I first heard about flaxseed, I was a little skeptical. How could such a tiny, hard seed offer such great health benefits? I learned about the benefits of flaxseed by looking at studies and from talking to people who included flaxseed in their successful programs that restore health. After learning about the protection this little seed offers, I wouldn't dream of not including flaxseed in my own program of daily prevention.

Just two tablespoons daily of freshly ground or soaked flaxseed may protect against hormone-related cancers. Flaxseed's cancer-fighting power comes largely from substances called lignans; flaxseed is, in fact, one of the richest sources of lignans. Clinical research published in the *Journal of Clinical Endocrinology and Metabolism* noted that flaxseed ingestion had a measurable effect on the menstrual cycle, and suggested that lignans from flaxseed in the diet play a role in the actions of sex steroids (hormones), and even possibly in hormone-dependent cancers.

Plant lignans, like those found in flaxseed, are converted by intestinal bacteria into mammalian lignans, which block estrogen's activity. Lignans are also anticarcinogenic, antifungal, antiviral, and antibacterial.

Although human studies began only in mid-1997 in Canada, numerous animal studies had already shown that giving flaxseed to animals with mammary tumors *reduced the size of the tumors as much as 67 percent.* Flaxseed was effective at preventing tumor formation (in animals) if it was administered before cancers were chemically induced. There is no reason to believe that flaxseed and flaxseed oil don't have the same anticancer effect in humans as they do in animals.

The North American diet, depleted in nutrient and fiber-rich foods but high in processed foods, promotes estrogen's activity and production. Excess estrogen often leads to early puberty, as well as shorter, more frequent menstrual cycles, which result in an increased lifetime exposure to estrogen, hence, a higher risk of breast cancer. As a result, women in North America have one of the highest rates of breast cancer in the world. Breast cancer patients, as well as people at high risk for both breast and colon cancer, have been found to make and excrete far fewer lignans than other people. Of all the high-fiber foods tested, flaxseed produces the highest amount of lignans in the intestines; it generates more lignans than any other fiber source.

The antiestrogenic actions of flaxseed and flaxseed oil can help neutralize the excess estrogen that can contribute to the development of breast and other cancers. Even the Food and Drug Administration has endorsed lignan-rich flaxseed for disease prevention. For just a few cents a day, flaxseed can be made part of your own program for health.

> TIP: To encourage benefits from flaxseeds and flaxseed oil, eliminate French fries, potato chips, candy bars, and corn chips. Foods made with junk fats contain trans-fatty acids, which displace essential fatty acids within the body, making it difficult for them to protect our health.

Some Facts About Flax

Flaxseed has been used to treat a wide variety of conditions all over the world. In Europe and elsewhere, it has been used to treat diabetes because it makes insulin control blood sugar levels much more efficiently. While flaxseed alone is not a cure for such a complex problem as diabetes, it can be a primary tool in lessening dependence on insulin. Insulin-dependent diabetics, of course, need to work closely with their doctors in employing flaxseed.

Researchers at the University of Ontario have used flaxseed to treat patients with lupus nephritis. Lupus, which mostly affects women, is an autoimmune disease—in other words, a disease in which the body begins to destroy itself. If the kidneys become involved, as they do in lupus nephritis, it can be fatal. These researchers found that 1.05 ounces of flaxseed daily improves kidney functions. Kidney inflammation decreased and clogging of the blood vessels within the kidneys was halted, indicating that the lupus had been brought under control.

Robert Roundtree, M.D., a practitioner in Boulder, Colorado, who works with patients experiencing environmental illness, has found that flax lignans help these patients detoxify and lessen their symptoms.

Flaxseed, which is rich in omega-3 fatty acids, discourages the production of prostaglandins that result in the symptoms of PMS and menstrual cramps while helping to produce soothing prostaglandins. Menstrual cramps result from contractions of the uterus in response to prostaglandins produced by omega-6 fatty acids. Too much omega-6 in the diet can result in increased contractions, and therefore in worse cramping.

Omega-3 fatty acid from flaxseeds and flaxseed oil help to reduce the symptoms of menopause. Ingesting the proper balance of essential fatty acids can correct an imbalance in prostaglandins that regulate estrogen's actions within the body.

There are good reasons to consume flaxseeds as well as flaxseed oil. Less than 5 percent of the lignans in flaxseed make it to the oil during processing, while over 97 percent of the lignans remain in the ground seeds. If you want flax lignans, you must obtain them from the seeds, not the oil.

Flaxseeds are an excellent source for adding both bulk and softness to the stool. To treat or prevent constipation, simply grind 2–3 tablespoons of flaxseed in a nut or seed grinder. Soak in a cup of water for 1 hour. Stir and drink. The mucilage from soaking the flaxseeds is a wonderful, natural way to prevent or remedy constipation. The soaked and stirred flaxseeds can also be added to health shakes or fresh vegetable juices. (To avoid constipation in general, I also strongly advise adding a daily acidophilus supplement, and be sure you are drinking at least 6 glasses of water daily.)

Studies show that flaxseed, because of rich levels of alpha-linolenic acid (omega-3), protects the heart by keeping platelets from collecting in the arteries, reduces bad LDL cholesterol, and raises protective HDL cholesterol. Both hyperactivity and attention deficit disorder (ADHD) have been linked to omega-3 essential fatty acid deficiency in children. These children have lower levels of DHA, an omega-3 fat. It was found that more boys are affected by ADHD, suggesting that boys may require more omega-3 not only after birth but also possibly prenatally. It's clear that omega-3 deficiency causes many health problems for both adults and children.

The Best of Three Cultures for Breast Health

For a breast health program, combine benefits of three different cultures: Utilize flax seed and oil from Northern Europe; soy foods from Japan; and extra virgin olive oil from Greece and the rest of the Mediterranean.

Superfoods: Flaxseed and Flaxseed Oil

Tips on Usage

Julian Whitaker, M.D., author of *Dr. Whitaker's Guide to Natural Healing*, points out, "Because flax oil is a highly polyunsaturated oil, it is extremely susceptible to damage by heat, light, and oxygen. Once damaged, the oil is a rich source of toxic molecules known as lipid peroxides. These molecules can actually do the body harm and should not be ingested."

Healthful ways to use flaxseed include:

• **Grinding.** Grind 2 tablespoons of flaxseed in a small coffee, nut, or seed grinder. Consume by mixing in water or juice. Seeds must be ground or they will pass through the body intact and benefits will be lost. (*See* Resource Guide for flaxseed grinders.)

• **Soaking.** Cover 2 tablespoons of ground flaxseed with filtered water. Soak 20 minutes. This helps soften the seeds to aid in digestion. Soaked seeds work well with health shakes. I prefer to consume ground flaxseed in drinks, shakes, or sprinkled on foods. (*See* the Resource Guide for ordering organic flax seeds.)

A general recommendation is to consume 3 tablespoons of seeds or 1 tablespoon of oil. Ann Louise Gittleman recommends about 1 tablespoon of flaxseed oil daily. Udo Erasmus recommends that we take enough flaxseed oil until our skin feels soft, and points out that most people need more in the winter. If your skin feels soft, it means that your internal organs have received enough benefits from the oil, since the organs receive those benefits first.

I use both seeds and oil, and always have both on hand. Flaxseed oil is a convenient and delicious way to increase the healthful omega-3 content of your diet. Flaxseed oil is especially delicious drizzled on organic eggs, as well as combined with extra virgin olive oil, or used by itself, in vinaigrettes. Some important tips on storing and using flaxseed oil are:

Refrigerate.	Never store at room temperature. Use within 2 months. Flaxseed oil can be frozen for up to 1 year.
Never fry, sauté, or heat flaxseed oil.	I have seen several cookbooks mistakenly recommend that flaxseed oil be used for sautéing. Harmful substances are created when you heat flaxseed oil. Potentially healing benefits are destroyed when oil is heated. People are becoming more informed about flaxseed oil usage; for instance, *Fitness* magazine pointed out in September 1997 that we shouldn't cook with flaxseed oil because it's "destroyed by heat."
Enzymes help in oil metabolism.	Consume more enzyme-rich foods, such as salads, fresh juices, and raw garlic.

Flaxseed oil protects against cancer.	Since the 1800s, some European doctors have had excellent results using flaxseed oil mixed with protein to protect against cancer. Drizzle oil on organic eggs or yogurt.
Sulfur-containing foods protect.	Garlic, onions, leeks, scallions, chives, and shallots are all wonderful, flavorful foods that contain sulfur, which promote oil metabolism and protect against cancer. Use these foods often in vinaigrettes, with flaxseed oil.
Antioxidants protect against cancer.	Antioxidant-rich foods like cayenne, red pepper, turmeric, cinnamon, cumin, rosemary, thyme, and fennel help to prevent oxidation of fats and oils within the body.
Protect oils from heat and light.	Select flaxseed and other oils bottled in dark amber glass to protect from light and heat. Avoid oils bottled in plastic, as Paul Pitchford advises in *Healing with Whole Foods* and in *Goldbeck's Guide to Good Foods*. Oils should be bottled in amber glass.
Combine oils for more protection.	Combine flaxseed oil with extra virgin olive oil to create a blend with even greater breast-protective constituents. Vinaigrette, humus, pasta, and soups taste great when you use one-half olive oil and one-half flaxseed oil.

Be sure flaxseed oil is bottled in glass. In a 1994 article in *Science News,* Janet Raloff warned against using plastics, which increase harmful estrogens. The Canadian magazine *Alive* has also reported that Dr. Ana Soto, an endocrinologist at Tufts University, found that breast cancer cells reproduce very rapidly in plastic test tubes. Robert Haas, M.S., reported in *Permanent Remissions* (1997, Pocket Books) that scientists have questioned the safety of plastics for quite some time. The following chemicals, Haas points out, may leech from containers into foods:

Bisphenol-A caused men working the the plastic industry to develop breasts, from simply inhaling dust that carried the chemical. In the 1970s, researchers from Stanford University found bisphenol-A able to leech out of polycarbonate bottles.

Nonlyphenol has also been found to have estrogenic effects on breast tissue. Nonlyphenol is used to make containers more flexible.

Polycarbonate is another chemical used in plastic containers that is also suspected by scientists to be estrogenic.

Haas concludes that scientists don't know exactly how much of these chemicals end up in our food and beverages, nor has it been concluded definitively whether they cause breast cancer in humans. Isn't it prudent, nevertheless, to choose glass over plastic containers?

Adequate Sources of B6 Foods Are Important When Consuming Flaxseeds and Oil

Pyridoxine (vitamin B6) is important for the immune system, and is required for protein metabolism. Be certain that you are consuming plenty of vitamin B6-rich foods when supplementing with flaxseeds and oil. Some foods rich in B6 are:

Avocado	Salmon
Carrots	Watermelon
Lentils	Melon
Chicken	Walnuts
Soybeans	Hazelnuts
Sunflower seeds	Chestnuts
Tuna	Trout
Shrimp	Turkey
Beef	

CHAPTER 7

Soybeans Protect Against Breast Cancer

The beta receptor [where estrogen is absorbed] . . . turns out to be ten times as efficient . . . at binding up with a renowned plant estrogen called genistein found in soybeans and other beans and vegetables.
—Natalie Angier, "New Respect for Estrogen's Influence Throughout the Body," *New York Times,* June 24, 1997.

More than thirty studies have confirmed the ability of soybean isoflavones such as genistein to prevent cancer cell growth, especially in breast cancer.
—Dr. Ronald Klatz, Dr. Robert Goldman, "The Soybean Solution to Aging," *Total Health Magazine,* December 1997

It's no wonder that the National Cancer Institute is spreading the word about soy's ability to protect against breast (and prostate) cancer. Let's take a look at some of the reasons why. The phytochemicals in soy:

- Inhibit the growth of tumor cells.
- Convert cancer cells back to normal cells.
- Block the entry of estrogen into breast cells, which is beneficial in preventing cancer. Research also shows that soy isoflavones may protect against high levels of synthetic estrogen in the diet. Soy may even prevent the metastasis of cancer cells.

At the 1994 national meeting of the American Cancer Society in Washington, investigators presented research indicating that certain phytochemicals found in soy foods may be part of the reason Asians have such low rates of breast cancer. Nutritionist Patti Tviet Mulligan, M.S., R.D., believes the consumption of soy may help prevent hormone-related cancers because soy foods possess properties that have been shown to block binding of harmful estrogen by estrogen-sensitive tissues.

Women receive many benefits from soy that include hormonal regulation (which helps to alleviate discomfort from symptoms of PMS and menopause), prevention of osteoporosis (soy has bone-building ability), cholesterol reduction, and general immune support from its antioxidant properties.

Soy foods include: soybeans, tofu, tempeh, miso, soy sauce, soy milk, natto (fermented beans), and second-generation soy foods such as cheese, textured vegetable protein, and others (soy breakfast links, for instance). Frozen green soybeans called "edamame" are available in many Asian markets and can be added to soups or braised Chinese cabbage and scallions, flavored with soy sauce and grated ginger—delicious!

TIP: Consume a half-cup of tofu, tempeh, miso soup, or soybeans daily as a breast cancer prevention strategy. Soy isoflavones offer protection against breast cancer in women and prostate cancer in men.

Phytoestrogens are similar in structure, but far less potent than, the estrogen produced in the body. They compete for estrogen receptor sites, providing protection against the damaging effects of too much estrogen resulting from poor diet and environmental exposure. Phytoestrogens are thought to protect estrogen receptor sites in the breasts (and elsewhere in the body) from overstimulation, which could lead to abnormal tissue growth. In countries where women consume diets rich in soy foods—rich in phytoestrogens—the rate of breast cancer is much lower than in the United States, and women don't have symptoms of menopause. Mary Stewart of the Women's Nutritional Advisory Service believes that natural estrogens from plants are a substitute for hormone replacement therapy for women who can't or won't take it. At least thirty-eight studies have shown that soy phytoestrogens also help to lower bad cholesterol (LDL) and triglycerides.

Phenolic acids from soy bean foods protect cells against potential harm. Phenolic acids have antioxidant properties, protecting against cancer as well as viruses.

Some Phytochemicals in Soy and Their Properties

Research from the University of Alabama, the University of Cincinnati, and the University of Helsinki, Finland, has found soy isoflavones to discourage both the initiation and promotion of cancer. *Isoflavones* are a wide variety of plant substances that protect the breasts; their mechanism of action is similar to that of tamoxifan (a drug used to treat breast cancer). These plant estrogens block estrogen receptor sites in the breasts and prevent stronger, potentially harmful forms of estrogen from initiating cancer. Isoflavones also slow tumor cell growth by blocking the process of new blood vessel formation (called "angiogenesis"). This is significant, since tumors depend on new blood vessels for the oxygen and blood needed to nourish growth. Isoflavones are most concentrated in soy, alfalfa, and red clover. Because of their antioxidant activities, isoflavones have been shown to protect not only against cancer—by protecting against harmful free radicals that may attack DNA, thereby initiating cancer—but also against atherosclerosis and coronary heart disease. There are more than ten isoflavones in soy, with genistein and daidzein being the most significant. *Genistein* limits the growth of breast and other tumors. Research shows that genistein can block cancer-creating enzymes and limit the blood supply necessary for tumor formation. Genistein is also an antioxidant that helps to protect cells from free radicals. A 1996 study from the University of Alabama found genistein specifically helps to prevent the growth of breast cancer. Genistein has been found to be even more potent than previously thought, as Natalie Angier reported in the *New York Times* in June 1997. A 1996 study from the University of Alabama found that genistein specifically helps to reduce the growth of mammary cancer in animals by 40 to 60 percent. Maybe this is why Japanese women have one-fourth the rate of breast cancer as American women, who eat very little tofu or other soy foods. As reported in *Total Health* magazine in December, 1997, genistein protects breast tissue in both peri-menopausal and post-menopausal women by preventing estrogen from causing malignant changes. (For more information, *see* Chapter 11, "Foods, Hormones, and Breast Cancer: What's the Conection?") *Daidzein* has been shown in studies to suppress the growth of cancer cells. It also battles osteoporosis by protecting against bone loss. *Saponins* are antioxidants that interfere with tumor promotion by preventing cancer cells from multiplying. Saponins have also been found to have cholesterol-lowering benefits.

Isoflavones are abundant in soybeans, but *not* soybean oil, because they are water soluble. Soybean oil may contain a small amount of isoflavones, but a richer source is tofu. Additionally, soybean oil is usually processed, and so possesses all the accompanying problems of processed, chemically treated oils.

Protease inhibitors can help protect DNA, and have strong anticancer benefits. They protect against inflammation, radiation, and the growth of breast cancer. Protease inhibitors can stay active in the body for months. A special protease inhibitor in soy foods, Bowman-Birk Inhibitor (BBI), has been found to be effective in blocking tumor growth in animals, and researchers at the University of Pennsylvania are studying it as a preventive agent for people at high risk of developing cancer. To protect the protease inhibitors in tofu, heat it gently, below the boiling point. Steaming, baking at 350–375 degrees, and simmering in soups or stews all preserve tofu's protease inhibitors.

Phytic acid in soy has been found to reduce tumor size and incidence significantly in mammary and colon tissues. Phytic acid's novel anticancer function lies in its "mineral binding ability," which was described in a 1991 study in *Carcinogenesis*. Susun Weed explains that "phytic acid is a plant-based phosphorus which prevents the formation of free radicals in the intestines."

Phytic Acid

Fiber-rich foods like oats; wheat; lentils; and Great Northern, white, soy, and pinto beans contain phytic acid or "phytates." People in the Middle East have traditionally consumed phytates in the form of unleavened wheat and flat breads and lentils, and Asians have traditionally consumed soy foods. These two cultures have always enjoyed lower rates of cancer and heart disease than Western cultures.

It is wise to rotate food selection, and avoid concentrating on mostly phytic acid-rich foods. I would never consider eliminating protective foods like soy, lentils, oats, and others, but I would avoid supplementing with bran as a fiber source when eating soy. Small amounts of phytic acid, on a daily basis, are a chelating agent that helps to bind heavy metals and eliminate them. Excessive consumption of phytates may present a mineral absorption problem because of their mineral-binding abilities. However, keep in mind that adequate consumption of phytates appears to have anticancer effects; phytic acid consumption may be one of the reasons a high-fiber diet is cancer protective. There are some phytic acid-rich foods that I don't recommend, mostly because I don't consider them to be whole foods, including puffed grain cereals (puffed oats or rice), bran by itself, or rice cakes. These processed foods were found in an animal study to bind nutrients in the gut and prevent them from being absorbed.

Nutritionist Joan Friedrich, who practices in Bronxville, New York, explains that, "Although dietary phytates may pose the risk of reducing bioavailability of minerals, to a large extent this concern can be addressed with dietary adjustments, such as proper food selection and broad dietary rotation."

Other Benefits of Soy for Women

Osteoporosis. Studies show isoflavones in soy protect bone mass and result in less urinary calcium excretion than animal protein produces. University of

Illinois researchers found that sixty-six postmenopausal women gained bone density from eating soy (as part of a low-fat, low-cholesterol diet) for six months. One-half cup of soybeans provides 232 milligrams of calcium.

Symptoms of menopause. Consumption of soy foods, which contain phytoestrogens, is believed to reduce or eliminate hot flashes and other symptoms of menopause. Asian women don't experience hot flashes, and it is believed that their soy rich diet is the reason. Consuming soy for just one month, as researchers reported at the University of Texas, helped premenopausal women to experience improved hormonal balance.

Symptoms of PMS. Moodiness, bloating, and cramps are relieved by soy foods.

Heart disease. Soy helps to reduce bad LDL cholesterol and raises good HDL cholesterol, thereby protecting us from heart disease. Soy also helps to prevent plaque formation in our arteries and reduces blood clotting.

Anti-Aging Benefits. A study conducted at the University of Nebraska found that animals fed soybean proteins lived 13% longer than those that weren't. Researchers determined that the antioxidants properties of soybeans help to protect cells from free radical damage and age-related diseases.

Gallstones. Did you know that cholesterol is the primary ingredient in gallstones? Because soy helps to dissolve and eliminate blood cholesterol, it may be helpful in disolving gallstones. In addition, people who consume diets high in animal protein and low in vegetable protein experience a higher incidence of gallstones.

In November 1996, the American Heart Association (in association with Gregory L. Burke, M.D., at the Bauman Gray School of Medicine in Winston-Salem, North Carolina) explored the effects of soy protein on forty-three peri-menopausal women between the ages of forty-five and fifty-five. After consuming a powdered supplement containing 20 grams of soy protein daily, these subjects' total cholesterol and triglycerides dropped 10 percent; LDL cholesterol ("bad" cholesterol) dropped 13 percent, while HDL cholesterol (the protective cholesterol) was unaffected. (Four ounces of tofu contain 8–13 grams of soy protein, and eight ounces of soy milk contain 4–10 grams.)

Times have changed with respect to soy. The newest *Joy of Cooking*, released in late 1997, contains a dozen recipes using soy; the 1963 edition contained only two. More than 700 studies examining the effects of soy on health have been published in recent years. People who consume soy foods regularly, like some vegetarians and semivegetarians, have been found to have lower rates of breast, uterus, colon, and prostate cancers.

Eating tofu once a week is three times more protective against breast cancer than eating tofu once a month, according to a study of nearly 1,600 Asian American women living in Hawaii and California. Daily servings of soy foods help to provide maximum protection. Select from tofu, tempeh, soy milk, miso, natto, green soybeans, second generation soy foods (also known as textured soy protein), and okra (made from soy milk and available in burgers and sausages).

Silken Tofu and Leeks with Sweet and Sour Garlic Miso Sauce on Noodles

(Serves 4)

🍎   *The secret of this dish is not to overcook the leeks or herbs. Fresh, simple ingredients and crispy-tender leeks ensure a dish redolent with unexpected flavors. Balance this meal with a large salad.*

> several romaine lettuce leaves
> 2 leeks, carefully cleaned and finely minced
> 1 lb soft tofu
> 1 8.8-oz package of udon noodles

> ### Sauce:

> 3 tbsp of sweet white miso
> juice from 1 ½–2 lemons
> 6–8 cloves of finely minced garlic
> 1 cup of chopped, reconstituted sun-dried
>   tomatoes, or equal amount of chopped fresh
>   seasonal tomatoes
> 3 tbsp extra virgin olive oil
> 3 tbsp flaxseed oil
> 4–5 tbsp minced fresh basil, dill, or
>   marjoram, to taste

Place cleaned lettuce leaves on the bottom of a stainless steel steam basket. Arrange minced leeks evenly over lettuce. Spoon tofu over leeks in an even layer.

Combine sauce ingredients, except oils and herbs, in a blender. After sauce ingredients are puréed (minus the oils and herbs), pour over tofu.

Place steamer basket containing food into large pot with 2 inches of gently boiling filtered water. Cover with lid. Steam over low boil for about 40 seconds. Turn heat down to medium-low and steam for about 8 minutes, until the tofu is heated through. Uncover and sprinkle minced herbs over sauce and continue to cook for 30 seconds more. Remove basket from pot. Set in sink to cool for 1-2 minutes.

Prepare udon noodles according to directions on the package and drain. Spoon noodles on each plate with half of the oils. Add herbs over noodles. Drizzle remaining oils and garnish with a little minced, uncooked herbs. Toss thoroughly and serve.

Update on the Politics of Soybeans: Will Quality Be Sacrificed for Commercial Purposes?

Several U.S. chemical companies have combined genes from undesirable organisms such as viruses and bacteria to form a genetically engineered soybean, sometimes called a herbicide soybean.

There are many unanswered health questions about genetically engineered foods, and because the government doesn't require testing or labeling of new biotech products, consumers need to be alert. Many scientists are aware that genetic modification creates entirely new strains and species of life. Suspected problems associated with these genetically engineered foods include decreased nutritional value, increased toxicity, and hidden allergens. The British Retail Consortium and nine other European trade organizations have protested genetically engineered crops by insisting that genetically engineered produce be distinguished from foods that are natural, including U.S. imported genetically engineered foods.

Since it's difficult to distinguish between natural soybeans and the genetically engineered ones, it's not uncommon for farmers to mingle the two when harvested. Because of this, the many products in supermarkets and health food stores that utilize soybean derivatives as basic ingredient—drinks, breads, snack foods, soy sauce, soy protein, and many others—should clearly state if they are "certified organically grown."

For more information on genetically engineered soybeans and other foods, visit the Citizens for Health website at www.citizens.org or call 1-800-357-2211.

Be sure your soy products are from companies that use only organic soybeans. Be aware, and question both your health food or grocery store and the product's manufacturer.

Fermented Soy Foods Are Especially Beneficial

Soy foods such as miso, natto, and soy sauce contain the strongest anticancer properties. Research has shown that the benefits of soy are especially potent when fermented, as these foods are.

Soy sauce is made from soybeans, water, sea salt, and wheat. *Tamari* contains no wheat; it is made from soybeans, water, and sea salt. Use either on vegetables, with fresh-squeezed lemon juice, in vinaigrettes with ginger, herbs, and sesame oil, or in marinades. I especially like to marinate lemon sole in this type of marinade:

> ¼ cup organic shoyu or tamari sauce
>
> 2 tbsp mirin (Japanese sweet rice cooking wine, excellent for balancing the salty taste of soy because of its subtle, sweet flavor)
>
> 3 tbsp grated ginger juice *or* grated horseradish juice juice from 1 lemon
>
> 1 tbsp minced, seeded hot pepper (peppers are a source of powerful antioxidants)
>
> 4-8 cloves of minced garlic, depending on taste

This marinade also works well for scallops or shrimp. To turn it into a vinaigrette, just add sesame oil and minced chives.

Natto takes some getting used to—either you love it, or you just can't eat it. I encourage you to try this food several times. Be sure you mix it together with organic mustard and plenty of minced scallions. It is available in the frozen food section, in little plastic tubs. Store it in your own freezer, and defrost several hours before use.

> TIP: Try *natto miso chutney*—a flavorful relish that contains protein, minerals, and enzymes, made from soybeans, barley, sea salt, kombu, ginger, and barley malt—with vegetables, fish, tofu, noodles, or grain dishes. *(See* Resource Guide.)

Tempeh is a wonderful food that people generally learn to enjoy. This fermented whole soy food has its origins in Indonesia, and it is frequently served with peanut sauce. I recommend you use it to stuff peppers, or in mock tuna salads, or braised with plenty of spices and herbs.

Basic tempeh salad: Add your favorite raw, grated vegetables. Don't be concerned about exact amounts; experiment with the ingredients and have fun.

8 ounces tempeh
clove of garlic
shoyu or tamari sauce
minced carrots, celery, and red onion
chopped parsley
tahini
umeboshi vinegar
mellow white miso

Cut tempeh into thin slices. Simmer with garlic and a small amount of filtered water and tamari for 20 minutes. Mash tempeh with remaining ingredients. Mix well, and serve. (For more tempeh recipes, *see* Resource Guide.)

The Magic of Miso: Folklore Was Right

Whoever would think that fermented soybean paste pureed in hot water would not only taste savory and satisfying, but would also contain multiple health benefits? The Japanese have possessed this knowledge for 2,500 years. Although miso was first discovered in China and later brought to Japan, it's so much a part of daily life in Japan that the average housewife has 365 different recipes for miso soup.

Zybilcolin, another substance in miso, expels toxins such as nicotine, radiation, and other pollutants from the body. The *Proceedings of the National Academy of Science USA* reported in 1993 that "Miso may prevent cancer, according to new scientific findings."

A Blood Cleanser and Builder

Miso not only protects against cancer and cleanses the blood, but also offers many other nutritional benefits.

1. Enzymes present in miso from the fermentation process hold powerful health benefits. They act as "spark plugs" for the entire body, helping to break down and digest proteins, carbohydrates, and fats. Digestive enzymes made from miso are marketed in Japan as supplements.

2. Lactic acid bacteria, necessary microflora that live in the digestive tract, are replenished by miso. Penicillin and other antibiotics destroy this friendly flora that is so vital to the digestive process. A cup of miso soup a day when on antibiotics restores the bacteria that are lost.

3. Hatcho miso, the darkest miso available, is excellent for protecting against candida and other yeast. Hatcho miso cleanses the body and restores friendly microflora destroyed by years of antibiotics taken to "control" yeast infections.

4. Soybeans, the main ingredient in miso, contain 34% protein, 31% carbohydrate, and 18% fat. The protein content of soybeans in miso is eleven times higher than milk, and as high as meat or fish. The fermentation process that creates miso encourages the body's use of these nutrients.

5. The fermentation process of miso also allows a superior absorption of the calcium, phosphorous, iron, and other materials contained in miso.

6. Miso aids in preventing arteriosclerosis and high blood pressure. Linoleic acid and lecithin contained in miso dissolve cholesterol in the blood and soften blood vessels.

7. For boosting stamina, miso is an excellent source of energy.

8. Dense with minerals and other nutrients, miso richly nourishes the skin and hair and aids in the regeneration of cell and skin tissue.

9. For weight loss, a cup of miso soup at breakfast encourages a boost in metabolism, as is recommended in macrobiotics.

10. Miso soup is one of the quickest ways to alkalinize the blood. After a night of overindulging in wine, a restorative swim in the ocean can eliminate fatigue, headache, and nausea, because the salty ocean water alkalizes the system efficiently. A steamy cup of rich, salty miso soup garnished with an emerald green fragment of sea vegetable holds the same alkalizing benefits as the ocean it so poetically reflects.

Miso Tips

• Use unpasteurized, organic miso.

• Transfer miso immediately from plastic containers to glass, enamel, or wood. In the highly respected nutritionists' reference book *Health with Whole Foods*, Paul Pitchford emphasizes that, "Miso has the ability to absorb toxins from plastic containers and should be transferred into glass for storage. The same holds true for other fermented foods and oils."

• There are many varieties of miso, depending upon the region of Japan you purchase it from, like wine from France. Basically, an experienced cook works with four to six types of miso, varying from light (chickpea) to dark (soybean or hatcho). The salty, dark misos are recommended in the winter. Lighter misos—such as garbanzo, millet, mellow, corn, and sweet white—are sweeter and less salty; they combine well with shallots or garlic, lemon juice, and herbs for sauces. Traditionally, lighter misos are in the spring and summer. Light and dark misos can be mixed. All misos contain fermented soybean paste.

• Since miso is a live food, boiling destroys the beneficial enzymes. When making healing soups, add miso to preparations a minute or two before removing from heat.

Miso Broth

(SERVES 1)

🍎 *This is a quick, easy broth full of the many benefits of miso.*

2 tbsp chopped scallions
1–2 tsp barley miso
1/2 cup cubed tofu
1 cup of hot water

Purée scallions and miso. Gradually add hot water, stirring constantly. Drink immediately.

> TIP: Michio Kushi, in *Macrobiotic Home Remedies,* recommends drinking a miso-scallion drink in the early stages of a cold or headache. It activates circulation and induces sweating, which helps to eliminate allergens and bacteria.

Miso Soup Suggestions

Any one of the following soups can be flavored with puréed miso. You can even add a lighter barley miso to chicken soup and no one will be the wiser.

- Vegetable soup with wakame or dulse seaweed.
- Tofu-miso soup: Add cubed tofu to miso.
- Bean-vegetable miso soup: Cook leftover beans in vegetable soup until creamy.
- Combine miso with leftover grains such as brown rice or millet.
- Purée squash and/or other sweet winter vegetables in soup.
- Noodle vegetable soup with udon noodles.
- Add leftover steamed green vegetables such as broccoli or kale, chopped fine.
- Garnish soups with chopped scallions, grated ginger, or chopped parsley.

CHAPTER 8

Nutrient-Dense Green Vegetables: Protective and Cleansing

I recommend that people I counsel include dark, leafy greens in their diets every day. Greens are a great source of a wide variety of important, breast-protective nutrients and fiber. *The darker green vegetables are, the richer they are in protective carotenoids, potential cancer inhibitors.* In May 1997, Jane E. Brody reported in her *New York Times* health column that women who routinely eat the most vegetables have a 54 percent lower risk of developing breast cancer. A study from Italy published in *The Lancet* in 1996 noted that a diet high in vegetables reduced the rate of breast cancer by 30–60 percent.

Some of the nutrients found in greens that create breast health are: carotenoids, antioxidants, folic acid, flavonoids, lutein, chlorophyll, and if gently boiled, vitamin C. Cruciferous green vegetables also contain indoles, which help to regulate cancer-promoting estrogen.

TIP: Select from the following greens and have two servings daily: kale, bok choy, turnip and collard greens, dandelion greens, watercress, mustard greens, dark green lettuce, broccoli, Brussels sprouts, Chinese cabbage, broccoli rabe, and nettles.

Greens clean the inside of the body by helping to eliminate undigested foods. The chlorophyll in green plants helps to rid the body of toxins from within the body (from the bowel) and from the environment (secondhand smoke or chemicals).

Bernard Jensen, D.C., Ph.D., described the many benefits of chlorophyll at the 1997 Medicines from the Earth Herbal Conference. He explained that chlorophyll helps to prevent bowel toxemia, which can be a result of undigested foods. "Bowel toxemia can affect every organ," Jensen pointed out. "For instance, bowel toxemia can cause a weakness in the heart. The greatest deterrent to weak organs comes from removing toxins both outside the body and inside the body," he concluded.

In addition to greens, herbs, particularly nettles, are also excellent sources of chlorophyll. Stinging nettle is a perennial that is rich in trace minerals and potassium as well as chlorophyll. (Wear gloves when picking them, and steam lightly before eating to avoid their stinging hairs!)

> TIP: Organic stinging nettles are available in seed packets from the Strictly Medicinal catalog. *(See* Resource Guide.) Nettles are a rich source of minerals and chlorophyll.

Green vegetables are also a rich source of calcium. Asian women do not eat dairy and they suffer from much lower rates of osteoporosis than do Western women. In fact, the *New York Times* reported on August 30, 1997, that the Japanese have the longest life expectancy in the world. I suspect both these facts are due in part to all the different types of vegetables the Japanese eat daily, with green vegetables playing a major role in their diet.

Greens can be simply prepared and served as a side dish. Dress with one or more of the following condiments: soy sauce, umeboshi vinegar, lemon, and brown rice vinegar. Drizzle with fresh, organic flaxseed oil or olive oil for added flavor and health benefits.

> Brussels sprouts and broccoli contain glucosinolates that help the body to eliminate cancer-producing substances. The process of chewing assists this phytonutrient by releasing an enzyme in the vegetable. For the most protection from vegetables, don't overcook them or leave them sitting around for long periods of time after they are cooked. Cook green vegetables until just emerald green and tender, and consume immediately. Overcooked Brussels sprouts have no protective phytonutrients. Fresh Brussels sprouts, in contrast, possess considerable carcinogen-detoxifying effects.

Water-Sautéed Vegetables

1 bunch kale
1–2 carrots
1 medium onion
filtered water
1 tsp tamari
small pieces of ginger
2–3 pinches of sea salt, to taste
Flaxseed, walnut, or extra virgin
     olive oil

Scrub carrots and cut into diagonals. Cut the diagonals into matchsticks. Rinse the kale and cut the stems into 1/2-inch pieces. Break the leaves up into pieces with your hands. Peel and thinly slice the onion. Using a deep stainless steel skillet, heat ½ inch of water along with tamari and 1 tsp of ginger juice. Add the kale and stir over medium-high for 4 minutes.

Add the carrots, stir for a couple of minutes. Turn down and cook for 5 minutes. Add onion slices and sauté for 3 more minutes. Add sea salt and a drizzle of your favorite oil, unheated.

Tips on Preparing Greens

• Once greens are cut, oxygen may affect taste and nutrients, so don't wash or cut them until right before cooking.

• Before cooking, discard discolored leaves and wash greens in a pot of water; drain.

• Dry greens by patting them with a clean dish towel.

• Cut off tough stems. Slice large leaves right down the middle, through the stem, then cut into thin strips for faster cooking.

• Plant kale in the late summer, and you can harvest it in the fall and winter. Kale is amazingly hardy and will grow as long as the ground doesn't freeze.

Purslane

If you are lucky enough to find purslane (its Latin name is *Portulaca oleraceae*) in your garden, I might be able to inspire you to include this wonderful, crunchy plant in salads.

Purslane's Exceptional Nutritional Profile

• Purslane is an extremely rich source of omega-3 fatty acid. You can obtain a day's supply of omega-3 fatty acid from less then 1 cup of this green vegetable.

• Purslane is a rich source of vitamin E. Researchers have found food sources of this protective antioxidant to be far superior to supplementing with vitamin E.

• Purslane also contains vitamins C and A.

• Purslane is a rich source of fiber.

• Purslane is commonly used in salads in France, Italy, Greece, and Turkey.

Purslane has a subtle, refreshing, tangy taste. It is mucilagineous in texture when chewed, and looks a little like a jade plant, with rich, green, succulent leaves, rather paddle-shaped, with a sturdy little stem. The early settlers of America regarded purslane as an antiscurvy herb because of its high vitamin content. (*See* Resource Guide to order organic purslane seeds.)

CHAPTER 9

The Hidden Power of Plant Foods

Vegetables, fruits, grains, nuts, seeds. and legumes all possess "chemoprotective qualities"—the latest scientific buzz phrase indicating that people
who consume a plant-based diet gain protection against illness. Researchers
all over the world now acknowledge that people who eat large quantities of
vegetables and fruits have reduced cancer risks, including breast cancer risk.
This effect is most probably related to the presence of literally hundreds of
nutrient and nonnutrient chemical substances in plants. Nutritionists and
researchers have come to realize the wisdom in not isolating single nutrients
and taking them as supplements, but consuming them in their whole foods
form. Because there are so many unknown compounds present in foods that
offer powerful, "chemoprotective" biological effects, the best nutritional plan
is to obtain these benefits from a wide variety of foods. For example, beta-
carotene, together with the forty other carotenoids in food, is more effective
than beta-carotene supplements. As Jane E. Brody reported in the *New York
Times* in October 1997, "It is the combination of food-borne nutrients and
other substances in plant food like fiber and various plant chemicals, that
may provide specific benefits."

Antioxidant Properties

Certain plant-based substances have the remarkable ability to regulate
oxidation reactions in the body—caused by environmental pollution; too
much sun; or from fats in the body, among other causes—which can generate

excess so-called free radicals—unpaired electrons—capable of causing molecular damage to cells, which can ultimately lead to disease. These so-called antioxidants are receiving a lot of attention for their promise in preventing cancer.

Carotenoids

Carotenoids are a huge family of phytochemicals (*phyto* is Greek for "plant"), including alpha- and beta-carotene, lycopene, and lutein. Over 600 have been identified so far.

Recent studies show carotenoids to be powerfully effective in cancer prevention, and a 1993 study specifically linked carotenoids with the prevention of breast cancer. Other research found that women with the highest levels of carotenoids had 20 percent fewer breast malignancies. *It is interesting to note that this protection came from whole foods rich in carotenoids, not from vitamin supplements.* Additionally, two studies from the University of Arizona Cancer Center reported that beta-carotene supplements may reduce blood levels of vitamin E—a nutrient that is even more important than beta-carotene in preventing disease.

TIP: When foods rich in beta-carotenes and related antioxidant phytochemical carotenes are cooked, they are up to five times more effective at cancer prevention than if eaten raw. *Flaxseed oil helps to assimilate carotenes, so when you steam kale or other greens, dress them with flaxseed oil.*

Two such carotenoids, alpha- and beta-carotene, have been found in more than 70 international studies to protect against cancer. "Breast cancer patients exhibit decreased levels of beta-carotene in their blood and breast tissue," the *American Journal of Obstetrics and Gynecology* reported in 1989. Over twenty-five years ago, international research showed conclusively that people who consume foods rich in beta-carotene have lower incidences of cancer, while recent studies show that alpha-carotene also possesses powerful antioxidant activities. Beta-carotene generates vitamin A more efficiently than alpha-carotene (50 of the 563 identified carotenoids can be metabolized into vitamin A), but alpha-carotene is ten times more efficient at inhibiting some cancers. Research shows that carotenes can stop already-present cancerous growths from enlarging, especially liver tumors. Carotenoids may be able to stop cancer growth because they cause cells to mature, or differentiate; cancerous cells are undifferentiated. Dietary sources of alpha- and beta-carotene (and other carotenoids) are yams, carrots, sweet potatoes, winter squash, pumpkin, lamb's quarters, shallots, spinach, dandelion greens, turnips, kale, collards, beet and mustard greens, bok choy, scallions, parsley, broccoli, cantaloupe, mangoes, apricots, and papaya.

> TIP: Beta- and alpha-carotene can also be found in fatty-rich fish and eggs.

Beta-Carotene Supplements? No Thanks!
The Journal of the National Cancer Institute reported in May 1996 that supplementing with beta-carotene may interfere with the utilization of carotenoids and other phytochemicals. Studies indicate that there are important biological interactions between carotenoids. Beta-carotene seemed the most promising cancer-preventive until researchers discovered in 1996 that carotenoids (which include beta-carotene) seem to work best in unison. *(See* the Resource Guide for a beta- carotene supplement that also includes other carotenoids of plant origin.)

In the 1997 *New York Times Book of Health,* Jane Brody noted, "In fact, supplementing with beta-carogene can cause high levels to build up in blood and tissues, actually creating oxidation, instead of guarding against it." Brody recommends eating carotene-rich foods over taking "a high dose supplement."

It seems that vegetables work in many ways to prevent disease and increase immunity, so consume bright orange, yellow, and dark green vegetables often.

> TIP: Red bell peppers possess nine times more beta-carotene and twice as much vitamin C as green bell peppers, which are picked before they're ripe.

Lycopene is similar to beta-carotene, but this carotenoid surpasses all others in protection against free radicals. In fact, lycopene quenches free radicals twice as effectively as beta-carotene. Lycopene is also significantly more active against tumor formation than the other caretenoids. A 1997 animal study showed that lycopene helps to prevent mammary cancer. Rats injected with a carcinogenic chemical were protected from cancer by a simple tomato extract. Both tumor size and frequency of tumors were significantly reduced when the animals were treated with the tomato extract. Interestingly, other animals treated with beta-carotene (in another part of this study) were not protected against developing breast cancer.

Foods rich in lycopene include tomato juice, tomato paste, tomato sauce, watermelon, pink grapefruit, and dried apricots.

Another carotenoid, lutein, also offers more protection against free radicals than beta-carotene. Dietary sources of lutein include green leafy vegetables, algae (chlorella), citrus rind, apricots, peaches, plums, apples, and cranberries.

OPCs

A powerful group of antioxidants is called *oligomeric proanthocyanidins* (OPCs). They allow wine to ripen and delay the wrinkling of a peach's skin. Practically all plants have the ability to create OPCs. Known by the American Indians, discovered and researched by Dr. Jack Masquelier, professor emeritus at the University of Bordeaux, France, OPCs are available in a supplement, owing to an extraction process patented by Dr. Masquelier in 1987.

How Do OPCs Benefit Health?

OPCs:

- Protect against the risk of developing cancer from exposure to radiation, chemical toxins, or biological agents.
- Protect DNA and RNA.
- Possess powerful antioxidant properties.
- Protect capillaries.
- Protect vascular walls, thereby protecting the lymphatic vessels.
- Protect eyes.
- Protect against edema (inflammation or swelling), which can occur after breast cancer operations.

Most of the studies on OPCs have been done in Europe, and some experts feel more information is needed before red grapes can be touted as a miracle food. In the meantime, it's not a bad idea to add red grapes (and their seeds), as well as raisins, to your diet.

Fruits containing OPCs include red grapes, blueberries, blackberries, cherries, and raspberries.

For studies on the many benefits of OPCs for cancer prevention and healing, such as tumor prevention, protection against radiation and chemicals, protection of DNA from free radicals, and reduction of edema (swelling) after breast cancer surgery, see *OPC in Practice: The Hidden Story of Proanthocyanidins, Nature's Most Powerful and Patented Antioxidant* (Alfa

Omega Editrice, Italy, 1995), written by Masquelier with Bert Schwitters. Schwitters explained to me that, in order for OPCs to work optimally, good diet and exercise are fundamental for maintaining health, and it's also important to be selective when buying OPC supplements. (*See* the Resource Guide for Dr. Masquelier's formula.) Schwitters made the following recommendations for supplementing with OPCs:

- General health (prevention of disease): 100 milligrams daily
- Preventing recurrence of breast cancer: 150-200 milligrams daily
- Reducing post-surgical edema (swelling): 200 milligrams daily
- Treating varicose veins (used for this condition in France for decades): 100-250 milligrams daily
- Reducing swelling after facial cosmetic surgery: 200 milligrams daily

> Vegetables are better than supplements in lowering the risks of colon cancer, according to researchers at Dartmouth Medical School. Antioxidants found in vegetables and fruits had a much more protective effect than antioxidant supplements, they reported in 1994 in the *New England Journal of Medicine*.

Vitamin A helps prevent altered cells from becoming cancerous; it also guards against tumor formation resulting from chemical carcinogens. Sources of vitamin A include carrots, sweet potatoes, spinach, dandelion greens, broccoli, tomatoes, asparagus, cantaloupe, peaches, cherries, and apricots. Foods rich in vitamin A also contain many other carotenoids, including lutein, alphacarotene, and lycopene.

> TIP: One cup of dandelion greens contains 1400 international units (IUs) of vitamin A.

Twelve studies of diet and breast cancer were reviewed at the Canadian National Cancer Institute, where it was concluded that *vitamin C* significantly lowers the risk of breast cancer. Vitamin C stimulates the production of protective cells that destroy cancer cells; helps prevent the formation of carcinogens in the body; detoxifies the blood; and protects collagen in skin, blood vessels, bones, and teeth. To preserve vitamin C, steam or simmer vegetables gently for no longer than 10 minutes; overcooking destroys this important vitamin. Sugar also depletes the body of this important nutrient.

Dietary sources of vitamin C include red and green peppers, broccoli, kale, tomatoes, potatoes, Brussels sprouts, cabbage, cauliflower, strawberries, spinach, oranges, grapefruit, melon, papaya, and other fresh fruits. Megadosing on vitamin C possibly increases blood iron levels in people with genetic conditions such as thalassemia and hemochromatosis. It is not advisable to consume large doses of vitamin C when undergoing chemotherapy for breast cancer.

TIP: For a healing, relaxing bedtime beverage rich in antioxidants, try lemon balm tea.

Vitamin E protects the essential fatty acids in the body from oxidation and free radicals. It has also been found to prevent tumors produced by carcinogenic substances and helps to form red blood cells. It's important to consume plenty of vitamin E-rich foods when consuming olive, flaxseed, and other protective oils. Dietary sources of vitamin E include dark green vegetables, tomatoes, fresh vegetable oils, whole grains, oatmeal, peanuts, sunflower seeds, almonds, peaches, and prunes. Freezing destroys vitamin E.

TIP: When supplementing with vitamin E, look for a combination of alpha-, gamma-, and delta-tocotrienol. A recent study has emphasized, once again, that the whole nutrient complex is more powerful than isolated, single ingredients for inhibiting the spread of breast cancer.

An arsenal of vitamins, minerals, and protective phytochemicals found in *sea vegetables* is specifically beneficial in the treatment of breast cancer. As long ago as 1981, an article in *Medical Hypothesis* showed seaweed to be protective against breast cancer. A daily two-ounce serving of seaweed has been found to have antitumor activities, preventing both initiation and recurrence. Alginic acid, found in seaweed, protects the body from heavy metals, radiation, and chemicals. Seaweed is also rich in antioxidants and selenium. Choose from among wakame (the most protective), kombu, nori, hijiki, and arame.

TIP: Use wakame daily in 1 cup boiling water with 1 teaspoon pureed barley miso for a quick, healing broth. Reconstitute a 2-inch strip of wakame in a small amount of water for 10 minutes. Discard the rib, and add to miso broth.

Other Phytonutrient-Rich Substances

Chlorella

Chlorella, a single cell algae, contains carotenoids, magnesium (in general, Americans have lower-than-optimal levels of this mineral), and chlorophyll, which is a super detoxifier and possesses many other well-documented health benefits.

Chlorella's anticancer properties are beginning to be acknowledged by the National Cancer Institute. Laboratory research has shown chlorella to offer protective benefits against mammary tumors. Chlorella contributes to the manufacture of superior quality RNA/DNA, which is linked to cellular growth, renewal, and repair.

Chlorella encourages normal growth, without stimulating the growth of tumors. The protein in chlorella is easy to absorb, and helps to balance blood sugar levels, which is beneficial in reducing sugar cravings. Chlorella stimulates the body to make protective interferon and macrophages (protector cells). Rich in omega-3 fatty acids, chlorella also contains:

- Vitamins A, B-2, B-6, B-12, C, K, E; calcium; iron; zinc; phosphorus; iodine; and 19 of the 22 essential and nonessential amino acids.
- Carotenoids.
- Chlorophyll; a super detoxifier, which eliminates toxic metals such as cadmium and uranium.
- Magnesium, important for immune function, blood sugar balance, and heart function.

> TIP: I consume a teaspoon of chlorella daily, mixed with water, in the morning. Some people like to mix it with juice, which I occasionally do as well. After drinking chlorella, I notice that I feel a calm sense of renewed vitality.

Royal Jelly

Made by worker bees to feed the queen, royal jelly is a major source of panothenic acid and contains biotin, folic acid, inositol, and vitamins B-1, B-2, B-3, B-6, B-12, A, C, D, and E. This concentrated food is also a source of acethylcholine, as well as seven minerals, all the essential amino acids, fatty acids, enzymes, 10-hydroxy-delta-2-decenoic acid (which may protect against cancer), and hormones believed to enhance the female reproductive system.

Royal jelly is used at The Gefion Cancer Clinic in Denmark, one of several treatment centers in that country which utilize both conventional and alternative practitioners and treatments. An article in the *Townsend Letter for Doctors and Patients* (July 1997) described methods of treatment used for fourteen cancer patients at The Gefion Clinic over a two-year period. Thirteen of the patients had previously received conventional cancer treatment. After the two-year program at The Gefion Clinic, eight of the fourteen cancer patients tested negative for cancer. This project was supported by the Danish Health Insurance Fund, which published its results in Denmark. Royal jelly was among the preferred treatments for these fourteen patients.

Additional Nutrients That Have Been Found to Be Protective

Selenium disrupts the initiation of cancer, protects DNA mutation from chemicals, and nourishes the immune system and enzymes. A study conducted by Harold Ladas, Ph.D. (published in *Holistic Medicine* in 1989), concluded that the more selenium in the blood, the lower the rate of breast cancer. This anticancer mineral is much more abundant in organic foods. Foods high in selenium are garlic, onions, greens, whole grains, mushrooms, and brazil nuts. Garlic and onions grown in soil with high levels of selenium "contain bioactive selenium compounds, which may have higher cancer preventive influence." than vegetables grown in low-selenium soil, according to Jeffrey S. Bland, M.D. Brazil nuts with shells have approximately ten times more selenium per nut than nuts that have been shelled.

Early research on selenium was convincing. Dr. Raymond Schamberger published the first information about selenium's important role as an anticancer nutrient in 1965. In the 1970s, he noted that cancer rates are actually higher in areas of the country where soil levels of selenium are lower. Studies from China verify that selenium levels in soil are linked to cancer incidence.

Selenium helps to protect the body against cancer in several ways. It:

• Causes cancer cells to die before they grow and spread, by encouraging "apoptosis" or programmed cell death.

• Helps to repair damaged DNA molecules. If enough selenium is present, damaged DNA is actually repaired. Selenium thereby protects against free radical damage.

• Helps to encourage the body's production of glutathione, a powerful antioxidant that the body needs for its detoxification processes.

In fact, women with the most selenium in their blood are five times less likely to develop ovarian cancer than women with the lowest levels of selenium.

TIP: Selenium aids in production of glutathione, nature's powerful protector.

Folic acid deficiency makes cells more susceptible to cancer-causing agents, and studies at the University of Alabama have shown the importance of folic acid in preventing cancer. When the blood level of folic acid is low, cancer cells seem to be more active. When the level is high, there is protection against cancer cell activity. Chromosomes break apart when there is a deficiency of folic acid, increasing the risk of cancer. Folic acid can also help to eliminate dysplasia (groups of precancerous cells). Foods rich in folic acid include leafy greens, whole grains, bulgur wheat, citrus fruits, broccoli, Brussels sprouts, asparagus, dried beans, peas, mung bean sprouts, and orange juice. As Marian Burros noted in the *New York Times* in September 1997, "Fortification and supplementation would be unncessary if Americans ate adequate amounts of foods in which folate occurs naturally."

A March 1996 article in the *National Council Against Health Fraud's Newsletter* recommended wariness about "synthetic folate, or folic acid used to fortify foods and vitamin supplements" and encouraged consumption of "food derived" folate.

TIP: Megadosing on high-potency, isolated nutrients may decrease the vitamin's effectiveness and throw other nutrients out of balance. A nutrient-dense, whole foods diet is the best source of vitamins such as folic acid. However, supplementing with a lower-potency, food-based multivitamin is an option worth considering (see Resource Guide). According to current nutritional research, folic acid deficiency is associated with heart disease. Supplementing with folic acid while undergoing cancer treatment with methotrexate is not advisable; folic acid interferes with the effectiveness of the drug.

Glutathione, a powerful breast ally, is a protective enzyme that has been found to offer specific protection against cancer. Although glutathione was first identified in 1888, it wasn't until a century later that scientists began to realize the importance of its links to cancer, the immune and endocrine systems, as well as to heart disease, joint problems and other chronic illnesses. More recent research has revealed glutathione to be an important natural antioxidant, and many experts in the field suspect that it is of vital importance in helping to prevent breast cancer. The abbreviation used for glutathione that you might see in the health food store is GSH. For in-depth information on glutathione, see Dr. Alan H. Pressman's *The GSH Phenomenon: Nature's Most Powerful Antioxidant and Healing Agent, Glutathione.*

Glutathione has many actions. It protects against free radicals, helps to remove metabolic waste and toxins from our bodies, and helps to strengthen cell membranes. Glutathione is also helpful in transporting valuable amino acids to cells throughout the body.

Because the liver plays such a strong role in the prevention and healing of cancer (and other diseases), it's important to know that glutathione helps to detoxify the liver, and helps to remove environmental toxins and waste. In the *Townsend Letter for Doctors and Patients*, Anna MacIntosh Ph.D., N.D., points out that glutathione detoxifies pesticides and herbicides, and acts as an enzyme-catalyzed antioxidant.

Cysteine-rich foods, important for making glutathione, are beans and whole grains. If you are healing breast cancer, consider supplemental cysteine in the form of N-acetyl-L-cysteine capsules (NAC is the abbreviation for this supplement). Let your nutritionist, physician, and oncologist know about the current studies on glutathione (refer to the References for this chapter).

Glutathione-rich foods are raw spinach, parsley, asparagus, avocados, cauliflower, broccoli, tomatoes, squash, potatoes, walnuts, pears, watermelon, and apples. Cruciferous vegetables stimulate glutathione production. Shallots, chives, garlic, onions, leeks, and all members of the allyl sulfide family, help increase the utilization of glutathione. These foods are best to consume raw, since they are damaged by heat. In Chile, scientists found that silymarin, a flavonoid found in milk thistle seeds, increases the glutathione content of the liver. (*See* the Resource Guide to order milk thistle seeds.)

TIP: Other foods that contain antioxidant-rich nutrients that aid in the metabolism of glutathione are: avocados and purslane, rich in vitamin E; carotene-rich foods such as sweet potatoes, dark leafy greens, and carrots; tomatoes and watermelon, rich in lycopene; and kale, turnip greens, and spinach.

For proper synthesis of glutathione (to encourage the excretion of carcinogens and to halt the reproduction of tumor cells), be sure you are eating plenty of calcium-rich foods.

Calcium has been found in laboratory studies to offer specific protection against breast cancer. Foods rich in calcium are sesame seeds, yogurt, sea vegetables, dark leafy greens, mint, nettles, dandelion, and red clover. Most people associate calcium consumption with dairy. It is true that dairy contains calcium, but there are many other food sources of calcium as well. For example, because Norwegian brisling sardines have soft, edible bones, one can (3.5 ounces) provides 382 milligrams of calcium, while a glass of milk only provides 297 milligrams.

Calcium Content of Selected Foods
(mg per 3.5 ounces)

Almonds	234	Kukicha tea	720
Sesame seeds	1,160	Bancha tea	440
Broccoli	103	Salmon	213
Kale	179	Collard greens	156
Mustard greens	183	Skim milk	123
Parsley	203	Low-fat yogurt	183

And for some adventuresome eaters, check out sea vegetables:

Nori	260	Dulse	567
Wakame	1,300	Arame	1,170
Hijiki	1,400	Agar agar	400

Co-enzyme Q10: Although CoQ10 is produced by the body in small amounts, levels decrease with age. This so-called nonessential nutrient is a powerful antioxidant that has been found to be beneficial for women with breast cancer. CoQ10 also contributes to breast health by enhancing the immune system and strengthening cellular structure. Because it promotes the conversion of starches and sugar into cellular fuel, it also provides energy for the body. CoQ10 is tied to many systems in the body. It helps our immune systems and is profoundly heart protective, which is especially important for women to know. Women with breast cancer are known to have low levels of CoQ10. Although there are foods that contain CoQ10, nutritionist Robert Crayhon, author of *Nutrition Made Simple*, suggests taking between 30-100 milligrams a day of CoQ10 before breakfast. The *Townsend Letter for Doctors and Patients* reported in its August-September 1997 issue that a dose of 390 milligrams of CoQ10 may be considered in the treatment of some cases of breast cancer. Foods rich in CoQ10 are spinach and peanuts.

Magnesium helps to build strong bones, relieves headaches, and helps to reduce sugar cravings. Magnesium deficiency can contribute to liver damage, insomnia, leg cramps, and even hair loss. Mildred Seelig, M.D. (adjunct professor of nutrition at Emory University and the University of North Carolina, Chapel Hill), has documented the importance of magnesium for reducing risks of both heart disease and osteoporosis. Magnesium is of vital importance to supplying the organic substance that protects bones from becoming brittle with age. Plant foods rich in magnesium include whole grains, nuts, curry powder, seaweed, potato skins, leafy greens, burdock, parsley, red clover tea, avocado, black beans, kidney beans, peas, bananas, apricots, tofu, and soybeans. All unprocessed foods contain magnesium.

Pyridoxine B6 is essential for rebuilding cells and body tissue. It is also important for carbohydrate-fat-protein metabolism and red blood cell formation. Earl Mindel points out in *Soy Miracle* that even a mild B6 deficiency can hamper the normal functioning of the immune system. Plant foods rich in B6 include: dried beans and lentils, whole grains, peas, parsley, broccoli, avocado, cabbage, filberts, sunflower seeds, carrots, salmon, tuna, shrimp, and cantaloupe. Alcohol, tobacco, and coffee deplete vitamin B6.

Vitamin D works together with calcium and phosphorus to strengthen skeletal mass. Research shows that ultraviolet rays from the sun work together with skin oils to produce vitamin D. Cancer specialist Dr. Joanna Budwig utilized sunlight (approximately twenty minutes a day) as part of the treatment program in her Natural Cancer Clinic in Europe. A study from the Northern California Cancer Center in Union City reported that those women who had the most sun exposure had a 30–40 percent reduced risk of breast cancer. Try to get at least ten minutes of sunshine daily and to consume foods containing vitamin D. (For more information on sunlight, *see* Personal Care Guide.)

Vitamin K: Since strengthening bones to prevent osteoporosis is a concern for all women, especially those undergoing conventional treatment for breast cancer, it's important to recognize vitamin K's contributions to our health. In addition to protecting bones, vitamin K helps protect liver function. To aid in calcium absorption, be sure to include foods containing vitamin K, which include green tea, kelp, dark leafy greens, broccoli, cooked spinach, cauliflower, nettles, soybeans, and polyunsaturated oils.

Zinc helps to make more white blood cells. A low level of zinc has been linked to a significantly higher rate of cancer. Protect your liver from free radical damage and strengthen your immune system by including more foods rich in zinc. Foods containing zinc include nuts, and pumpkin and sunflower seeds.

It is essential to consume a wide variety of vegetables and fruits for the many breast-protective nutrients they contain. However, many of these nutrient substances originating in plant foods can also be found in certain meats, seafoods, and in eggs. For example:

• *Vitamin A* can be found in the oils from salmon, halibut, sardines, mackerel, eel, rainbow trout, and cod. It is also found in egg yolks and beef liver.

- *Vitamin E* can be found in shrimp and other seafoods.
- Dietary sources of *alpha-* and *beta-carotene* include fish oils and eggs.
  - Egg yolks are also rich in *lecithin* and *lutein*.
- *Cysteine* can be found in lean red meats, poultry, and eggs.
- Lean red meat also contains *lipoic acid*, a powerful antioxidant that aids in excreting harmful substances such as lead and cadmium from the body. Lipoic acid also helps to synthesize glutathione.
- *Conjugated linoleic acid (CLA)* is especially rich in lamb. In animal studies, CLA has been shown to lower the risk of both cancer and heart disease.
- Foods rich in *CoQ10* include sardines, mackerel, tuna, and organ meats.
- *Magnesium* can be found in fish and shellfish.
- Foods rich in *vitamin B6* include chicken, fish, and seafood.
- Vitamin D can be found in brisling sardines, salmon, herring, liver, eel, end egg yolk.
- Cold-water, fatty-rich fish also contain *vitamin K*.
- *Zinc* can be found in oysters, other seafood, dark poultry, eggs, lean red meats, and liver.

Prevention: Variety Is Key

Phytochemicals

One reason scientists are so excited about phytochemicals is their apparent ability to stop a cell's conversion from healthy to cancerous at so many different stages.

—American Institute for Cancer Research

Even though the National Institutes of Health and the National Cancer Institute recommend eating at least five different types of vegetables and fruits a day, the reality is that only 9 percent of the population follows that advice. In fact, nearly half of all Amencans recently polled said that they had only one vegetable a day, and that vegetable was French fried potatoes! Herbalist Susun Weed points out in *Breast Cancer? Breast Health! The Wise Woman Way* that fruits, vegetables, beans, and whole grains contain substances that protect against the development of cancer in numerous ways. The phytochemicals in these foods protect the DNA in cells, strengthen the immune system, stop carcinogenic substances and free radicals from causing damage, and encourage the production of anti-cancer enzymes.

The breast cancer rate for American women is eight times higher than that of Korean women, and twenty-two times higher that of Thai women. Japanese women also have a much lower rate of breast cancer than American women. The Tokyo School of Medicine recommends consuming at least thirty different fruits and vegetables each day! The school studied a group of Japanese farmers over an eighteen-year period and found that health improved dramatically when they increased the variety of fruits and vegetables they ate each day from eleven to twenty-three.

Diane Mills, at the Institute for Optimum Nutrition, agrees with the Japanese approach. "You need all the compounds that a variety of foods can offer so that the body can work efficiently," she says.

Phytochemicals, the nonnutrient substances responsible for giving fruits, vegetables, nuts, and grains their smell, color, and taste, also provide an incredible arsenal of weapons for cancer protection. Over 900 phytochemicals have been identified to date. Consuming a variety of foods—the greater variety, the better—is the common-sense approach to obtaining maximum benefits from these incredible substances.

In her *Health Wisdom for Women* newsletter, Dr. Christiane Northrup has explained how phytochemicals work. The chronic inflammation and tissue irritation that result from free radical damage—caused by pollution, tobacco smoke, excess sun, excess alcohol, trans-fatty acids, and stress—are believed to release nitrous oxide into cells. Nitrous oxide, in turn, damages the cell's DNA. Some phytochemicals have been shown to inhibit the chronic inflammation that begins this cycle and, as a result, help to prevent cancer.

TIP: Fruits and vegetables that are allowed to ripen on the vine contain more beneficial phytochemicals than produce that is harvested unripened. Remember how much easier it used to be to find vine-ripened tomatoes? It is just not cost-effective for commercial growers to allow tomatoes to reach their natural maturity on the vine and turn a natural red. Lycopene, the powerful antioxidant in tomatoes, isn't formed until the tomatoes ripen—just one more reason to purchase organic produce.

Some important phytochemicals with "chemoprotective qualities" include:

Protease inhibitors: Found in potatoes, rice, and soybeans, protease inhibitors may be capable of neutralizing the effects of a wide range of cancer-causing agents such as radiation and noxious fumes like diesel exhaust. Ann Kennedy, Ph.D., from Harvard University, found that the effects from protease inhibitors can last up to 45–135 days, and can "reprogram" precancerous cells back to their normal state.

> TIP: Organic potatoes are incredibly sweet and delicious. For those evenings when you are too tired to prepare anything complicated, simply bake a potato and top with poached eggs. Drizzle flaxseed oil on top, and season with delicious natural Herbamare, available in the spice section of most health food stores. Lightly steamed spinach or a simple salad completes the meal.

Indoles: Found in cruciferous vegetables such as broccoli, Brussels sprouts, and cabbage, indoles help to prevent breast cancer. Chris Beecher, Ph.D., professor of medicinal chemistry at the University of Illinois in Chicago, and Jon Michnovicz, M.D., Ph.D., author of *How to Reduce Your Risk of Breast Cancer,* are among several researchers who have confirmed this finding. Women who are athletic and eat many cruciferous vegetables have more protective estrogen in their blood, a condition that helps guard against reproductive cancers. (To read about protective estrogen, refer to Chapter 11, "Food, Hormones, and Breast Cancer: What's the Connection?")

The *Journal of the National Cancer Institute* reported that indole-rich foods (containing indole 3 carbinol, or I-3-C) doubled the amount of protective estrogen produced. The protective effects continued over an extended period of time.

Other protective substances in cruciferous vegetables are *isothiocyanates* and *sulforaphane.* Sulforaphane, a naturally produced isothiocyanate, helps the body to produce more detoxification enzymes to neutralize the effects of exposure to carcinogenic chemicals such as like pesticides and exhaust fumes. Sulforaphane also helps glutathione to eliminate harmful substances from the body.

As Dr. Michnovicz points out in *How to Reduce Your Risk of Breast Cancer,* cruciferous vegetables contain hundreds of protective phytochemicals in addition to I-3-C and sulforaphane.

> TIP: Sulforaphane increases the body's detoxification enzymes. When we eat cruciferous vegetables, sulforaphane is released into the stomach. Broccoli sprouts, three-day-old broccoli plants that "look like alfalfa or bean sprouts," have been found to be up to fifty times richer in isothiocyanates, according to a report by Natalie Angier in the *New York Times* (September 16, 1997). Extracts made from the sprouts were found to greatly reduce the frequency, size, and number of mammary tumors in rats.

The following cruciferous foods offer many benefits. Consume them often, and avoid overcooking. Steam, blanch, or water sauté lightly to protect heat-sensitive phytochemicals.

Bok choy	Collard greens
Broccoli	Horseradish
Broccoli rabe	Mustard seed
Brussels sprouts	Radishes
Cabbage	Swede
Cauliflower	Rutabaga
Turnips	Savoy cabbage

TIP: Brussels sprouts and savoy cabbage contain the most indoles.

Bioflavonoids (or "flavonoids") are a very large group of phytochemicals (more than 800) found in every plant we consume. Dr. Michnovicz states that eating a few servings of fruits and vegetables a day delivers 1,000 to 2,000 milligrams of these compounds. Research has shown that bioflavonoids:

• Inhibit enzymes that produce cancer.
• Increase production of protective enzymes.
• Protect the liver.
• Detoxify harmful estrogen (*see* Chapter 11, "Food, Hormones, and Breast Cancer: What's the Connection?").
• Increase immunity.

Some common sources of anticancer flavonoids are green tea, soybeans, cereal grains, cruciferous vegetables, celery, parsnips, carrots, winter squash, parsley, tomatoes, artichokes, eggplant, peppers, flaxseeds, turmeric, citrus fruits, red grapes, strawberries, blueberries, and herbs such as rosemary.

TIP: To utilize organic lemon or orange peels, try grating a small amount into a rice salad. Combine long-grain brown rice with chopped parsley, chives, peanuts, lemon juice, and extra virgin olive oil, with a touch of lemon peel.

Limonene or D-limonene is found in organic lemon and orange peels. According to *Science News* (May 1993), this phytochemical has been found to be especially effective in preventing breast cancer. Michael Gould and his team from the University of Wisconsin Clinical Cancer Center have found limonene interferes with cancer cells' utilization of protein in cellular growth. When rats with mammary tumors were fed limonene, more than 80 percent of the cancers disappeared. Limonene is also found in mint, dill, caraway, and celery seed.

Tangeretin and *nobiletin*, two chemicals in tangerines which migrate to different types of breast cells, are up to 250 times more powerful than genestein (from soybeans) at squelching breast cancer, according to research findings reported at the 208th Meeting of the American Chemical Society in Washington, D.C. (1994). It was also found that these phytochemicals actually increased the effectiveness of the breast cancer treatment tamoxifan. Tangeretin is also being tested in University Hospital, Gent, Belgium, on mice with liver cancer. Oranges contain the flavonoid *hesperitin* and grapefruit contains *naringenin* (another flavonoid) that have also been found to help stop the spread of breast cancer. These phytochemicals help prevent tumors and aid the body in eliminating carcinogens. *Terpenes,* another phytochemical in citrus fruits, blocks the growth of mammary cancer cells in animal studies.

> Tangeretin and nobiletin, found in tangerines, inhibit the growth of breast cancer cells, according to a recent study from the Center for Human Nutrition at the University of Western Ontario, Canada.

Nomilin has been shown to prevent stomach cancers. Nomilin is a fruit chemical that can cause bitterness in fruit juices. An important benefit of this compound is that it increases the activity of the detoxifying enzyme glutathione by as much as threefold.

Quercetin, one of the most protective flavonoids, inactivates a cancer-causing mold. Quercetin is found in cruciferous vegetables, onions, shallots, yellow squash, apple skins (make sure they are organic), and berries, and offers powerful protection against tumor growth by protecting DNA from damage. Quercetin has potent antiinflammatory properties and is an anti-oxidant.

Resveratrol is found in grapes, especially concentrated in grape skins, and contains antimutagen and antioxidant properties. It inhibits carcinogens and encourages detoxification. The chemoprotective activity of resveratol was described in *Science* magazine in January 1997.

Saponins help to protect us from cancer by protecting genetic material in our cells and preventing cancer cells from multiplying. Saponins are found in beans, soybeans, garlic, and onions. A diet rich in saponins also offers cancer prevention by protecting against excessive amounts of damaging saturated fats in our diet.

Ellagic acid is available in grapes, raspberries, strawberries, and pomegranates; it protects us from potential carcinogens in substances like air pollution and cigarette smoke by blocking cancer-causing agents. Gary D. Stoner, Ph.D., at the Medical College of Ohio, Toledo, has found that ellagic acid works best when added to the system before exposure to cancerous chemicals. Ellagic acids strengthen connective tissue, which may keep cancer from metastasizing.

Perillyl alcohol, which belongs to a class of phytochemicals called terpenes and is found in lavender and cherries, helps tumor cells to switch to a less malignant type.

Foods high in naturally occurring *laetrile* are almonds, lima beans, garbanzo beans, and millet.

Polyphenols are antioxidant-rich phytochemicals found in all plants that act in both the initiation and promotional stages of cancer development. Plant polyphenols, which protect against cellular damage, are currently of great interest to the scientific community. Polyphenols are found in all fresh fruits and vegetables, but particularly rich sources include green tea, soybeans, garlic, ginger, and flaxseeds.

Allyl sulfides, found in onions, shallots, garlic, scallions, and leeks, inhibit the action of cancer-causing substances and slow tumor growth. In Vidalia, Georgia, where the world-famous onions are grown, stomach cancer rates are said to be two-thirds the national rate, and one-half of the rate found in the rest of Georgia. Researchers at Pennsylvania State University reported in late 1997 that potent carcinogens that form in the breasts, nitrosamines, can be blocked by onions and garlic. Research is also revealing that the strongest-flavored onions contain the most protective sulfur compounds.

> TIP: Consuming garlic and onions offers many healing benefits. The cancer-protective effects of garlic have been found to intensify when eaten with red, green, and chili peppers. *Capsicum* has been found to help the body detoxify carcinogens. One of my favorite breakfasts (or lunches) is my own version of *huevos rancheros.* Water-sauté onion, garlic, and red pepper (I like the small hot ones) for 3–5 minutes. Add several pinches of sea salt, and serve with poached or soft-boiled eggs. Drizzle with a little flaxseed or olive oil, and enjoy.

Isothiocyanates offer special protection for DNA in breast tissue. Eat plenty of the following foods, rich in isothiocyanates, to increase beneficial enzymes: radishes, daikon radish, kale, horseradish, Brussels sprouts, cabbage, and broccoli. Broccoli sprouts contain concentrated amounts of isothiocyanates.

Phytochemicals help to detoxify cancer promoters, boost immune response, reduce the risk of cancer from excessive hormone levels, and act as powerful antioxidants.

One hundred of the world's leading cancer experts evaluated over 4,500 international studies and reported that eating the right foods, exercising, and maintaining a healthy weight could help women reduce breast cancer risk by as much as 50 percent. This report, issued in December 1997 by the World Cancer Research Fund and the American Institute for Cancer Research, recommended we eat ten servings of a variety of vegetables and fruits each day.

CHAPTER 10

Herbs, Spices, and Mushrooms: Potent Enhancers of Flavor and Health

I've always had an avid interest in herbs, spices, and mushrooms. Isn't paprika deliciously aromatic, and how delectable garlic smells when roasted! And mushrooms, in their infinite variety, are infinitely flexible in how they can be utilized. As a child, I loved to watch my mother make soup. Barley mushroom soup was my favorite, made with just a touch of beef and lots of herbs. Another favorite dish, which inspired many similar grain pilafs in this book, is my mother's rice and mushrooms.

When I became interested in whole foods cooking as an adult, my fascination with herbs, spices, and mushrooms grew when I discovered scientific studies showing their multitude of health benefits. Herbs have been used for thousands of years in traditional medicine—garlic is even mentioned in the Old Testament.

Scientists writing in the *Journal of the National Cancer Institute* in 1995 described the protective effects of rosemary, parsley, and basil. The antioxidants present in these herbs protect against free radicals, particularly when combined with unheated olive oil, the *Journal of the National Cancer Institute* report showed, and they are protective against colon cancer. Rosemary, parsley, and basil, which are used frequently in Mediterranean cooking, have also been found to help prevent lung cancer. Researchers at Rutgers and the University of Illinois found rosemary to be particularly effective at helping prevent mammary cancer in mice. Women living in the Mediterranean countries have a lower incidence of and mortality from breast cancer than women living in Northern America or Europe, and fresh herbs are part of Mediterranean women's daily diet. In laboratory experiments at Rutgers University, many different types of herbs and spices were found to have antioxidant properties, neutralize free radicals, and suppress cancer growth. Garlic, for instance, increases antioxidant levels by helping to increase vitally important glutathione, according to the *Nutrition Reporter* (1997).

Mushrooms contain polysaccharides, which stimulate the body's immune system. Maitake mushrooms are thought to thwart tumor growth and even "prevent the initiation of new cancers," as *Better Nutrition* reported in March 1997. Women from Asia consume mushrooms frequently, and they have lower rates of breast cancer than women living in North America and Europe.

Herbs, spices, and mushrooms have been found to be helpful in strengthening the immune system and lowering the risk of breast and other cancers. It is time to become more familiar with these wonderful foods.

Herbs and Spices: Season Your Food for Health

Garlic is a profoundly protective food. Did you know that just half a clove of raw garlic a day increases natural killer cells and that the National Cancer Institute acknowledges its effectiveness in the prevention of cancer? Russian doctors prescribe it to treat cancer, and research has shown it to cure mammary cancer in mice. Compounds in garlic can modify certain biomarkers related to breast, prostate, and many other cancers, *Better Nutrition* editor James Gormley reports.

According to Earl Mindell, M.D., author of *Garlic: The Miracle Nutrient*, solid research indicates that garlic has "antitumor activity." Dr. Mindell reports that raw garlic, garlic powder, and cooked garlic all yield benefits. It is believed that grinding garlic and consuming it shortly thereafter offers particular health benefits. If you wait too long to eat garlic after it is crushed, important enzymes are lost, so I like to prepare vinaigrettes right before eating, using fresh garlic. It has been reported that garlic may prevent damage to the liver, an important organ in hormone-related cancers. Garlic is also rich in selenium, which is important for the production of white blood cells and protects against the effects of radiation.

Garlic is antibiotic, antiviral, and antifungal; it helps protect against colds, flu, and yeast infections.

Rosemary has antioxidant, antitumor properties. Researchers at both Rutgers and the University of Illinois found that rosemary has preventive effects against mammary cancer in mice. I like to keep a pot of rosemary right on my kitchen windowsill all year long. Use rosemary in vinaigrettes on salads, like blanched green beans on a bed of mixed lettuce, as well as in stews. I particularly love roasted chicken with rosemary (*see* Roasted Chicken in Parchment, page 322). Lamb also goes very well with this aromatic and breast-healthy herb. Use rosemary in cannellini bean soup for a taste sensation, or with fava beans and onion. Most frequently, I use rosemary with garlic, lemon, and extra virgin olive oil for vinaigrettes drizzled over steamed vegetables and salads. This profoundly protective herb is a member of the mint family.

Basil contains enzymes called "monoterpenes," potent anticancer sub-stances. Use basil leaves broken into a bibb lettuce salad for a refreshing change. Basil, tomatoes, and onions are often used together in Southern Italy and France, dressed with delicious, fresh, extra virgin olive oil and lemon. Use basil with salmon or squid in salads. Basil is a member of the mint family.

TIP: *Gremolata,* a favorite in Milan, is a combination of three healthy, breast-protective foods. Make a fresh combination of three pro-foundly protective foods: finely chopped garlic, parsley, and organic lemon zest. Use gremolata to garnish soups, chicken, or lamb. A similar garnish, popular in the Middle East, is grated garlic and raw potato, which is truly delicious.

Mint contains potent cancer-blocking agents. Mint, a member of the laven-der family, contains breast-protective limonene. Although limonene is usually associated with lemon and orange peels, this powerfully protective, breast-friendly phytochemical is also found in mint. Mint also is a rich source of calcium. I developed such a strong enjoyment of mint while traveling in the Middle East, I will forever crave it, and use it to garnish many aromatic dishes, such as stuffed cabbage rolls, and in freshly prepared vinaigrettes with lots of lemon.

Be creative with this healthy and delicious herb. Explore mint in vinai-grettes over salads; tossed through bulgur, with plenty of chopped parsley, lemon, olive oil, and garlic (for tabbouleh salad); add chopped mint to boiled new potatoes with olive oil, garlic, and lemon; flavor chilled kukicha tea with mint in the summer.

Dill also contains limonene, the breast-protective phytochemical. I love fresh dill, especially combined with the unexpected flavors of mellow or sweet white miso, garlic, and lemon, as a sauce over fish. A touch of fresh dill adds flavor and sophistication to your favorite fish recipe.

Parsley is a rich source of immune-strengthening magnesium. Use parsley in every way you can. This woodsy, grassy, simple herb contains "phytosterols which specifically hinder recurrence of breast cancer," says herbalist Susun Weed in *Breast Cancer? Breast Health! The Wise Woman Way.*

Parsley also contains cancer-protective glutathione in abundance. We've learned a great deal in recent years about glutathione being protective to the body against toxins, as well as its being a powerful nutrient. *New York Times* food columnist Molly O'Neill describes parsley as having healing benefits associated with it throughout the ages. Medical folklore, O'Neill points out, has touted parsley as an effective cure for rheumatism, swelling, and lethargy. When I was in the Jordan, I learned that people used parsley, particularly the stems, for dissolving kidney stones.

Parsley has grown all over the world for thousands of years. I love the refreshing flavor it imparts. Parsley can improve almost any recipe. After visiting Jordan, I began to appreciate parsley as a defining flavor instead of simply a background herb.

Mediterranean Potato Salad

(SERVES 3–4)

1 lb boiled new potatoes
2 cloves minced garlic
2 tbsp sea salt
½ cup lemon juice
3 tbsp extra virgin olive oil
¼ cup finely chopped purple onion
¾ cup minced flat leaf parsley

Cut boiled potatoes into small pieces. In a big bowl, pound garlic and salt together with a wooden pestle. Add lemon juice and oil. Mix in potatoes, onions, and parsley.

> TIP: Parsley can be utilized in many ways. Consider the following suggestions: parsley, garlic, and olive oil with linguine; parsley combined with basil, olive oil, and pine nuts for pesto sauce; parsley, purple cabbage, and green onion in a pressed salad; parsley blended with cucumber, lemon, dill, and olive oil for coleslaw.

Sage is a member of the mint family and contains breast-protective antioxidants. I like to use this aromatic herb as a garnish on roasted poultry and in stews.

Tarragon is a wonderful herb that is frequently used to flavor vinegars in France. I love to combine tarragon with potato, green bean, or beet salads, and also use it in vinaigrettes.

Cilantro has a chelating effect. It binds to heavy metals and moves them out of the body, holistic practitioner Robert Roundtree, M.D., told *Nutrition*

Science News. Cilantro has a captivating, aromatic flavor that complements such diverse dishes as guacamole and chicken salad, and is wonderful in vinaigrettes for salads with plenty of summer-fresh tomatoes. Make a puree from cilantro, garlic, and olive oil, and drizzle into Spanish-style soups.

Thyme is another of my favorite herbs. It combines well with rosemary, and is frequently used in the French Mediterranean. Gently roast onions on parchment lightly rubbed with extra virgin olive oil, seasoned with thyme and balsamic vinegar. Combine thyme with cabbage, a dash of vinegar, and a few pinches of sea salt.

Marjoram, also used frequently in the French Mediterranean, blends well with assorted, delicate lettuce leaves and tomatoes for a flavorful salad. I love to use lots of marjoram and garlic with a touch of rosemary to flavor lamb.

Oregano, another member of the mint family, contains many protective anticancer polyphenols, phytosterols, and flavonoids. I like to use fresh oregano when preparing seafood. I briefly steam delicate, fresh scallops and then dress them with a light vinaigrette of shallots, garlic, lemon, oregano, and olive oil. I serve the scallops and vinaigrette over mesclun greens surrounded by asparagus and tomato wedges. Try oregano in a vinaigrette with the juice from a blood orange, extra virgin olive oil, chopped black olives, and a little vinegar over endive, blood orange, and thinly sliced Spanish onion salad.

All herbs have antioxidant benefits, and contain many protective, anticancer phytochemicals. I like to rotate my use of fresh herbs, and encourage you to do the same. This assures that you receive the variety of nutrients and plant chemicals that are offered by all herbs. The following quick vinaigrette is delicious over steamed vegetables or tossed salads. Substitute any fresh herb for mint.

Mint Vinaigrette

2 tbsp chopped fresh mint
½ cup extra virgin olive oil
1 tsp natural mustard
¼ cup minced shallots
¼ tsp sea salt
juice from 1 fresh lemon

Combine ingredients in a suribachi or small food processor. Adjust seasonings, and serve, drizzled over salad for vegetables with some freshly ground black pepper.

TIP: A variety of fresh seasoning herbs contains many breast-protective, antioxidant phytochemicals. Utilize fresh herbs daily; combine them with extra virgin olive oil in delicious vinaigrettes for added breast cancer prevention.

The following spices have been shown to help prevent cancer:

Turmeric has a long history of use in the treatment of cancer and is a much stronger antioxidant than vitamin C. *Curcumin*, the active principle in turmeric (and cumin), is a potential antimutagenic agent; its activity against cancer is being studied. Curcumin can help in preventing cancer in a couple of ways. It can help the liver to detoxify carcinogens and also helps to protect against environmental carcinogens. Liver-protective turmeric is helpful for women on tamoxifan or undergoing chemotherapy. Turmeric has been prized for thousands of years as a powerful medicine. Use turmeric mixed with other spices such as roasted and ground mustard and cardamom seeds for curry, or as a seasoning in fish dishes, grains, or tofu. Turmeric is also delicious in chicken salad made with grapes, celery, and yogurt.

TIP: The flavor and aroma of freshly ground spices are irresistible, probably because natural compounds and phytochemicals within the spices are released when freshly ground. You can grind your own fresh spices by purchasing a small spice/seed/nut grinder. *(See the Resource Guide.)*

Celery seed contains strong, breast-protective limonene. I have become accustomed to using a light sprinkle of celery seed in tuna salad with yogurt instead of hydrogenated mayo, or "healthy" canola mayonnaise. Combine minced vegetables, like onions and celery, with tuna, yogurt, lemon, and sea salt; serve with tomatoes and lettuce. This creates a wonderfully different, tasty salad rich in breast-protective ingredients, including celery seeds.

Cumin protects DNA from cancer. Use it in sauces, soups, and stews. To make the Indian yogurt condiment raita, combine yogurt, chopped carrots and cucumber, lemon, and cumin for a salad dressing or a refreshing sauce for chicken.

Paprika is a rich source of antioxidant vitamin C. I love paprika and garlic with roasted potatoes. It is also delicious sprinkled liberally on chicken with garlic before roasting. Paprika adds a wonderful dimension to vegetarian casseroles. Try it with tempeh and sauerkraut with onions for a Hungarian or Northern French flavor.

Ginger has many protective properties. Paul Schulick strongly recommends using only ginger and ginger products that are certified organic, to assure that the remarkable anticancer properties of ginger are not diminished or destroyed by potential chemical contamination. In *Ginger: Common Spice and Wonder Drug*, Schulick describes research on the many benefits of ginger, including its antimutagenic, antioxidant, and protein-digesting enzymatic abilities. Benefits are available from numerous formulations of ginger, including, "fresh, dried, syrup, capsules, and extract," according to Schulick. I encourage you to use freshly grated ginger (my favorite) over fish and in miso soups, or on fresh vegetables like steamed broccoli, or with winter squash to emphasize the sweetness. Ginger can also be added to banana bread and pumpkin pie.

> TIP: Larger ginger roots have stronger flavor; smaller ginger roots are less pungent.

Galanga root is a member of the ginger family, and has also been found to have similar protective properties. Galanga has a slightly sweet and spicy flavor, and can be purchased in the frozen food section of Asian markets. I use it for Thai cooking.

Lemon grass, used frequently in Thai cuisine, is a strong antioxidant that contains cancer-emulsifying agents. Add it to fish dishes, for instance, to "refresh" the flavors right before serving.

> TIP: Simply peel off the outer leaves of lemon grass and mince the inner core to use this herb in preparing steamed vegetables, vinaigrettes, soups, fish, and other dishes.

Hot peppers contain capsicum, a phytochemical, as well as carotenoids, flavonoids, essential oil, and vitamin C. The strong antioxidant properties make hot peppers a healthy addition to your cuisine. Choose from among a wide variety which includes such peppers as jalapeño and Scotch bonnet. Dried cayenne pepper is best used toward the end of cooking to avoid overheating.

> TIP: Wear rubber gloves to protect your hands from burns while handling Scotch bonnet and other hot varieties of peppers.

Mushrooms for Immunity

The large molecules in some of the food mushrooms and many of the hard, medicinal mushrooms from Japan and China are called polysaccharides. Andrew Weil, M.D., points out in the May-June 1996 issue of *Natural Health* that "polysaccharides found in mushrooms may enhance cellular immunity, increasing defenses against viral infections and cancer."

Along with polysaccharides and other beneficial plant chemicals, mushrooms also contain selenium and antioxidants. Use them regularly, especially in soups, to stimulate immune function.

Maitake: Studies with animals show maitake mushrooms to be the most effective in preventing tumor growth. Maitake supplementation, with extract of maitake, has been found to help women prevent breast cancer by stimulating immune strength. It was reported in *Better Nutrition* (March 1997) that women undergoing chemotherapy benefited from consuming maitake. Positive results were reported in both tumor size and blood tests. (*See* the Resource Guide for sources of maitake mushrooms.) Dried maitake mushrooms are readily available, while fresh ones are still a rarity in this country. For prevention, include just a few grams daily in soups, stews, and other dishes. Don't forget to use the leftover soaking water for stews or soups.

Reishi: This tough little mushroom, best used in slow-simmer soups, has been found in clinical studies to eliminate and shrink tumors; and increase T-cell and alpha-interferon production.

> TIP: For a version of an immune tonic soup (the original version is in Christopher Hobbs's book *Medicinal Mushrooms),* try the following: Fill a medium pot two-thirds full with filtered water. Combine 1 reishi and 1 shiitake mushroom with 5–7 sticks of astragalus (a powerful herb also containing immune-enhancing polysaccharides). Bring to a boil and cook for 20 minutes. Add a combination of your favorite vegetables (collards, savoy cabbage, carrots, onions, leeks). Cook for another 20 minutes. Season with barley miso, approximately 1 tsp per cup of liquid, and serve. Garnish with minced scallions and/ or grated ginger juice, or grated fresh garlic.

Shiitake: In Japan, shiitakes are used in treating breast cancer. The Chinese and Japanese use shiitakes to increase resistance to disease. Shiitakes increase the production of *protective macrophages* (cells that eliminate foreign substances); and they aid in vitamin D production and utilization.

I prepare both dried and fresh shiitakes frequently. Dried shiitakes are best used in soup, stocks, and broths. Use reconstituted shiitakes in unexpected ways, such as in chicken soup, for a delicious surprise. As with maitakes, use the leftover soaking broth.

TIP: To reconstitute dried shiitakes, heat water almost to the point of boiling. Combine with soy sauce (4 parts water, 1 part soy), and soak dried mushrooms for 15 minutes. Use shiitake mushrooms in soups (like miso, minestrone, and chicken), stews, vegetable dishes, and sauces (like tomato sauce).

CHAPTER 11

Food, Hormones, and Breast Cancer: What's the Connection?

It is exciting to realize that food can be a powerful aid in producing a natural balance of the protective hormones that are so important for breast health. Food selection can also be a tremendous aid in helping to prevent PMS, symptoms of menopause, endometriosis, fibrocystic breasts, depression, and other hormone-related problems. Mothers can help their daughters, in terms of building a healthy hormone system, by selecting and preparing healthy foods, and by encouraging exercise. A nutrient-dense diet helps women of all ages to create protective hormones for breast health.

In a 1984 report, the Mayo Clinic offered a theory of how cancer is initiated, and how we can actually influence its promotion, and its progress, by modifying our diets.

The Three-Phase Theory

Initiation. The combination of inherited risk factors, such as a family history of breast cancer, with environmental factors, such as chemicals (like pesticides), creates a situation in which cancer can develop.

Promotion. This phase follows the initiation phase and develops over many years. It is, however, reversible. Harmful forms and excessive amounts of estrogen (in pharmaceuticals, such as birth control pills and hormone replacement therapy [HRT], as well as estrogen in our food supply), along with alcohol and saturated fat, can promote the development of breast cancer.

Studies have shown that diet modification can help prevent breast cancer by reducing estrogen levels in the body. For example, indole-3-carbinol found in cruciferous vegetables, genistein, and other phytochemicals found in soy foods, and lignans in flaxseeds have the ability to protect the body against potentially dangerous forms of estrogen.

Progression. The final phase, before cancer spreads, is influenced by diet and its effect on the immune system and our hormones. *There is much we can do to prevent the progression of tumors with antioxidant rich vegetables, flaxseeds and flaxseed oil, fatty-rich fish, and herbs.*

There are two kinds of risk factors related to breast cancer: controllable and uncontrollable. Uncontrollable factors include a women's menstrual, reproductive, and family history, while controllable risk factors include diet, exercise, emotional well-being, weight control, and exposure to certain chemicals. The majority of women with breast cancer (70-80%) fall into the controllable risk category. For these women, their disease cannot be linked to genetic predisposition or reproductive history. This is exciting information that provides encouragement to do as much as we can do for ourselves: We can improve our diets and try to reduce exposure to chemicals. Exciting, too, is the knowledge that regular exercise plays such a profoundly important role in creating breast health.

Estrogen-Sensitive Breast Cancer

The hormone estrogen stimulates breast cells to grow, divide, and spread. Basically, breast cancer is an exaggerated, uncontrolled proliferation of breast cells. About 50-70 percent of all breast cancers are estrogen-receptor-positive. Cutting off the estrogen supply to tumors stops their growth. In older women, estrogen-receptor-positive (ER positive) breast cancer is more common. As women age, they usually have lower levels of progesterone. Adequate levels of progesterone are needed to balance or inhibit levels of estrogen.

Progesterone—The Protective Hormone

Progesterone plays an important role in all stages of a woman's life. Progesterone regulates and modifies the actions of estrogen.

• Progesterone and estrogen are the two most significant hormones produced by a woman's ovaries. Because of the estrogen in our food supply (in dairy, meat, and eggs) and environmental sources of xenoestrogens from chemicals, a woman's levels of estrogen are often excessive. When the amount of estrogen is higher than that of protective progesterone, problems such as

PMS, endometriosis, and breast cancer can occur. (See chart on estrogen and progesterone.)

• Progesterone is made by corpus luteum right before ovulation, and goes into rapid production directly after ovulation, during the last two weeks of the menstrual cycle.

• Smaller amounts of progesterone are produced by the adrenal cortex in women (and men).

Increasing Progesterone by Food Selection

• Good-quality dietary cholesterol supports healthy hormone production. Hormones are made from cholesterol, so we can influence the quality of our hormones by the quality of the cholesterol we ingest. Flaxseed oil supports healthy hormone production; cholesterol from processed fats, poor-quality oils, and saturated fats does not.

• Free radicals from rancid, bottled salad dressings and other rancid oils and processed foods may play a role in harming the corpus luteum, thereby depleting progesterone production.

• Nourish the adrenal glands with sweet vegetables such as turnips, rutabagas, and carrots. Eliminate sugar and coffee to support adrenal function.

Progesterone's Protective Role During Pregnancy

• If pregnancy occurs, progesterone is essential to the survival of the embryo. It is so necessary to the fetus that progesterone synthesis is taken over by the placenta.

• Progesterone prevents miscarriage during pregnancy, and is responsible for the sense of "well-being" during the second trimester. (Most miscarriages occur during the first trimester of pregnancy, when estrogen is high and progesterone levels are low.)

Progesterone Also Plays a Protective Role in Reducing Symptoms of PMS

Progesterone deficieny contributes to PMS. Unhealthy prostaglandin production is also a factor.

Prostaglandins are the tiny, hormone-like substances that influence every cell in our body. Unfriendly prostaglandins are responsible for menstrual cramps and bloating. To increase production of friendly prostaglandins, include fatty-rich fish such as tuna, Norwegian salmon, rainbow trout, and sardines in your diet. Studies show fish oils from fatty-rich fish help to reduce painful menstrual cramps and bloating. Fresh, organic flaxseed oil also helps to build protective prostaglandins.

ABNORMAL

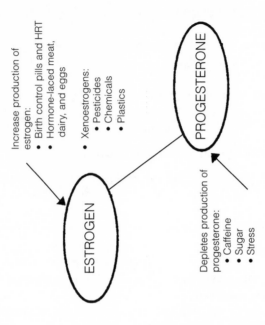

Increase production of estrogen:
- Birth control pills and HRT
- Hormone-laced meat, dairy, and eggs

- Xenoestrogens:
  - Pesticides
  - Chemicals
  - Plastics

ESTROGEN

PROGESTERONE

Depletes production of progesterone:
- Caffeine
- Sugar
- Stress

The following conditions are a result of an excessive level of estrogen and a decrease in progesterone:

Estrogen-receptor-sensitive breast cancer, uterine and endometrial cancers, endometriosis, fibroid tumors, increased copper retention, stroke and embolism, breast cysts, breast pain, PMS, irregular periods, menstrual flooding, and thyroid problems (low thyroid).

NORMAL

A balance of estrogen and progesterone helps to prevent breast cancer and other health problems

ESTROGEN _____ PROGESTERONE

Increases production of progesterone:
Proper EFA consumption to nourish adrenal glands; flaxseed oil and fatty-rich fish.

Sugar increases symptoms of PMS. Sugar interferes with adrenal gland function. Because adrenal gland disturbances have been found in studies to contribute to PMS, eliminating sugar is an important option.

Perimenopause

Excessive levels of estrogen (and low levels of progesterone) contribute to the perimenopausal problems many women experience, such as irregular periods and menstrual flooding. Perimenopause is the five years before menopause.

Progesterone Offers Protection During Perimenopause

• Helps to eliminate menstrual "flooding" due to fluctuating estrogen levels.

• Chronic progesterone deficiency interferes with the body's ability to shed the uterine lining uniformly each month, which can cause endometrial hyperplasia. This is an abnormal thickening of the uterine lining, and it can lead to uterine cancer.

Progesterone Offers Protection During Menopause

• Increases libido.

• Rebuilds bone mass. Progesterone tied to "osteoblastic" function actually rebuilds bone mass, instead of temporarily halting the disintegration of bone, as does supplemental estrogen. New information on estrogen receptor beta also correlates this recently identified form of estrogen with osteoblastic function.

TIP: Udo Erasmus pioneered a blended oil (see the Resource Guide) that contains rice bran oil, which relieves menopausal symptoms. Rice bran oil contains gamma-oryzanol. Studies show that gamma-oryzanol supports pituitary function, which encourages endorphin release by the hypothalamus. An added bonus of gamma-oryzanol is that it is helpful in keeping cholesterol and triglyceride levels low.

Ask Your Doctor About Natural Progesterone Cream

Natural progesterone products are available. Progesterone converted from yams and soybeans is similar to the hormone made by the female body, and is manufactured into a cream. Progesterone cream can used as an adjunct to diet and exercise in treating symptoms of menopause and PMS, and in preventing osteoporosis. This cream is an option for women who do not have breast cancer. For more information on natural progesterone compared to progestins, refer to *Natural Progesterone. The Multiple Roles of a Remarkable Hormone* by John Lee, M.D.

Progesterone and Breast Cancer

Breast cancer research has shown progesterone deficiency to be the most consistent finding.

At least nine different studies have reported that women with breast cancer excrete lower levels of progesterone in their urine. In perimenopausal women, high estrogen levels are coupled with progesterone deficiency. Estrogen dominance has been reflected in many studies, and this imbalance of estrogen and progesterone, with estrogen excess, begins early in our culture. A diet high in saturated fat, sugar, and junk food initiates this imbalance in puberty. Low levels of progesterone and excessive levels of estrogen can cause PMS, painful menstrual cramping, fibroid tumors, endometriosis, fibriotic breast disease, hypothyroidism, depression, and symptoms of menopause. This progesterone-estrogen imbalance also sets the stage for breast, uterine, and endometrial cancers.

TIP: Vitex (or "chaste tree") is a wonderful, progesterone-enhancing herb that has been used for more than 2,000 years with great success for women going through menopause. Vitex agnus-castus may take three to four weeks for effects to be noticeable, but it can reduce and eliminate hot flashes, mood swings, and flooding, and it gently lowers estrogen levels. Vitex helps to guard against reproductive cancers, headaches, and osteoporosis. *(See* the Resource Guide for information on a convenient, one-capsule-a-day supplement of this protective herb.)

Early Menarche and Late Menopause: Longer Exposure to Estrogen, Which Stimulates Cell Growth, May Contribute to Breast Cancer

In countries where the breast cancer rate is low, such as China, girls begin menstruating at age seventeen. Breast cancer researchers suggest that women who begin menstruating at age twelve have a 100% greater risk of breast cancer than women who begin menstruating at age thirteen or older. In fact, scientists have found that early menarche may set estrogen levels higher throughout life.

> Puberty now begins at an earlier age. Some girls show development as early as three to seven years of age. We need to examine what aspects of our diets, lifestyles, and environment contribute to this earlier development.

When the menses start (unless pregnancy occurs), there is a surge of estrogen, followed (hopefully) by a strong surge of progesterone that courses through the blood to the breasts. The hormones stimulate breast cells to divide and create glands and ducts for milk production. Because pregnancy doesn't usually occur, cells die at the end of each cycle. Researchers believe that modern reproductive patterns have distorted the body's natural hormonal patterns. Later menopause has also been associated with increased breast cancer risk.

Changing Reproductive Patterns: A Link to the Increase of Breast Cancer

Women had fewer menstrual cycles 100 years ago than they do today. Because of factors such as diet and environment, women did not begin menstruating until much later than they do today. For example, at the turn of the century, women began menstruating at approximately age seventeen. Women married and began their families at a much earlier age, as well. Typical families were much larger 100 years ago; having six to ten children was not unusual. Breastfeeding was the norm. Because the average woman at the turn of the century was often either pregnant or nursing, she had fewer menstrual periods over the course of her lifetime than women do today.

A menstrual period every month, with no break for pregnancy or breastfeeding, puts many women at risk for breast cancer. Since the eighteenth century, it has been noted that nuns have a very high rate of breast cancer. It is also true that other childless women are at a higher risk. The solution isn't for every woman to have a large family, but instead to make changes that offer protective effects similar to those of pregnancy—increasing the body's protective hormone progesterone, while decreasing exposure to potentially damaging effects of estrogen from diet and environment. A reduction in breast cancer risk is also seen in women who have their first pregnancy at an early age and women who breastfeed.

Importance of Diet Begins *In Utero*

Intrauterine influences may contribute to chances of breast cancer in adulthood. Studies show certain growth processes during pregnancy may affect the risks of breast cancer. Babies born in Japan and China, where the rates of breast cancer are considerably lower than they are in the West, weigh 150 grams less than babies horn in the United States. The Seventh European Nutrition Conference reported in May 1995 that birth size is influenced by dietary intake and pregnancy hormones.

Early in life, a high calorie and fat intake may also contribute to breast cancer risk in adulthood by affecting the number of mammary stem cells formed. Even adult height, as well as age at menarche, are thought to be affected by fat and calorie consumption early in life. There is a great deal of epidemiologic evidence positively associating adult height with breast cancer.

Breast Cancer Prevention

Reducing the amount of food we eat offers protection against breast cancer. Animal studies show that caloric restriction, with adequate vitamin and mineral intake, produced smaller animals with a lower rate of breast cancer. Researchers at the American Institute for Cancer Research have suggested that maintaining a balance between the amount of calories consumed and the calories used could be a neglected but important part of protecting against cancer. They even suggest that an imbalance between the calories consumed and those burned might *increase* the risk of developing cancer.

Xenoestrogens: Estrogenic Substances Have Increased Greatly

Naturally occurring estrogens made in a woman's body are not like the artificial estrogens found in much of our food supply and environment. Artificial estrogens, or xenoestrogens, can be found in produce and other foods treated with pesticides; in plastics and dry-cleaning fluids; and in pesticides in water. These sources of xenoestrogens may contribute to the estrogen overload, and may have a special significance when exposure to these chemicals occurs before and during puberty. Many researchers are concerned about the harmful effect these chemicals have when they are combined. Researchers are also concerned about the *cumulative* effects of lifetime exposure to pesticides and other chemicals.

As many as sixty cancer-causing pesticides can be legally used to grow our food.

The *New York Times* reported on October 30, 1997, that a study led by Dr. David J. Hunter, an epidemiologist at the Harvard School of Public

Health, found that DDT (a pesticide) and PCBs (chemicals thought to be carcinogenic) are not linked to an increase in breast cancer. Contradictory results have been found in other studies. The use of DDT pesticide was banned in 1972; PCBs (polychlorinated biphenyls) were banned in 1977. Julia Brody, a representative from the Silent Spring Institute in Newton, Massachusetts (an advocacy group concerned about the environment and women's health), pointed out that the new study is by no means definitive, noting, "This is a study of two chemicals out of 80,000." Dr. Hunter also acknowledged that the results of the HSPH study "by no means exonerated all environmental chemicals."

Dr. Mary S. Wolf, a chemist at the Mount Sinai School of Medicine in New York City and co-author of the study, had some reservations about abandoning the DDT/PCB breast cancer link. Dr. Wolf told the *Times*, "It may be important in some groups of women and it may be not only how high the levels are but the time of life in which they occur. Maybe it's even different for different kinds of breast cancer, like pre-menopausal and post-menopausal."

Alklphenol ethoxylates (APEs), banned in Switzerland and on the way out in other European countries, are estrogen mimickers used in many laundry detergents.

Men living on Long Island who have prostate cancer have been found to have high levels of xenoestrogens in their blood. (Xenoestrogens have also been linked to a lower sperm count.) One in two men in the United States will develop prostate cancer. The same foods that help to prevent breast cancer also can help to prevent prostate cancer, both hormone-sensitive cancers. I like to point this out to women I meet in my workshops or lectures: *What helps to create breast health also helps to create prostate health.* Help yourselves, and help your husbands at the same time.

"World Breast Cancer Forum Blames Environmental Ills," New York Times Reports

Speakers at the First World Conference on Breast Cancer focused concern on industrial chemicals and other pollutants in fighting breast cancer, Anthony DePalma reported in the *New York Times* in July 1997. Speakers pointed out that researchers might be influenced to "play down" environmental factors by corporations that manufacture chemicals. Representatives from countries such as Guyana, India, and Ghana pointed out that their rates of breast cancer have increased in relation to the degree of industrial development in their nations. A global plan developed through this conference, outlining recommendations to change policies (such as prohibiting the export of industrial chemicals to developing countries), will be presented to the United Nations. Dr. Sandra Steingraber, an ecologist at Northeastern University, expressed her belief that enough evidence of the impact of environmental chemicals on the development of breast cancer exists to act right away.

For more information on the dangers of other estrogenic substances in our environment such as plastics, pesticides, and other chemicals, visit the Health Web Site on the Internet:

http://easyweb.easynet.co.uk/~mwarhurst/oestrogenic.html

The Body's Ability to Produce Progesterone, the "Protective" Hormone, Has Dramatically Decreased

Modern dietary habits (i.e., fast food) and our hectic lifestyle deplete the body's supply of progesterone. Having adequate levels of progesterone to protect the body against potentially dangerous forms of estrogen can protect women from breast cancer.

Twelve Things You Can Do to Protect Your Daughter Against Breast Cancer

The Harvard Medical School recommended that "preventive efforts should be focused on young girls because it is young breasts that are most vulnerable to molecular damage that can accumulate over the years."

• Encourage your daughter to express her feelings and to honor them; learning self-expression early will help her develop valuable feelings of self-worth.

• Keep your daughter slim—obesity is increasing in children, and in young girls is linked to an increase in estrogen. Feed your daughter fewer calories, and encourage her to consume calories from nutrient-dense foods, so she does not develop deficiencies in protective nutrients like folic acid, calcium, and essential fatty acids. Many studies show that adolescent girls do not consume the recommended daily allowance of many vital nutrients.

• Encourage her to eat organic yogurt, found to reduce breast cancer significantly if eaten before puberty (*see* Chapter 18, "Secrets of a Healthy Kitchen").

Heavy girls tend to menstruate earlier. Two hundred years ago, before the breast cancer epidemic, the average age of menarche was seventeen.

- Encourage her to exercise. Physical activity decreases levels of estrogen and may delay menarche.
- Feed her a fiber-rich diet, which decreases excessive levels of estrogen. Include lots of vegetables for both fiber and phytochemicals, with special emphasis on cruciferous vegetables like broccoli, turnips, Brussels sprouts, and savoy cabbage.
- Make sure she consumes protective fats (flaxseed and extra virgin olive oils, and fatty-rich fish), and eliminates trans-fats (in processed vegetable oils and hydrogenated products) and fried food to encourage absorption of protective fats. Harel Zeev, M.D., at Brown University Medical School in Providence, Rhode Island, found these foods to benefit teenage girls suffering from PMS. Sloan Kettering also recommends fatty-rich fish as an optimum source of protective fish oils to prevent menstrual cramps.
- Include soy foods in her diet. Phytoestrogens have the ability to even out hormone levels, and to protect estrogen receptors in the breasts from potentially harmful forms of estrogen. Soy foods consumed before puberty have been found to be particularly protective against breast cancer.
- Purchase only organic meat, dairy, and eggs for your daughter (and yourself).
- Try to purchase organic produce, or rinse produce to remove pesticides (*see* Chapter 18, "Secrets of a Healthy Kitchen").
- Purchase chemical-free paper products; avoid plastics; use natural cleaning products and natural detergent; avoid the use of bleach in your home; and purchase a water filter. *Less than 10-15 percent of all breast cancers are hereditary.* The environment may have a bigger role in breast cancer than we think.
- Encourage your daughter to sleep in a darkened room to increase levels of melatonin.
- Discourage smoking, a habit that unfortunately begins in the teenage years. There is a 60 percent increase in the risk of breast cancer in women who have smoked cigarettes for more than thirty years.
- Discourage alcohol consumption, another habit that can begin in the teens. Some studies linking alcohol to an increased risk of breast cancer reflect that the risk is limited to women who begin drinking before age twenty-five.
- Discourage the use of birth control pills, which have been linked to an increased risk of breast cancer when older. A study published in *The Lancet* (September 24, 1994) and reported in the *Townsend News Letter for Doctors and Patients* (August-September 1997) emphasizes the need to eliminate birth control pills. Researchers in the Netherlands found that women who'd taken the pill when they were in their teens were up to three-and-one-half times more likely to get breast cancer than women who hadn't, and women who were over thirty-six and had taken the pill for less than four years had a 40

percent increase in risk. The synthetic progesterones in birth control pills inhibit the body's ability to manufacture progesterone of its own, and actually worsen the symptoms of PMS.

For in-depth information on healthy child-raising, read Lendon H. Smith's book *How to Raise a Healthy Child (see* "Suggested Reading" in Resource Guide).

The Liver: Hormone Modulator

The liver is the most significant organ in terms of hormone balancing. It weighs approximately three to four pounds, is the largest organ in the body, and performs more functions than any other organ.

The liver converts potentially toxic forms of estrogen (either from the environment or those created by the body) into safer forms of estrogen. Since estrogen is so significant in the development of breast and other hormone-sensitive cancers, it is of vital important to ensure the health of the liver, which:

• Detoxifies environmental toxins, chemicals, and drugs that get into the bloodstream.
• Cleanses the system of metabolic waste created by the body (by-products of internal functions).
• Digests deenergized red blood cells.
• Produces bile for digestion and absorption of fats.

> Failure to eliminate estrogen by the liver is caused by alcohol, chemicals, protein deficiency, and slow thyroid. The liver plays a vital role in metabolizing breast-protective omega-3 fats.

For liver health, include lots of dark, leafy greens, especially dandelions, parsley, watercress, and mustard greens; minimize saturated fat; and eliminate junk fats and oils. Beets, radishes, cruciferous vegetables, fresh vegetable juices, unroasted organic nuts and seeds, and adequate, good-quality protein should also be consumed. Fresh fruits to include are grapefruit, pears, apples, and lemon juice (as a condiment on vegetables, soups, and so on). Liver-protective umeboshi vinegar can be added to vegetables and salads. Adequate water intake (6–8 glasses daily) encourages the liver to filter out toxins.

Foods rich in B vitamins help the liver break down estrogens and help protect the heart by helping the body to break down homocysteine, which damages blood vessels. Include the following foods in your diet: salmon, tuna, shrimp, soy beans, whole grains, brewer's yeast, eggs, legumes, chick peas, kidney and navy beans, lentils, almonds, sunflower seeds, filberts, avocados, beets, parsley, broccoli, carrots, cabbage, potato skins, spinach, Brussels sprouts, root vegetables, turnip greens, orange juice, and bulgur wheat.

Alcohol, fried, greasy foods, all artificial fats, oils (margarine, partially hydrogenated and hydrogenated fats and oils), trans-fats, sugar, rich foods (like butter and ice cream), and artificial ingredients (food colorings, preservatives) are damaging to liver health. In fact, avoiding any food with a label will ensure the freshest, whole-foods diet possible. Exposure to pesticides can also be damaging to the liver. An herbal tonic containing dandelion milk thistle compound is protective for the liver. (*See* the Resource Guide for Herb Pharm. Refer to Chapter 16, "Power Teas," for instructions on how to brew dandelion tea, which helps protect the liver.)

Because the liver works so hard, we can "lighten its load" by selecting specific foods that can detoxify potentially dangerous forms of estrogen. Cruciferous vegetables protect the liver by converting potentially dangerous forms of estrogen into a safer form. Cruciferous vegetables contain the phytochemical indole-3-carbinol, which helps to facilitate this process.

Sulforaphane, another protective phytochemical in cruciferous vegetables, increases the liver's supply of detoxification enzymes.

Eat lightly while cleansing the liver. Include dandelion greens in your salad. And be sure you are consuming at least five different vegetables a day!

Jon J. Michnovicz, M.D., Ph.D., author of *How to Reduce Your Risk of Breast Cancer,* and director for the Foundation for Preventative Oncology, has researched the transformative powers of cruciferous vegetables and potentially dangerous forms of estrogen. For more information on the importance of cruciferous vegetables, I highly recommend his book (*see* "Suggested Reading" in the Resource Guide).

Fiber and Hormones

A diet rich in vegetables not only offers breast-protective phytonutrients, but is also an important source of fiber. Fiber is extremely important in lowering all cancer risk. With breast cancer, it is especially significant; with a low-fiber diet, waste can take up to three times longer to pass through the body than it does on a diet containing adequate fiber. The liver sends estrogens into the intestines to be eliminated, and women excrete estrogen each day in stools. The more estrogen that is eliminated, the more protection for the breasts.

Many studies have found the relationship between high stool fiber content and lower estrogen levels linked to protection against breast cancer. However, if the diet does not contain enough fiber, these intestinal estrogens may not be eliminated as quickly as they need to be. The greater the amount of fiber eaten, the more quickly this estrogen waste can be eliminated; this prevents estrogen from being reabsorbed into the bloodstream. Because breast cells need estrogen to grow, a diet high in fiber prevents intestinal estrogen from returning to the bloodstream to stimulate breast cell growth. There are two types of fiber:

• **Soluble fiber.** Dissolves in water, and is important in the digestion of food. Food sources include agar, pectin from apples, dried beans and other legumes, citrus fruits and vegetables, and whole grain foods such as oats and barley.

• **Insoluble fiber.** Does not dissolve in water, and provides bulk, hastening the transit of wastes through the colon. It has the ability to dilute cancerous substances that may be in the large intestines, and also protects against the harmful effects of estrogen. Sources of insoluble fiber include brown rice, fruits, and vegetables.

> Ground and soaked flaxseeds are a source of both soluble and insoluble fiber.

The American Institute for Cancer Research recommends that most Americans double their fiber intake to reach the 20-35 grams recommended daily. Since all fruits and vegetables contain not only fiber, but also breast cancer-protective antioxidants, multiple benefits can be obtained from consuming more of them.

> In 1970, Dr. Denis Burkitt published a study which pointed out that, in countries where diets included large amounts of fiber, there are fewer cases of cancer and heart disease. Since then, scientific research has focused on fiber.

Foods high in fiber also contain protective antioxidants and phytonutrients. *Glucarates,* a phytochemical in some fruits and vegetables, can prevent a woman's bloodstream from absorbing intestinal estrogen. Some fiber-rich foods include raspberries, apples, kidney beans, raisins, brown rice, and flaxseeds.

If you aren't used to a high-fiber diet, you may want to introduce fiber-rich foods gradually to reduce gas and bloating. Drinking more water will also help. The following substances will help to decrease the gas and bloating that may accompany adding more fiber to the diet.

- **Acidophilus.** I use PB8 acidophilus. It contains bifidus, which promotes colon health, and acidophilus (*see* the Resource Guide). Take two capsules in the morning. Also, organic, unflavored yogurt, about ½ cup daily, supplies natural acidophilus (*see* the Resource Guide).
- **Digestive Enzymes.** Digestive enzymes from a broad-spectrum plant-based enzyme supplement can be a great digestive/intestinal aid. For more information on increasing enzymes in your diet, *see* Chapter 5, "Raw Foods and Juices Provide Protective Enzymes."
- **Dried Beans and Legumes.** I recommend small portions of beans. For information on cooking with beans, *see* Chapter 18, "Secrets of a Healthy Kitchen."

In addition, chew food thoroughly to help the body break down fiber for easier digestion. In macrobiotics, it's recommended that you chew each mouthful at least thirty times. Saliva contains beneficial enzymes and solutes which begin the digestive process and help to buffer chemicals. Most people "eat on the run," swallowing food as quickly as possible and not chewing each mouthful completely until the food is liquid. Not chewing properly creates a variety of problems: indigestion, poor absorption of nutrients, bloating, gas, constipation, and low energy.

Fiber should be obtained from whole foods that have not been processed. The less processed a food is, the greater the power its phytonutrients and phytochemicals possess. For instance, I would recommend whole oats, or steel-cut oats, for breakfast instead of cold, dry bran cereal. In the October 1997 *Health* magazine, Walter Willett, a professor of epidemiology and nutrition at the Harvard School of Public Health, explained that fiber-rich carbohydrates, like whole grains, keep blood sugar at safer levels because they are digested more gradually (compared to mashed potatoes or white bread), and pointed out that, "unground whole wheat is better for you than ground whole wheat." Willett also noted that the fiber, perhaps because it is accompanied by important nutrients such as vitamins, magnesium, and other minerals, can slow the absorption of carbohydrates, which is desirable for general health. For information on how starchy foods may be linked to breast cancer, *see* Chapter 12, "Preventing Carbohydrate Overload: A New Equation for Health." For a selection of herbal teas that can help to reduce gas and bloating, *see* Chapter 16, "Power Teas."

Sample Menus
How to Increase Your Fiber

One of the advantages of consuming unrefined and unprocessed foods is that you don't have to worry about counting fiber grams. For instance, selecting brown rice instead of white rice provides three times as much fiber, and whole fruit offers more fiber than stewed fruit.

Breakfast

2 capsules of acidophilus to prevent gas and bloating
Fresh fruit such as grapefruit, pear, or apple (with skin), organic yogurt, as a source of acidophilus (and protein), ground flaxseed added to water *or,* Steel cut oats, sunflower seeds, and soft-boiled egg with flaxseed oil

Lunch

Spinach salad "Niçoise" with tomatoes, mild onions, potatoes (with the skin), sardines, and hard-boiled egg *or,* Fresh raw vegetables with humus or lentil soup

Dinner

Salad, brown rice, poached fish, Brussels sprouts, and carrots

Dessert

Raspberries or red grapes

Thyroid and Estrogen

The thyroid gland is butterfly-shaped, and lies on either side of the windpipe. Alan Cohen, M.D., of Milford, Connecticut, explains why an underactive thyroid, or "hypothyroidism," is often related to breast cancer: Thyroid problems can begin in childhood. Teenage girls who have irregular or heavy periods (or no periods) are often put on birth control pills to regulate their periods artificially. *Artificial estrogen interferes with thyroid hormone.* Natural progesterone helps to facilitate thyroid hormone action. Low thyroid contributes to general immune problems, thereby contributing to breast and other types of cancer.

Hypothyroidism (underactive thyroid) manifests in the following symptoms: weight gain, thinning hair, depression, cold hands, infections, low energy, irregular menstrual periods, and infertility.

Blood tests are notoriously inaccurate for detecting thyroid problems, Dr. Cohen explains. Find an M.D. who is experienced in using basal body temperature. See the Resource Guide for the Brodha Barnes Foundation in Connecticut; its counselors can help you find a doctor in your area who is experienced in using basal body temperature for diagnosing thyroid problems. This method is recommended by Dr. Cohen as being the most accurate.

Because symptoms of hypothyroidism include depression, nervousness, and fatigue, women are often given Prozac instead of identifying the real problem and treating it naturally.

Food can be very beneficial in promoting a healthy thyroid. Foods for hypothyroidism include:

• Protective fats, such as fresh organic flaxseed oil, extra virgin olive oil, and avocado.
• Saltwater fish (the richest source of iodine; may reduce the risk of breast cancer).
• Vegetables.
• Organic foods (pesticides and hormones increase estrogen overload).
• Sea vegetables or sea vegetable supplements.

Breast Cancer Studies: More on Diet, Hormone Levels, and Breast Cancer Risk

Two UCLA doctors, David Herber and John Glaspy, have found that diet directly impacts hormone levels. In a 1990 study of postmenopausal women who had followed a diet low in saturated fat, high in omega-3 oils (from fish oil), and high in fiber, the women's estrogen levels dropped in only four weeks. In 1995, Dr. Glaspy developed a diet for women with breast cancer as part of his special program:

• 15% fat—avoidance of saturated fats (solid fat found mostly in animal foods).
• Avoidance of margarine and vegetable shortening.
• Avoidance of corn, safflower, and soybean oils.
• Heavy on whole grains, fruits, and vegetables.
• High fiber.

- Light on dairy products and meats.
- Nonfat frozen yogurt is forbidden (sugar turns to fat).
- Fish oil.

It was found that breast cells in women with breast cancer were very high in omega-6 before dietary changes. After just one month of a changed diet, omega-3 began replacing omega-6 in breast cells.

> Avoidance of processed omega-6 oils, in conjunction with inclusion of plenty of omega-3 fatty-rich fish, flaxseeds and oil, soy, and whole foods, clearly impact hormone levels.

Not All Estrogens Are Created Equal

There are three types of estrogen: estrone, estradiol, and estriol. Estradiol is actually a thousand times more powerful than estriol, and is the most stimulating to the breast. Estrone is a little weaker than estradiol, and estriol is much weaker. Estradiol and estrone are thought to promote cancer. In *Breast Cancer Research and Treatment, 1992*, it was pointed out that estradiol-17-beta is associated with breast cancer. Estradiol and estrone are also linked to uterine bleeding, thyroid and liver problems, swollen breasts, and heart palpitations. (Estradiol is the form of estrogen used in birth control pills and hormone replacement therapy.) Marcus, Laux, N.D., author (with Christine Collins) of *Natural Woman, Natural Menopause*, pointed out that nearly every study showing that estrogen increases the risk of cancer has studied Premarin and other, similar drugs. Premarin, formulated from estrone (which the body converts to estradiol), is the estrogen most implicated in increased risk of breast cancer, according to Dr. Laux. Estriol, on the other hand, "has cancer prevention properties" and is "the form of estrogen that is most dominant during pregnancy," he notes. Furthermore, estriol has particular benefits for women who are at risk of breast cancer and need hormone balancing and replenishment. *See* the Resource Guide for information on natural vitamins, then share the material with your OB/GYN.

> The September 1994 issue of the *American Journal of Clinical Nutrition* reported that women who ate 60 grams of soy protein daily (the equivalent of one pound of tofu) had changes in their estrogen levels similar to those induced by tamoxifan. Also, it was noted that although the women in the study ate soy protein just for one month, they

experienced increases in their menstrual cycle lengths due to changes in their hormone levels.

Radical New Findings on Estrogen Reveal Soy Foods Ten Times More Protective Than Previously Thought

For many years—decades, in fact—it was thought that there was only one type of estrogen receptor and that not all organs and tissues in the body contained them. Now a second receptor labeled "beta" (the original is labeled "alpha") has been identified and found, generally, to exist in the body where alpha does not. Even though these two receptors are similar in the way that they both readily bind to the most powerful estrogen, estradiol, the beta receptor has the astounding characteristic of being ten times more effective in binding to the plant estrogen genistein, which is abundant in soybeans, other legumes, and some seeds (such as sunflower). It is the beta receptor's affinity to genistein, one theory suggests, that preempts its binding with estradiol, serving to keep this more aggressive form of estrogen in check. With the discovery of the beta receptor, tumors, previously diagnosed and treated as nonestrogen type, based on the absence of the alpha receptor, will now have to be examined in light of this groundbreaking discovery. Moreover, the discovery of additional estrogen receptor sites where none was formerly thought to exist suggests that estrogen plays a much greater role in creating or destroying health than anyone previously suspected.

Transformative Power of Foods: Foods That Protect Against Potentially Dangerous Forms of Estrogen

1. Cruciferous vegetables—in particular, savoy cabbage, Brussels sprouts, and broccoli—are rich in indole-3-carbinol. I-3-C is a phytochemical that the *Journal of the National Cancer Institute* reported can reduce breast cell growth and breast cancer by encouraging the transformation of estrogen into an inactive form.

2. Phytoestrogens in soy are adaptagenic. This simply means that if you have too much estrogen in your body, phytoestrogens will bind to your estrogen receptor sites and prevent them from being overly stimulated. This helps to protect against abnormal cell growth. Phytoestrogens also help to alleviate symptoms of PMS or menopause. *The Lancet,* Britain's esteemed medical journal, has reported that Japanese women have infrequent hot flashes because their diets are rich in phytoestrogens from soy. In 1991, the *Journal of the National Cancer Institute* reported that women consuming a diet containing 200 milligrams of isoflavones from soy products experienced a reduction in both vaginal dryness and irritation.

> Be sure to include a variety of phytoestrogenic foods, such as lentils, tofu, burdock root, flaxseeds, dried beans, sweet potatoes, fermented soy foods, and red clover tea in your diet to ensure healthy production of desirable forms of estrogen. The *Australian Journal of Medical Herbalism* reported in 1995 that these foods contain compounds with estrogen-like activity: alfalfa sprouds, fennel seeds, beans (mung, red, and split peas), oily seeds and nuts, rhubarb, apples, and members of the cabbage family.

3. Plant lignan precursors, found in flaxseed, are compounds that are converted during digestion into phytoestrogens. *Women's Health Advocate* reported in June 1996 that phytoestrogens are "thought to protect against a number of hormone-mediated conditions, ranging from hot flashes and fibroid tumors to breast and ovarian cancer."

There is evidence of a link between early childbearing and high urinary estriol and, in turn, low incidence of breast cancer.

The October 2, 1995, *Journal of the National Cancer Institute* published information confirming that dietary changes (i.e., reducing saturated fat and increasing fiber) can decrease estradiol and estrone.

> TIP: A nutrient-dense, whole foods diet can convert potentially dangerous forms of estrogen—estradiol and estrone—into a weaker, more protective estrogen, estriol. Estriol is converted from estradiol and estrone in the liver.

Update on a New Breast Cancer Supplement: Calcium D-Glucarate Is Also Available in a Common Food

There's a new supplement for breast cancer prevention and treatment on the horizon: calcium D-glucarate. CDG helps to metabolize excess estrogen in the body. A process called glucoronidation gets rid of excess estrogen by passing it through the liver, where glucuronic acid helps to pass it out of the body with the stool. This prevents the estrogen from being reabsorbed into the body. CDG is nontoxic, and is naturally made by the human body. Two studies show that when CDG is combined with vitamin A, it can inhibit cancer growth. I'm inclined to focus on foods as my source of nutrients, so I was delighted to find that yogurt is a source of calcium D-glucarate.

> TIP: Just three tablespoons of yogurt each day provides the protection of Calcium D-glucarate for breast health. Organic, plain yogurt is recommended.

Even the pharmaceutical companies want to provide women options other than ERT for maintaining bone density and lowering cholesterol, as well as providing antiestrogen effects. Raloxifene, a new drug under development in 1997 by Eli Lilly, will offer another option to women who may be concerned about breast cancer and want to avoid ERT and its estrogen-promoting effects.

Flaxseed: Estrogen Regulator

Flaxseed contains 100 times the levels of lignans found in other foods, and those lignans provide flaxseed with much of its cancer-fighting power. Flax lignans help to regulate estrogen levels by binding to the estrogen receptors in breast tissue and protecting against the stimulation of estrogen. Canadian studies have shown that giving flaxseed to animals with mammary tumors can reduce the size of the tumors as much as 67 percent. For more information on flaxseed, *see* Chapter 6, "Flaxseed and Flaxseed Oil: Nature's Superfoods for Breast Health."

Measuring Hormone Levels

Even though saliva testing for hormone levels isn't currently the standard practice, it is becoming increasingly popular. About 500 doctors nationwide use saliva testing to determine hormone levels. Numerous studies conducted in recent years support this more accurate form of testing, and its popularity is expected to grow. Because hormone levels fluctuate in premenopausal women, it is optimum to test at the same time of day for two or more tests. Hormone levels vary according to the time of month as well as time of day. According to the *Women's Health Advocate* newsletter (September 1996), unless blood is drawn at the same time of day for each test, the results may not accurately reflect hormonal changes over time, or response to supplementation.

Advantages of saliva testing:

• The saliva test is easy for women to do themselves, at home, with the sample collected at the optimal time of day.

• Multiple tests can be performed easily. This can be helpful if your doctor is trying to fine-tune your dosage of homones. (*See* the Resource Guide for saliva test kits.)

Natural Menopause

Information on menopause without relying on hormone replacement therapy (HRT) is important, since HRT may increase the risk of breast cancer. Menopause without medication can be a healthy choice.

A very important report examining the effects of postmenopausal hormone therapy in the Nurses' Health Study was published June 19, 1997, in the *New England Journal of Medicine*. It revealed an increase in deaths from breast cancer among long-term hormone users, and concluded that the survival benefit of HRT diminishes greatly over the years because of the increased risk of developing breast cancer. At least seven studies have shown a correlation between HRT and increased risk of breast cancer. The Reuters news agency reported October 10, 1997, that the most comprehensive and conclusive survey to date on HRT studies, which examined about 160,000 women from fifty-one studies in twenty-one countries, found that HRT does increase breast cancer risk. Dr. Valerie Beral of the Imperial Cancer Research Fund, who directed the study, said in a news conference that, "While women are using HRT, there is an increased risk of breast cancer, and the risk increases the longer women take HRT. When they stop taking HRT, this risk disappears."

In the recent past, doctors have urged women to begin taking HRT as soon as they go through menopause to guard against bone loss. More current research indicates that a woman can wait ten years or more to begin a program of estrogen therapy for the reduction of bone thinning and fractures. In a study conducted at the University of California, San Diego, of 700 women aged sixty to ninety-eight, it was found that women who started taking estrogen eighteen years after menopause, and had been on the hormone only nine years, had the same bone density as women who began estrogen therapy around the time of menopause and had been taking it for twenty years. This is important information, because it means that women can begin a program of HRT for bone loss at a much later age than previous thought. This option is not to be taken lightly. In June 1997, it was reported in the *New England Journal of Medicine* that long-term use (ten years or more) of HRT increased risk of breast cancer. An editorial accompanying the report, "Post Menopausal Hormone Replacement Therapy: Time for a Reappraisal?" questioned long-term use of HRT, based on the new study's findings.

Baby boomers are approaching menopause. It is our generation that will be looking toward alternatives, and asking more questions than generations past. Is HRT the only way to eliminate hot flashes and vaginal dryness, and to prevent osteoporosis and heart disease? It is not. For information on perimenopause, *see* Louise Gittleman's book *Before the Change (see* the Suggested Reading in the Resource Guide).

This discussion of natural alternatives for women entering the change-of-life addresses a profound deficit in the conventional wisdom regarding menopause. Here are the basic facts:

• The key role of progesterone during menopause has been virtually ignored by conventional practitioners. The focus has been exclusively on estrogen deficiency when in reality it is the balance of these two hormones that is so important.

• Estrogen refers to a group of hormones including estradiol, estrone, and estriol. The *Journal of the American Medical Association* notes that healthy women produce estriol in the liver from the more active forms, estradiol and estrone. Research show that estriol is protective against breast cancer. Japanese women who eat a traditional diet high in soy foods have much lower breast cancer rates. These women also have higher estriol levels.

• Progesterone is manufactured in the adrenals, where it serves as a precursor for the production of estrogen and other hormones. Chronic stress overworks our adrenals and upsets our estrogen-progesterone balance.

• It is clear that both the liver and the adrenal glands require our special focus in addressing natural approaches to menopause because of the vital role they play.

By introducing a little food for thought into our lives, women can leave conventional wisdom about menopause behind forever, and embark on a new way of thinking that will truly shape the experience of change-of-life for the better.

Natural Foods—The Foundation of a Healthy Menopause

Many American women enter menopause in a state of nutritional depletion, after a lifetime of consuming a diet high in saturated fat, sugar, protein, sodium, and phosphorus. This type of diet does not support our general state of health and particularly depletes adrenal health. Our diet and high-stress lifestyle set the stage for menopausal problems. Women following traditional Japanese lifestyles have fewer hot flashes and much lower rates of osteoporosis, heart disease, and breast cancer compared to women in the United States.

1. Nourish the liver and adrenal glands. Sour foods and condiments such as grapefruit, sauerkraut, umeboshi vinegar, and lemon are important for liver health. Bitter foods such as artichokes and dandelion greens or tea (from the root) help to regenerate the liver. Coffee, sugar, and stress deplete the body of much-needed minerals for properly functioning adrenal glands. Adrenal vitality will increase sexual energy and ease the transition from cycling to noncycling.

Dandelion Leaf and Mixed Vegetable Salad:

Invigorate Your Liver

½ cup chopped dandelion greens
1 cup thinly sliced purple cabbage
½ cup grated carrots
½–¾ cup thinly sliced radishes
⅓ cup sliced scallions
½ tsp sea salt
2–3 tsp umeboshi vinegar, to taste
juice of ½ lemon
⅓ cup sunflower seeds

Wash vegetables. Scrub carrots and radishes with natural vegetable scrubber, available in health food stores. Chop vegetables. Placed mixed vegetables on a large plate. Spread out on plate. Mix salt and umeboshi vinegar uniformly throughout the vegetables. Place another plate of the same size on top of the vegetables. Put a 5-pound weight on top of the second plate to press vegetables. Press until liquid extraction occurs—at least 10 minutes, or up to 6 hours, according to taste. Remove vegetables from plate. Drain liquid. Garnish with lemon juice and sunflower seeds.

Comment: Organic sunflower seeds are a rich source of healthy omega-6 and vitamin E.

TIP: Artichokes help the liver to produce more bile. Cynarin, an active ingredient in artichokes, encourages the production of bile, which is necessary to break down fats. Artichoke is closely related to milk thistle.

2. Eat according to climate and season. Many of the foods we eat tend to appear at every meal in every season. Thinking about seasonal change is a great way to incorporate more variety in our diets. Food selection (and life) are about change and flexibility, which are never more important than during and after menopause. If you were born and raised in Maine and relocate to Southern California, that would require major changes in food selection and preparation. In the warmer climate of Southern California, you would want lighter foods, like salads and fruit, more frequently.

Living in a warm climate, and during the summer, we should increase our intake of raw foods and fresh vegetable juices. In hot weather, we require less oil, less animal food, and smaller quantities of bean dishes. Emphasizing raw foods for their cooling effects will alleviate hot flashes and ease constipation, both of which are common menopausal complaints.

Trying to select seasonal foods also ensures that our fruits and vegetables will be fresher. Frequent farmers' markets, and if possible, think about planting a small garden.

3. Eat *whole* foods. Select *unprocessed, unrefined* whole grains such as brown rice, quinoa, millet, and oats. Modern processing has reduced grains from a nutrient-dense food to a depleted one.

A diet rich in whole foods is a good source of fiber, which helps to eliminate excess estrogen. A higher-fiber diet reduces the entry of toxins and prevents the eventual damage at various sites, specifically (but not exclusively) at the breast.

Whole grains are a good source of B-complex vitamins, the antistress vitamins that nourish the adrenal glands and are so important for women in menopause. Adding phytochemical-rich herbs and vegetables to grains to reduce serving size helps to reduce the glucose levels that too much grain can cause.

Herbed Rice in Radicchio

1 cup of long-grain brown
   basmati rice
1¾ cups of water
½ tsp sea salt

¼ bunch parsley (2 tbsp minced)
¼ bunch chives (2 tbsp minced)
¼ bunch cilantro (2 tbsp
  minced)
1 tbsp extra virgin olive oil
2 tbsp flaxseed oil

Combine rice, water, and salt in a pot. Bring to a boil and reduce heat. Simmer on low heat, covered, for about 40 minutes. Do not stir. Remove pot from heat and let contents steam for additional 15 minutes. Combine rice with remaining ingredients. Serve on a leaf of radicchio or arugula for bitter taste.

4. Adequate servings of high quality protein are especially important at menopause. When women are tired, they crave sugar to maintain their energy levels. Refined sugar then depletes mineral levels, further stressing overworked adrenal glands. This contributes to a vicious cycle of sugar craving. Vegetarian women may be especially prone to these symptoms. Adequate, but not excessive, protein intake will help women in menopause feel better and break this cycle. Organic chicken, fatty-rich fish, tofu, tempeh, and organic eggs will greatly improve energy levels. Fish—such as albacore tuna, mackerel, lemon sole, and salmon—can be prepared three to four times a week. Organic chicken and turkey breast, and organic, lean cuts of beef and lamb are additional options for meat eaters. Adequate amino acid intake also helps to reduce food cravings, and to revitalize sluggish metabolisms, thereby encouraging the burning of calories.

5. Emphasize soy foods. Soy foods are high in phytoestrogens, which reduce symptoms of menopause and are protective against reproductive cancers. Isoflavones in fermented soy foods are particularly beneficial for menopause. Foods rich in isoflavones such as tempeh, soy sauce, and natto are especially recommended.

Braised Tempeh:

Increase Your Intake of Phytoestrogens

½ block (8 oz) of soybean tempeh cut into thin slices
2 tbsp of mirin
2 diced cloves of garlic
2 diced shallots
a splash of shoyu
1 cup of arugala or mixed bitter greens of your choice

2 scallions
wedge of lemon
umeboshi vinegar to taste

Place tempeh, mirin, garlic, and shallots in a small pot filled with 1-1/2 inches of filtered water. Bring to a low boil; cover and simmer for 4 minutes. Then add shoyu and continue to cook for 2 more minutes. Place on a bed of selected greens and scallions. Dress with lemon and umeboshi vinegar.

6. **Vegetables, vegetables, and more vegetables!** Lightly steamed or blanched, calcium-rich, dark, leafy greens such as bok choy, kale, or collard greens are great choices. Chlorophyll-rich leafy greens facilitate calcium absorption. Bitter greens such as dandelion greens and escarole help to improve liver function. Root vegetables such as daikon radish, turnips, rutabaga, and carrots are particularly nourishing to the adrenals and kidney.

Blanched Mixed Greens with Tofu:
Calcium-Rich Energizer

2 cups chopped Chinese cabbage
2 cups of chopped watercress
¼ tsp (8 oz) sea salt
½ block of firm tofu cut into
   chunks
¼ cup thinly sliced Spanish
   onions
¼ tsp rice vinegar
¼ tsp shoyu

Wash greens and put aside. Bring 4 inches of salted, filtered water to a low boil in a pot. Add tofu and cabbage. Cook for ½ minute; add watercress and onions. Then quickly remove all ingredients and place in a bowl. Season with vinegar and shoyu, toss, and serve.

Option: Toss ingredients into cooked udon noodles with minced garlic, a squeeze of lemon, and a teaspoon of olive oil.

Comment: This recipe features light cooking for easy digestibility.

7. **Fat-free foods are detrimental in the menopause.** Essential fatty acids are as important as vitamins and minerals; they cannot be manufactured by our bodies and must be provided by diet. The essential fatty acids, including

both omega-3 and omega-6, are vitally important at this time. A deficiency of essential fatty acids will cause or contribute to symptoms of dryness including dry skin, brittle hair and nails, dry eyes, and sexual discomfort (from a lack of vaginal secretions). Reported improvements from essential fatty acid supplements include relief from poor memory, depression, fatigue, weight gain, and constipation.

Foods that are high in EFAs include flaxseeds, untoasted sesame and sunflower seeds, walnuts and the oils made from them. Pumpkin seeds and almonds are also rich sources.

To achieve optimal health, oils should be fresh, organic, and unrefined. *Keep in mind that these oils are living foods; their freshness ensures their powerful benefits. Refrigerate your flaxseeds and oils. Buy oils that are dated and bottled in dark glass.* (For more on fresh, unprocessed oils, see Chapter 18, "Secrets of a Healthy Kitchen.")

Lemon Vinaigrette with Pumpkin Seed Oil:

Include Essential Fats

⅓ cup mirin
½–1 tsp minced garlic, or 2 tsp ginger juice or minced shallots
3 tbsp pumpkin seed oil
⅓–½ cup Bragg's Liquid Aminos (nonfermented natural condiment) or shoyu
½ cup fresh lemon juice

Heat mirin in a small pot until it just reaches a delicate boil. Reduce heat and simmer for 3 minutes. This removes the alcohol. In a suribachi or small bowl, crush garlic and slowly add the rest of the ingredients.

Optional: For a thicker dressing, add chickpea or mellow white miso. Also, any finely minced fresh herbs, such as cilantro or rosemary, work well in this basic mixture. Create your own favorites, and be creative in your selection of unrefined oils.

TIP: Pumpkin seed oil, rich in phytosterols, can be helpful in creating healthy hormones. For men, pumpkin seeds and oil help to prevent prostate cancer. Pumpkin seeds are a source of immune-enhancing zinc.

8. Be selective with dairy. If you eat dairy, make sure your sources are organic. Hormones, pesticides, and antibiotics collect in saturated animal fats.

9. Enzymes are vital for healthy digestion. If you eat a healthy diet, you still may not be getting the nutrients you need if digestive enzyme production is low. The older we get, the fewer enzymes we produce. *See* Chapter 5, "Raw Foods and Juices Provide Protective Enzymes," for more information about enzymes.

10. Be aware of the xenoestrogens in our food. Foreign estrogens in our food and environment may have deleterious effects. Xenoestrogens appear in pesticides, industrial chemicals, and chemicals used to manufacture certain plastics. They also appear in food, food additives, animal feed, and our drinking water. **These environmental estrogens, may react more dangerously when combined and may contribute to our estrogen overload.** While studying breast cancer cells, Professor Ana Soto of Tufts University noted that xenoestrogens released from plastic test tubes caused the breast cancer cells to multiply. There is widespread use of plastics to line food cans, which emit xenoestrogens when heated.

11. Eliminate sugar. When processed by the body, sugar causes depletion of many minerals and is particularly depleting to the adrenals. Sugar causes calcium to be released from bone, contributing to osteoporosis.

12. Beverages—a toast to good health! Switch to kukicha tea. For a sparkling beverage, choose San Pellegrino, St. Remo, or Apollinaris mineral water, which contain substantial amounts of minerals. Cola drinks, which are high in sugar, phosphorus, and dyes, have been shown to be a culprit in osteoporosis. Coffee, a calcium-robber, is best avoided. For more on coffee, refer to Chapter 15, "Alcohol, Coffee, and Sugar."

13. Table salt—put down that shaker. Table salt is full of additives to prevent sticking. Many valuable trace minerals are chemically removed and then sold to the chemical industry. Sea salt is full of rich minerals and lower in sodium than table salt.

14. A word about fruit. Tangerines, grapes, berries, melons, grapefruit, apples, pears, and kiwi fruit are excellent choices. Pomegranates are the highest source of plant estrogens. Did you know that organic lemon and orange skins can prevent hot flashes because of their high bioflavonoid content? The white, inner lining of grapefruit and orange peels is also a rich source of bioflavonoids, and can be consumed directly.

TIP: Mince citrus peels and toss with your favorite green salad, or steep in herbal teas for powerful breast-protective benefits. Citrus peels stimulate enzyme production in the body, which strengthens immunity—another bonus!

15. Avoid over-the-counter antiinflammatory drugs. Painkillers like aspirin and ibuprofen impair liver function, which in turn has a negative effect on the breakdown of estrogen. Be aware that acetaminophen, found in many common over-the-counter drugs (including cold and cough medications, and pain killers not identified as acetaminophen), has been linked to potential liver problems.

Herbs

Herbs contain phytoesterols, which can help regulate hormones. Phytoestrogens are plant compounds that specifically exert protective effects. By regulating hormone levels, herbs used for menopause also benefit the heart and the bones. Work with a qualified professional for a program designed specifically for you. See the Resource Guide for a naturopathic physician referral service.

Alcohol and HRT

It was reported in the December 4, 1996, issue of the *Journal of the American Medical Association* that women on hormone replacement therapy had increased blood levels of estradiol. Drinking half a glass of wine daily doubles estrogen levels in postmenopausal women on HRT. For more information on alcohol and breast cancer, see Chapter 15, "Alcohol, Coffee, and Sugar."

Homeopathy

Naturally occurring substances, taken in minute doses, can stimulate your own innate balancing powers to alleviate the symptoms of menopause. In Europe, where homeopathy has been used for centuries, it is not considered to be "alternative medicine."

TIP: Hylands Co. offers the following combination remedies: For general menopausal symptoms, try No. 13. For insomnia, try No. 23. For headache, try No. 7. For information on homeopathy, read Dana Ullman's book *The Consumer's Guide to Homeopathy (see* the Suggested Reading in the Resource Guide).

Aromatherapy

Don't underestimate the power of essential oils. These sweet fragrances offer powerful therapeutic value for the symptoms of menopause. Essential oils are strong, so use them with respect. For information on essential oils and aromatherapy, read Kathi Keville and Mindy Green's book *Aromatherapy: A Complete Guide to the Healing Art* (*see* "Suggested Reading" in the Resource Guide). Use essential oils:

- In your bath.
- As a massage oil.
- As a compress.
- On your pillow at night.
- In a ceramic diffuser (put water in your diffusers, then add essential oils).

Using these oils in multiple modalities increases their effectiveness.

These essential oil formulas are useful for the following complaints:

Hot Flashes
  Clary-sage
  Sage
  Lemon
  Geranium

Depression or Anxiety

  Geranium
  Bergamot
  Lavender
  Chamomile

Insomnia
  Clary-sage
  Valerian
  Vetiver
  Lavender

Day Sweats
  Grapefruit
  Sage
  Thyme
  Lime
  Peppermint

Fatigue

  Grapefruit
  Rosemary
  Ginger

TIP: In two ounces of a carrier (or base) oil, add no more than twenty-four drops of the essential oils you select, and enjoy a deliciously fragrant and profoundly therapeutic massage oil. For reducing hot flashes, sprinkle peppermint oil in a handkerchief and breath deeply whenever you feel a flash.

Women are conditioned either to accept life with a high risk of heart disease and osteoporosis, hot flashes, mood swings, and sleeplessness or to take hormone replacement therapy, with its attendant risks. A possible escape from this dilemma exists nowhere in the conventional wisdom about menopause.

But there is a way out. It is liberating to understand that the risks of hormone therapy can be avoided.

Osteoporosis is a disease of Western culture. The African Bantu women, who consume only 350 milligram of calcium per day, are essentially free of osteoporosis. Studies have shown that women's bone mass begins to decline in their mid-thirties. If estrogen alone were responsible, why would osteoporosis begin fifteen years before menopause? Anovulatory cycles with deficient progesterone production are common as women enter their thirties. Jerilynn Prior, M.D., while measuring estrogen and progesterone levels in athletes at the University of British Columbia, discovered that athletes with low progesterone and high estrogen had significant signs of osteoporosis. Progesterone is clearly an important and overlooked hormone in bone formation.

John Lee, M.D., who has studied the role of progesterone in bone, points out that in bone remodeling, progesterone is linked to bone formation whereas estrogen is linked to bone reabsorption. Studies show that estrogen slows but does not stop or reverse osteoporosis. In his book, *Natural Progesterone: The Multiple Roles of a Remarkable Hormone*, Dr. Lee notes that natural progesterone used with a program of diet, mineral, and vitamin supplementation and modest exercise can prevent and reverse osteoporosis. Hydrogenated oils and sugar deplete mineral metabolism necessary for bone health. Frequent use of antibiotics robs us of vitamin K, also very important for bone health, by depleting friendly bacteria in the intestinal tract. When the level of protective bacteria is low, so is vitamin K. Raw or steamed leafy greens provide vitamin K. Nuts and seeds provide added minerals. Stress depletes two other minerals important for bone health—magnesium and zinc.

Heart disease in this country has increased greatly since the turn of the century while at the same time cholesterol consumption has remained about the same. What has changed? Diet and lifestyle have changed drastically since the early 1900s. The consumption of processed foods and soft drinks began and flourished, while the consumption of whole foods and fresh produce declined. Our diets have become deficient in fiber, vitamins, and minerals while they've increased in refined sugar, pesticides, animal food, and *processed fats*.

Cholesterol is the building block for many hormones in the body. We need healthy forms of cholesterol during menopause. Our bodies cannot deal with the processed forms of cholesterol or related, processed fatty acids. New discoveries show that *oxidized cholesterol* and *oxidized fatty acids* are the culprits in cardiovascular disease. Cholesterol becomes oxidized because our diet contains foods that are aged, stored, whipped, and processed. Cheese, whipped cheese dips, processed vegetable oils, and whipped dessert toppings are all examples of oxidized fats and cholesterol. A good program for heart health includes *fresh, organic foods*, antioxidant supplements, and the elimination of sugar (where it interferes with antioxidant function), cigarette smoking, and coffee. Exercise and relaxation, by decreasing stress, will improve cardiovascular health.

What Protects Your Heart Will Also Help to Prevent Cancer

Did you know that heart disease claims the lives of more American women than breast cancer? Of women's deaths each year, 30 percent are from heart disease; 3 percent are from breast cancer.

In 1997, a report in the *European Journal of Clinical Nutrition* correlated the consumption of margarine and the danger of heart attack. In a study of 429 Italian women who'd had heart attacks, it was found that the more margarine these women ate, the higher the risk of heart attack.

Other studies have also shown that the larger the quantities of margarines and shortenings consumed, the higher the risk of heart attacks and cancer.

Because margarine contains hydrogenated vegetable oils, its use has been linked to elevated blood cholesterol. This is true even for margarines that are described as "natural," made from soy or safflower oils, and available from health food stores. The process of hydrogenation is generally harmful to the immune system.

For heart health, eating fewer carbohydrates and more protein have proven to be more effective than previously thought. According to research conducted by Dr. Bernard Wolf and published in the *Canadian Journal of Cardiology* in 1995, when some of their diet was replaced with more protein, twenty-one volunteers experienced a lowering of LDL cholesterol, an increase in protective HDL cholesterol, and a dramatic decrease in triglycerides.

Remember, increasing protein means choosing adequate protein, such as replacing a breakfast of dry cereal or a muffin with an egg or soy product (such as soy sausage), or nuts and seeds.

> A study reported in the *New York Times* October 16, 1997, found that calcium channel blockers, prescribed widely to women aged sixty-five or older for heart disease and to control high blood pressure, are thought to double the risk of breast cancer. The researchers, however, said the results "are far from conclusive."

As obstetrician-gynecologist Christiane Northrup, M.D., says in her book *Women's Bodies, Women's Wisdom,* "The cause of heart disease in women over fifty-five is commonly thought to be estrogen 'deficiency,' and estrogen replacement therapy (ERT) is thought to be the answer. Merely linking cardiovascular disease with lowered estrogen levels implies that cardiovascular disease is *caused* by lowered estrogen levels. But this theory has never been substantiated."

Since heart disease and osteoporosis may very well be prevented by proper nutrition, exercise, and lifestyle decisions (i.e., no smoking), vaginal dryness may be a reason many women want to take artificial hormones. Also, some women may experience urinary tract infections or irritation, and may consider HRT for those reasons. Another group of women who want to avoid HRT because they are concerned about breast cancer in their families could also be candidates for the new vaginal ring. Estring (by Pharmacia and Upjohn) is about the size of a diaphragm and delivers low doses of estrogen. Studies show it relieves both urinary tract infections and dryness. Minimal levels of estrogen get absorbed into the blood.

> TIP: Estriol cream, for vaginal dryness, is available from pharmacies that specialize in natural hormones. Because this type of estrogen does not bind with estrogen receptors within the cell structure, it does not cause a build-up of tissue inside the uterus. It is safe to use small amounts of estriol vaginal lubricant, even if there is a history of breast or uterine cancer. *(See* the Resource Guide for information on where to obtain natural hormones; be sure to discuss this issue with your physician.)

Case Study: Susan's Changes
The Benefits of Adding Oils for Perimenopause

I met Susan Kalev in New York City in January 1995 at a lecture I was giving at Gulliver's Macrobiotic Center. At the time, she was following a strict macrobiotic diet. She had been experiencing very severe hot flashes and aggravating cravings for sugar. Susan had a low-fat diet (the only oil consumed was small amounts for cooking/heating) that was high in whole grains, soy foods, some sea vegetables, and vegetables. I felt Susan needed to add essential fatty acids in the form of unprocessed organic oils drizzled on food before eating, and eliminate the heated oils. This would allow the protective benefits of the oils to be more easily metabolized. (Heated oils compete with unheated oils, blocking the effects of healing EFAs.) I also advised her to start eating salads (drizzled with flaxseed and extra virgin olive oil) to increase enzymes for oil metabolism, and to add more good-quality protein to help prevent sugar cravings. Susan was eating very little protein, no fat or oil, and her diet was extremely high in carbohydrates. It is especially important for women to eat adequate protein to help alleviate sugar cravings. A diet very low in proteins and protective fats, and high in starches—breads, pasta and even whole grains—encourages wicked sugar cravings. Although Susan began consuming sardines, she was hesitant about adding eggs because of her spiritual beliefs. I advised her that if she purchased organic, unfertilized eggs from a small farm at a farmer's market, she might feel as though she was supporting more humane methods of treating animals.

Currently, Susan is experiencing less frequent and less severe hot flashes, simply by having included flaxseed oil, Udo's Choice Ultimate Oil Blend, and more raw foods in her diet. Also, her sugar cravings subsided as she added protein to her diet. The guidelines I gave her were as follows: 30% of the food she consumes should be fat (in the form of fresh, organic, unprocessed oils from nuts, seeds, and avocados); 30-40% protein (tofu, tempeh, organic plain yogurt, organic unfertilized eggs, and fatty-rich cold water fish); and 30-40% complex carbohydrates (mostly vegetables, some fruits, and not more than 10% whole grains). Susan subsequently reported to me that, while on vacation for a couple of weeks, she eliminated the oil I had encouraged her to add to her diet. During that time, her hot flashes returned and were as disturbing as they'd been before she modified her diet, both in severity and frequency.

> A 1996 study in *The Lancet* from Italy shows that a low-protein, high-starch diet from pasta—a diet which also includes margarine and sugar, including sugar (fructose) from sweet fruit—is linked to the risk of breast cancer.

Beneficial Prostaglandins Are Made from Good-Quality Cholesterol

The Howell Study, a landmark investigation utilizing 224 studies between 1966 and 1994, laid to rest the erroneous assumption that dietary cholesterol was directly linked to blood cholesterol levels. Strict limitations on eggs for the general population have been lifted. Protective prostaglandins are made from good-quality cholesterol, which is provided by organic eggs. Eggs are also a source of good-quality protein, which helps to reduce sugar cravings.

Homocysteine and Heart Health

Many experts are beginning to believe homocysteine is more of a concern in heart disease and strokes than cholesterol. Homocysteine is created when the essential amino acid methionine is metabolized, and its levels in the blood rise as a result of consuming excessive animal protein like milk, meat, and eggs. When the diet is deficient in nutrients like B vitamins and folic acid, the body cannot break homocysteine down. Because homocysteine damages blood vessel walls, it is theoerized that cholesterol forms and collects in the damaged tissue. Because vitamin B6 is depleted when women who take birth control pills also smoke, Kilmer S. McCully, M.D., is concerned that their blood homocysteine levels become elevated, increasing their risk of blood clots and arteriosclerosis. Josephine Mahi, managing editor of *Total Health* magazine, reported that Dr. McCully also makes the connection between homocysteine and cancer. Dr. McCully points out that ". . . the growth pattern of cancer cells in culture resulted in the discovery that the sulfur atom of homocysteine thiolactone fails to react with oxygen to form sulfate in those cells." Unlike normal cells in culture, Dr. McCully explains in his book, *The Homocysteine Revolution*, cancer cells tend to accumulate homocysteine thiolactone.

Estrogen and Alzheimer's Disease

Media reports have promoted estrogen's ability to prevent Alzheimer's disease, but it's important to realize that women don't necessarily go into a steady mental decline without artificial estrogen. There are natural alternatives to artificial estrogen for memory enhancement. Consult with a nutritionist or physician experienced in complementary medicine for a nutritional supplement and herbal program. For memory aids, *see* Chapter 20, "Personal Care Guide."

Misuse of Demographics: An Argument for HRT?

Some proponents of hormone replacement therapy (HRT) argue that it is "unnatural" for women to live to seventy-seven, the average life expectancy of women today. Infant death, childhood disease, and childbirth deaths contributed to the forty-year-old life expectancy of women in the early 1900s. Even then, if women survived their childbearing years, many lived beyond menopause. After ovaries stop producing eggs at menopause, they continue to supply the type and amount of estrogen that women need. Today, each woman has the choice whether or not to take hormones. This choice should be made with her physician and determined by what is comfortable for her, as well as by her medical and family history.

CHAPTER 12

Preventing Carbohydrate Overload: A New Equation for Health

In terms of optimizing health, the emphasis placed on carbohydrates during the last two decades is coming under increasing scrutiny. Many nutritionists are recognizing that a diet high in carbohydrates and low in animal protein may not be right for most people. Still, the number of carbohydrate-rich recipes is disproportionately high in many health-oriented cookbooks, and magazines offer an abundance of grain, bread, and pasta recipes, emphasizing carbohydrate over protein consumption. Many women I work with believe they are eating healthy diets, when in fact, their diets are too high in carbohydrates. "What do you eat for breakfast?" I begin by asking. Nine times out of ten, a woman will say, "I eat something healthy, like a muffin and juice, or cereal and skim milk." These breakfasts are high in carbohydrates relative to protein. Carbobydrate-rich diets have been linked to breast, colon, and stomach cancers, and to diabetes.

An Italian study published in *The Lancet* in May 1996 presented the most direct evidence yet that a starchy diet may contribute to the risk of breast cancer. The study followed 5,000 women and concluded that the risk of breast cancer increased with increasing carbobydrate consumption through such foods as white bread, pasta, rice, crackers, and cookies. A study of 65,000 women linked carbohydrates from white rice, pasta, potatoes, and white bread to diabetes. Interestingly, high intake of unsaturated and polyunsaturated fats were associated with a decreased risk of cancer. Carbohydrates also have been found to lower protective HDL cholesterol (moderately), and increase triglycerides and insulin levels, all of which contribute, it is suspected, to an increased risk of heart disease in postmenopausal women. Excessive carbohydrates, because they raise glucose levels in the body, help to create an environment in which cancer may grow. Knowing about the carbohydrate-cancer connection encouraged me, for instance, to reevaluate the amount of pasta I was eating, and not only to reduce its frequency in my diet but also to substitute more vegetables in place of pasta's simple carbohydrates.

These findings encouraged me to make sure I was eating adequate amounts of good-quality protein at every meal, without carbohydrate overloading. According to Ann Louise Gittleman, M.S., C.N.S., carbohydrates should not exceed 40%, of total calories; good-quality fats and proteins should contribute 30% each (60% combined) to total calories. In trying to get enough protein from non-animal/fish sources, the tendency is to overload on carbohydrates. As a result, vegetarians must necessarily be more conscientious about diet and nutrition than nonvegetarians. I don't advocate one diet over the other; it's a lifestyle choice that every individual must make. It should, however, be an informed choice.

Traditional Diets from Asia and the Mediterranean

It may perhaps be useful to consider how people in Asia and the Mediterranean have been eating for centuries. As we have seen, women from this region of the world enjoy love incidences of breast cancer, as well as heart disease and osteoporosis. The consumption of small portions of meat and fish seems to help keep these women healthy.

Small amounts of protein, such as fish, organic meat, and eggs, can benefit the body in many ways by:

- Helping the body release energy more slowly and balancing blood sugar.
- Supplying the body with necessary amino acids for liver and immune function. Adequate amino acid consumption also helps to rejuvenate tired metabolisms, which encourages burning of calories.
- Supplying the body with the three essential amino acids needed to produce glutathione, a powerful antioxidant and neutralizer of dangerous free radicals.
- Supplying the body with B12.
- Helping prevent harmful effects of bacteria and viruses through improved antibody function.
- Helping to reduce sugar and carbohydrate cravings.
- Helping to create the guardian enzyme CP-450, which is low in women

The Traditional Healthy Asian Diet Pyramid

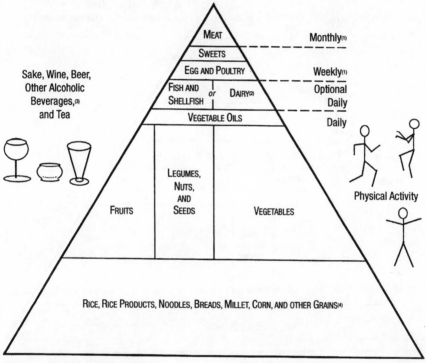

1. Or more often in very small amounts.　　©1995 OLDWAYS PRESERVATION & EXCHANGE TRUST
2. Dairy foods are generally not part of the healthy, traditional diets of Asia, with the notable exception of India. In light of current nutrition research, if dairy foods are consumed on a daily basis, they should be used in low to moderate amounts, and preferably low in fat.
3. Wine, beer, and other alcoholic beverages should be consumed in moderation and primarily with meals, and avoided whenever consumption would put an individual or others at risk.
4. Minimally refined whenever possible.

The Traditional Healthy Mediterranean Diet Pyramid

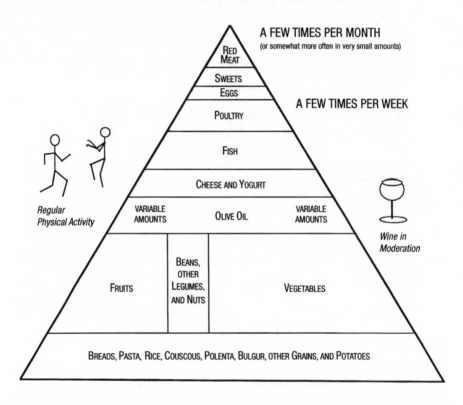

A FEW TIMES PER MONTH
(or somewhat more often in very small amounts)

RED MEAT

SWEETS

EGGS

POULTRY

A FEW TIMES PER WEEK

FISH

CHEESE AND YOGURT

Regular Physical Activity

VARIABLE AMOUNTS

OLIVE OIL

VARIABLE AMOUNTS

Wine in Moderation

FRUITS

BEANS, OTHER LEGUMES, AND NUTS

VEGETABLES

BREADS, PASTA, RICE, COUSCOUS, POLENTA, BULGUR, OTHER GRAINS, AND POTATOES

Author's Note: Oldways Modifications

Some women will feel better if they eat more frequent servings of meat, chicken, and fish than the pyramid indicates. This is fine, as long as portions are small (3–3½ ounces). I recommend consuming bread and pasta less frequently than suggested in this food pyramid, and that wine be avoided if you are healing breast cancer.

with breast cancer. Dr. Robert Crayhon explains in *Nutrition Made Simple* that CP-450 is an enzyme that neutralizes toxins. If inadequate amounts of protein are consumed, inadequate amounts of CP-450 are made. CP-450 also helps to eliminate many toxic, free-radical-producing substances.

Both meat eaters and vegetarians alike should take action to reduce intake of less desirable simple carbohydrates that are linked to cancer—found in pasta, cakes, muffins, and other baked goods—and replace them with foods rich in complex carbohydrates, such as vegetables and whole grains.

12 Important Meat Safety Tips

The following suggestions should be implemented when purchasing and storing meat to help reduce the possibility of infection with bacteria and protection against parasites:

• Select meat from a quality company, and be sure that there is a recent date stamped on the package.

• Return home immediately after purchasing meat so that you can refrigerate it right away.

• If meat or poultry is not cooked 24 hours after purchase, freeze it.

• Thaw frozen meat in the refrigerator, *not* on the counter at room temperature where bacteria can multiply.

• Keep raw meat and poultry separate from other foods.

• Immediately wash hands thoroughly after cutting and handling meat.

• Be sure your cutting board, knives, and sponges are kept clean. Replace sponges regularly.

• Cook hamburger well done (so that it's brown all the way through).

• Never let leftover meat sit out on the counter unrefrigerated. Bacteria multiply rapidly, so refrigerate leftovers immediately. This is an important reason for avoiding fast food hamburgers, chicken, and other meats, which can remain unrefrigerated for varying periods of time before or after cooking, increasing the likelihood of bacterial growth.

• Use fresh garlic for its antimicrobial qualities, and fresh ginger for its antiparasitic properties, on a daily basis.

• Eat small portions of meat (3½ ounces) with plenty of fresh salad and vegetables.

• Use clear vinegar for washing counters and cutting boards. Cutting boards may be scrubbed with a solution of ½ vinegar and ½ baking soda (for instance, 3 tbsp each vinegar and baking soda, depending on the size of the surface to be cleaned).

Does Irradiating Meat Pose Hazards to Our Health?

E. coli contamination has brought the issue of meat safety to the public, and health officials are attempting to increase the safety of the meat we consume. One of the methods of killing bacteria currently under discussion is irradiation. However, irradiating meat may pose other problems. Consider the following facts about irradiating meat:

- Irradiation destroys vitamins K, C, E, and the B-complex vitamins.
- Cobalt 60 and Cesium 137, which are used during the irradiation process, are nuclear toxins.
- Irradiating meat utilizes 100,000 rads of radiation which is equal to 10 million medical X-rays, as *Delicious!* magazine reported in December 1997.

Aren't there other ways of protecting the public from bacteria-tainted meat? Food & Water Inc., an organization dedicated to protecting health, suggests methods such as warm water washing and steam pasteurization offer effective options for stopping the growth of *E. coli* and other bacterial contaminants. (*See* the Resource Guide for Food & Water Inc.)

Do Farm-Raised Animals Suffer From Carbohydrate Overload?

Animals such as wild pigs, sheep, and rabbit are more muscular than farm-raised animals. Meat from wild animals is lower in saturated fat than meat from their more domesticated counterparts. Even in freezing northern climates, wild animals remain sleek, carrying very little extra body fat. Of course, wild animals are much more active than farm-raised animals, but diet also plays a big factor in keeping them slender. Farm-raised animals are fed carbohydrate-rich grain and wild animals feed on grasses. A diet rich in carbohydrates increases body weight.

Protein and Osteoporosis

Early studies linking diets high in protein consumption to osteoporosis are now considered questionable. Nutritionist Robert Crayhon reports that those studies used protein sources that were high in salt; excess salt causes calcium loss. A 1995 study published in the *American Journal of Clinical Nutrition* reported that a diet containing adequate protein does not cause calcium loss.

TIP: Spread protein intake throughout the day for optimum benefit, especially if you are involved in weight training. Two to three servings of protein daily, 3½ ounces a serving, is recommended.

Good Protein Sources and Their Benefits

• Select organic eggs and dairy, and the highest quality lean meat, fresh fish, and soy foods.

• Don't eat oxidized cholesterol, in the form of aged meat, cheese, or freeze-dried eggs (found in packaged cake mixes, for example).

For Meat Eaters

• Remove the skin from chicken or turkey.

• Don't eat red meat more than once or twice a week, and make lamb your red meat of choice.

• Avoid barbecued and charred meats. Heterocyclic amines, benzo(a)-pyrene, and other polynuclear hydrocarbons from burned fats have been found to contribute more to the risk of developing cancer than either the amount of meat consumed or the frequency of meat consumption. Roast meat instead.

• Consume smaller portions of meat. Balance with lots of fresh vegetables.

Cooking Meat

When meat is heated to high temperatures in the course of baking, roasting, broiling, and frying, carcinogenic substances are formed. Fat dripping onto the coals during barbecuing or grilling outdoors creates additional carcinogenic agents which are in the smoke and coat the meat. People who have cancer or who have a family history of cancer will need to be cautious about grilling. For safest grilling, cook meat medium-rare rather than well done. Grill as far away from the coals as possible (to avoid the charred spots), trim fat from meat, and use the leanest cuts of meat possible. Studies going back to 1964 have linked polynuclear hydrocarbons and other chemicals that are found in grilled meat to cancer. The amount of benzo(a)pyrene found in one charcoal-broiled steak is equal to that of approximately 600 cigarettes. Furthermore, the melted fat that drips down to the hot coals and turns to smoke contains polynuclear hydrocarbons that end up on the meat as the smoke rises. Oven roasting is recommended over charcoal broiling.

> TIP: If you feel you have to use the grill: Marinating chicken (in some combination of lemon, olive oil, garlic, mustard, and spices) and not overcooking it will eliminate 90 percent of the heterocyclic amines, according to a study conducted at the Lawrence Livermore National Laboratory.

TIP: Avoid consuming smoked, pickled, and salt-cured foods such as smoked salmon or bacon. These foods, which contain nitrosamines and hydrocarbons, have been found in both epidemiological and animal studies to be linked to cancer.

Avoid ground beef. The potential contamination from the animals' intestines (resulting from sloppy butchering practices) with dangerous forms of the *E. coli* bacterium has caused numerous outbreaks of food poisoning in the United States, some fatal.

For Vegetarians

- Eat a variety of breast-protective soy foods such as tofu.
- Consider adding free-range, unfertilized, organic eggs for an excellent nutrient-rich source of protein.
- Consider adding small amounts of breast-protective fatty-rich fish.
- Consider supplementing with protein-rich chlorella.
- Be sure you are getting plenty of green vegetables and protective fats such as organic flaxseed oil, avocado or extra virgin olive oil, as well as *adequate* (but not excessive) amounts of whole grains with your protein source to help reduce sugar cravings.
- Fermented soy foods like tempeh and natto are good protein sources.

Ginger Salmon and Rice "Homestyle":
Balance Carbohydrate-Rich Grain with Protein-Rich Fish

(Serves 4)

❦ *Vegetarians may want to consider adding a little fish to their diets. Salmon, rich in Omega-3 fatty acid, is a delicious and protective choice. The whole grain in this flavorful recipe is balanced by the vegetables and fish. The breast-healthy result is that less glucose is made than would be produced by consuming carbohydrates alone.*

2 carrots
2 tsp filtered water
1 tsp untoasted sesame oil

1 chopped medium onion
7-8 cloves minced garlic
7 sliced shiitake mushrooms
2 tsp sea salt
Herbamare organic seasoning
1½–1¾ cup broccoli florets
¾ cup of deboned, flaked, cooked salmon
1 ½ cups of cooked, fluffy brown rice
6 scallions, cut into small pieces on the diagonal
4 tbsp of freshly grated ginger root
2 tbsp flaxseed oil

Cut carrots on the diagonal, then cut into thin strips, approximately 1½–1¾ cup. In a large skillet, put 1 tsp of water and sesame oil. Do not heat on high. Add onions, garlic, and sliced mushrooms. Sauté until vegetables are tender, about 8-10 minutes on medium-low. Add a couple of pinches of salt and Herbamare.

Add carrots and broccoli, with several pinches of salt and Herbamare. Add another tsp of water. Continue to water-sauté gently on medium-low for 15–25 minutes. Cover with lid after cooking 5 or 10 minutes, stirring occasionally. Vegetables should be "crispy tender."

Stir in salmon, rice, and scallions. Cook for another 5 minutes. Add ginger juice by squeezing grated ginger over mixture. Discard ginger after squeezing juice out. Stir well, remove from heat. Adjust taste by adding a pinch or two of sea salt and/or Herbamare. Add flaxseed oil. Mix thoroughly and serve.

When I began to explore clay pot cooking, it was as if a whole new world opened up for me. Roman pot, or clay pot, cooking is a terrific way to prepare grains, combining them with fish, chicken, or soy foods (like Indonesian-style tempeh), casserole style. Any ethnic combination of herbs and spices may be used. For example, combine Israeli couscous, the large round variety, with skinned organic chicken breasts that have been marinated in lemon, extra virgin olive oil, tomatoes, onions, turmeric, and rosemary. Pour the marinade throughout the precooked fluffy couscous, add the chicken breasts on top, and roast in a water-soaked clay pot. Serve with a garnish of additional fresh herbs. The "heavy" dry-roasting technique is complemented greatly by clay pot cooking, a technique which creates a moister, flavorful dish.

Roman Pot Chilean Sea Bass and Rice with Cardamom

(SERVES 4)

❦ *You can convert your favorite recipe to clay pot cooking by simply increasing cooking temperature about 100° F and deducting one-half hour of cooking time.*

    1 lb Chilean sea bass
    1 cup yogurt
    4 cloves minced garlic
    juice from 1 lemon
    2 chopped and seeded serrano chilis (wear gloves when
       handling)
    ¾ tsp mustard seeds
    1¾ tsp cardamom seeds
    ½ tsp sea salt
    6 cups cooked long-grain brown rice
    2 tbsp sesame oil
    2 cups coarsely chopped, seeded, or skinned tomatoes
    1 cup minced shallots
    ¼ tsp turmeric
    ½ cup chopped fresh parsley

Completely immerse the entire clay pot in water for 15 minutes. *Do not preheat oven.*

Clean the fish and cut it into 4 slices. Combine yogurt, garlic, lemon, and 1 chopped chili and several pinches of sea salt in a suribachi (use a food processor or simply a bowl if you don't have a suribachi). Grind the garlic as much as possible, together with the yogurt mixture.

Next, roast the cardamom and mustard seeds gently over low-medium heat for several minutes in a small pan. Quickly put roasted spices in a spice-seed grinder and grind for a minute or so. Add ¾ of the spice mixture to the marinade. Pour marinade over fish and allow to marinate for at least one-half hour.

Remove the clay pot from the water. Combined the cooked rice, 2 tbsp sesame oil, tomatoes, shallots, turmeric, and additional chopped chili pepper with the rice, in the bottom of the clay pot. Add several pinches of sea salt.

Place the 4 pieces of fish on top of the rice. Pour the yogurt marinade over the fish and rice. Add a pinch of turmeric for color, and a little more sea salt.

Cover clay pot. Put into oven. Roast at 450° for 40 minutes. Remove from the oven; do not place on a cold surface (like a tile or marble counter), to avoid "shocking" the clay and causing it to break. Open the pot, add the minced parsley, adjust seasonings, and enjoy. Present with a garnish of thinly sliced lemon and avocado.

Making sure you have adequate protein at every meal will help to balance your blood sugar, reducing carbohydrate cravings. Fermented soy foods offer breast-protective phytochemicals and provide an excellent source of protein. Eating condiment-sized portions of meat or fish, as is done in the countries with the lowest rates of breast cancer (such as Mediterranean and Asian nations), balanced by plenty of vegetables, provides us with a healthy paradigm. Purchasing fresh, fatty-rich fish and consuming it the same day offers a superior source of protein rich in breast-protective fish oils. Organic eggs, five to six a week, is another nutrient-rich source of proteins.

Not All Carbohydrates Are Created Equal

A diet high in carbohydrates and low in fiber, is not recommended.

- Low-fiber carbohydrates like most bread, potatoes, and pasta, are foods that create a quick surge in blood sugar. These carbohydrates may lead to breast cancer, heart disease, and diabetes.
- Your body recognizes simple carbohydrates like mashed potatoes and pasta just as it recognizes sugar, because they have no fiber. Therefore, these starchy foods are utilized as if they were sugar.
- Bread with well-milled, finely ground whole wheat had the same effect on blood sugar as white bread. According to the October 1997 issue of *Health* magazine, Harvard School of Public Health researcher Walter Willett recommends consuming bread made with unground whole wheat instead of bread made with ground whole wheat. Research shows that the more whole grain a bread contains, the less likely it is to raise blood sugar. In fact, Willett recommends that potatoes and white bread be moved into the "sweets" category in the Food Guide Pyramid because they are the same as sugar metabolically.
- Vegetables, whole grains, nuts, seeds, and berries provide good sources of carbohydrates.

Consuming excessive carbohydrates lowers blood sugar and sets up cravings for sweets. It also encourages weight gain. The most serious concern is that it raises blood glucose, which encourages tumor growth.

The following guidelines are flexible. Everyone has different needs, and these needs change according to different stages in life and even different seasons of the year. For example, in the summer, people want more salads and less fat. In the winter, people need more protective fats (flaxseed and other protective, organic oils). Some people require more whole grains to help prevent constipation. Life is an always-changing process, but the following recommendations provide a *general guideline* for a healthy, balanced diet:

- 50% of total calories from complex carbohydrates: vegetables, salads, fruit, potatoes, beans, and whole grains.
- 25–30% from good-quality protein sources such as organic eggs, organic yogurt, tempeh, tofu, fish, organic skinless lean chicken and turkey, organic lean lamb and beef.
- 15–20% from healthy fats like unprocessed organic oils, avocados, and nuts.

This type of diet will create breast-protective prostaglandins, prevent fatigue, improve memory, help to burn fat, and greatly reduce cravings for sweets.

Ann Louise Gittleman, M.S., C.N.S., One of America's Leading Nutritionists, Discusses Protein's Significance in Creating Breast Health

The typical foods most women eat encourage high levels of glucose. For example, a breakfast of cereal, skim milk, and fruit; a lunch consisting of pasta and bread; and a dinner of stir-fried vegetables with maybe an ounce or two of chicken encourages the production of glucose. *Tumor cells thrive on glucose.* Nutritionist Ann Louise Gittleman warns, "Fat-free, high-carbohydrate foods raise insulin levels. Blood sugar rises. What seems to be 'quick fuel' also happens to be a source of glucose." In Gittleman's book *Your Body Knows Best* (Pocket, 1996), she warns that "commonly consumed carbohydrates such as pasta, bread, bagels, and potatoes quickly release sugar into the bloodstream." Gittleman recommends "Good, lean, high quality protein" (if meat is consumed, for example, it should be organic) and healing fats such as flaxseed oil. "When women reduce fats, we overeat carbohydrates. Overeating carbohydrates, because it raises glucose, encourages tumor growth." Gittleman emphasizes, "It is like throwing gasoline on a fire."

"Since people have been reducing fat and overeating carbohydrates, health has declined," Gittleman, who began writing about the importance of protective fats in 1988 in *Beyond Pritikin*, points out. Consider the decline in health. One in three Americans is overweight, which has increased from one in four

20 years ago. (Carbohydrates release sugar into the bloodstream. If not quickly used, the sugar is turned into body fat.) Type II diabetes has skyrocketed. More people than ever are experiencing heart attacks, viruses, and yeast infections. "I see many women in my nutritional practice who suffer enormous problems because of inadequate protective fats and carbohydrates overload," Gittleman said.

Gittleman dispels some popular myths. "Although I try to honor the moral and ethical concerns of my clients and readers, I make my dietary recommendations primarily on what seems to be best for the body. For example, although I am aware of the myriad of studies and research done on the health benefits of vegetarianism for women's health (to prevent osteoporosis, most specifically), I have simply not seen this evidenced in the new generation of vegetarians and vegans I have worked with over the years. In *Before the Change: Take Charge of Your Perimenopause* [Harper-Collins, 1998], I discuss problems regarding copper overload—often the result of a strict vegetarian diet." Gittleman continued, "The typical foods vegans eat daily—nuts, seeds, tofu, and avocado—are high in copper. I do a hair analysis in all of my clients. I always see excessive levels of copper reflected in the hair analysis in vegetarian women. Excessive copper is also increased when adrenal activity becomes depressed. Too much copper can be a factor in general immune-related problems. I feel that increased tissue levels of biounavailable copper, perhaps because it competes with zinc, may also be a factor in weakening the immune system, which can eventually lead to cancer. Copper is a mineral that is associated with estrogen." She suggests that if women are eating a high-copper diet, they should avoid copper in multivitamins and mineral dietary supplements. [Author's note: Copper can also leech from water pipes and be ingested in tap water. A point-of-use water filter can help to solve this problem. *See* the Resource Guide.]

With regard to protein, Gittleman recommends women "select mostly fermented soy products for breast health, and that vegans widen their protein choices so that soy is not consumed for breakfast, lunch, and dinner," because of her concern about copper overload and the estrogen connection. She thinks vegans would benefit by broadening their diets to include organic, free-range eggs several times a week (avoid eating just egg *whites*, she cautions—that can create allergies). Flaxseed oil on eggs is delicious.

It is also beneficial for vegetarian women to consider the inclusion of fatty-rich fish. "About 3 ½ ounces of protein per meal is a good general guideline for all women to follow," Gittleman recommends. "I think organic plain yogurt is a breast-protective source of protein. For women consuming meat, I recommend lean, organic sources of meat such as skinless, free-range, white meat chicken. Always cut the fat off, and be sure all sources of meat and dairy are organic. There should be no xenoestrogens in a breast-protective diet: no hormones, antibiotics, pesticides, or other damaging chemicals," Gittleman warns.

Another myth Gittleman was anxious to dispel is that skim milk is healthier than whole milk. "Skim milk is higher in sugar. It is not a healthy choice because it raises glucose levels," Gittleman emphasizes.

Ann Louise Gittleman's *Your Body Knows Best* is an excellent source of information about foods that rapidly increase insulin levels.

CHAPTER 13

Rejuvenating Your Immune and Lymphatic Systems: What You Can Do Now

If you are concerned about preventing breast cancer—or about preventing its recurrence—increasing nutrients and reducing exposure to harmful chemicals in your diet and environment can create the foundation for health. Providing a nutrient-dense diet supports this natural elimination of potentially harmful substances, as well as helping to repair tissues and rebuild DNA. Decreasing exposure to chemicals (as much as possible) also prevents the body's natural pollutant-discharging processes from becoming overwhelmed. The damage caused by exposure to harmful substances over the years is cumulative, but there is much you can do now to begin to limit it.

If permitted to, the body can heal itself, and we can support those efforts. Through the decisions we make every day, we can improve blood quality and help the immune system, liver, and kidneys to sustain or improve their vital functions. Increasing nutrients can help to revitalize your body's natural process of eliminating harmful substances, and also help to regenerate organs.

Nourishing Your Spirit Can Strengthen Immunity

Don't underestimate the power of the mind (and spirit), including deep breathing, positive imagery, and prayer or meditation, when it comes to maintaining well-being. Take the time to walk in the park, and to interact with supportive, loving friends and family. Research shows that the mind affects the immune system, and that relaxation and stress reduction are important to health. For information on the mind-body connection and its effect on the immune system, read *Minding the Body, Mending the Mind* by Joan Borysenko, Ph.D., and *Peace, Love, and Healing* by Bernie Siegal, M.D. *See* the Personal Care Guide for natural medicines to reduce anxiety.

> Studies show that when people are depressed, it is easier to pick up low-grade infections. When spirits are low, so is the immune system.

Reduce Overload on Internal Organs by Eliminating Harmful Substances

Begin nutritional support by reducing exposure to pesticides, chemical food additives, and other harmful substances such as trans-fats. *When the body doesn't have to work overtime detoxifying potentially harmful substances, it has much more energy to heal—especially when you are following a health-enhancing program that includes nutrient-dense foods.* Alcohol consumption (along with exposure to chemicals and pesticides) can cause liver overload. Protect your liver by eliminating these substances as much as possible. A complex of chemicals from milk thistle, known as "flavonolignans," are found in silymarin, a substance that has been intensively studied in Germany. Silymarin has been found to protect the liver against chemicals, alcohol, drugs, and even chronic hepatitis. In fact, this milk thistle extract has been thought to be liver-protective since the first century. *See* the Resource Guide to order milk thistle seeds; use them in a pepper grinder to season food.

An increasing number of studies show a correlation between hormone-sensitive cancers and chemicals used in farming, manufacturing, pest control, and industry. A study conducted in Israel showed that ten years after a 1976 ban on several types of pesticides, breast cancer decreased by 20 percent. Previous to that ban, Israeli women had one of the highest breast cancer mortality rates in the world, and concomitantly, Israeli mothers had much higher pesticide residues in their breast milk than did women in other countries. As we are now discovering, such substances may mimic estrogen in the body. Since it is impossible to avoid contact with chemicals completely, at least make sure produce, meat, and dairy are organic, and use only filtered water for drinking and cooking.

Never use plastic containers if glass is available, and certainly never heat or microwave food in plastic. Even the plastics that line food-containing cans are able to act like cancer-promoting estrogens when they enter the food supply, providing one more reason why whole foods are always best.

Tips for Rejuvenating the Body and Boosting Nutrients

The following recommendations may help strengthen your immune system and rejuvenate tissue, organs, and blood.

• Consume organic foods, when possible, to reduce exposure to pesticides.

• Eat foods that are natural and unprocessed to ensure high vitamin, mineral, and essential fatty acid content. Nutrients help the body to eliminate potentially harmful substances. A natural diet also has the advantage of not being a source of harmful substances such as food additives, colorings, fillers, and preservatives.

• Use filtered water to avoid exposure to metals from pipes (iron, lead, and copper), as well as pesticides and other lawn chemicals from ground water. Drinking clean water throughout the day aids the body's elimination processes. We are apt to avoid drinking adequate water if it has a metallic or plastic taste (like some spring water from the grocery store, bottled in plastic), or if it tastes of chemicals. Drinking adequate amounts of water—about six glasses daily—helps the body to eliminate harmful substances as quickly as possible.

• Increase fiber intake.

• Consume more flaxseeds and oil, and avoid harmful fats such as fried foods, rancid oils, and margarine. Flaxseeds and oil have the ability to discourage tumor formation, as well as help the body to eliminate cancer cells. Harmful fats and oils prevent flaxseeds and oil from penetrating tumor cell membranes and destroying the tumor cells.

• Utilize castor oil packs. (*See* the Personal Care Guide for details.) Castor oil has cleansing and regenerating properties that are discussed in detail in *The Edgar Cayce Companion* (by Edgar Cayce and B. Ernest Frejer).

• Increase raw foods and vegetable juices. They provide valuable enzymes that help to revitalize the body.

• Eat plenty of dark, leafy green vegetables. The chlorophyll in green vegetables helps the body to cleanse the colon and detoxify heavy metals.

• Add the super-food chlorella to your diet. Researchers have found biologically active substances in chlorella that assist with tissue reproduction and protect cells against some potentially harmful substances. There are many studies documenting chlorella's ability to support cell renewal and growth. I recommend a teaspoon of chlorella each morning, mixed with water or freshly made vegetable juice.

• Consume 5–10 different vegetables and fruits daily to obtain a wide spectrum of phytochemicals that help the body's detoxification processes.

• Eat sea vegetables. They contain alginic acid, which is known to absorb and eliminate some chemicals and heavy metals. Sea vegetables are also generally strengthening to the lymphatic system. To aid the detoxification process, consume delicate wakame or sturdy kombu in soups, and try delicious arame or hijiki with arugula for an exotic salad.

• Use specific nutrients. Work with a qualified nutritionist to design a personalized program.

• Reduce exposure to chemicals used on lawns and gardens. Explore horticultural oils, natural soaps, and natural pest control. Use natural cleaning products in your home.

Improving Lymphatic Vitality

The lymphatic system is a central component of the immune system and protects the body by draining and filtering out waste. Anything we can do to encourage vital and active lymph drainage is an important component of breast health.

The vessels of the lymph system, which were first identified in the mid-1600s, run throughout our body, paralleling blood vessels. Lymph fluid is transported through those vessels to the lymph nodes, which filter waste from it. The volume of lymph fluid in our bodies is actually three times greater than our blood volume; lymph fluid fills the space between the cells in the body. Since the lymph fluid eventually blends into the blood system, the quality of blood can be improved by encouraging lymphatic vitality.

It is very important in breast cancer prevention to safeguard the lymphatic system and lymph nodes. Breast cancer usually spreads to the lymph nodes first when it metastasizes.

When the lymph system cannot keep up with the level of waste within the body, the lymph nodes become tender and swollen.

Stagnation of the lymphatic system can occur when activity is reduced, as when traveling frequently, sitting for long periods, or eating heavy meals. You can improve lymphatic vitality by movement (i.e., exercise). Massage and body brushing also help to get stagnant lymph to move.

Because the lymph system is involved in fatty acid metabolism, the wrong kind of fat can impede proper functioning, causing tissues to swell because of fluid accumulation.

Margarine and other poor-quality fats can cause fluids to accumulate in the lymph system. This stagnant lymph fluid can overburden the lymphatic system, taxing our immunity. Because lymph fluid can develop a cottage cheese-like consistency, this condition is also linked to cellulite deposits right below the surface of the skin. Eliminating margarine and poor-quality fats and replacing them with health protective, freshly pressed flaxseed and other superior oils help to reduce toxic build-up in the lymph fluid.

TIP: The homeopathic remedy Silicea (6X) helps to revitalize the lymphatic system. The recommended dosage is four tablets, taken four times a day.

Increase Lymphatic Drainage

There are several points in the body to massage lightly to encourage lymphatic drainage:

- Under the arms
- Inside thighs
- Behind the knees
- The groin

Body brushing. I highly recommend daily body brushing, before showering or bathing. Once you become accustomed to body brushing, your shower won't feel complete without it. Body brushing increases circulation and encourages lymphatic detoxification. Refer to the Personal Care Guide for complete instructions for body brushing.

Self-lymphatic massage with protective essential oils and salves. Use organic almond oil as the carrier oil, and add several drops of the following essential oils, known for their lymphatic cleansing properties: tangerine (or mandarin), lemon, and bay laurel. Or try Organic Herbal Breast Massage Salves from Hygieia, which use fresh picked herbs, blossoms, and plants in infused olive oil salves. (*See* the Resource Guide.) Oil your body well, and stroke the lymphatic channels upward, beginning with the feet, moving all the way up toward the neck and jaw. Now reverse the stimulation, and stroke/massage the lymph downward, beginning from the jaw.

TIP: For a natural, herbal lymphatic massage, try a salve made in a base of dandelion, with either evergreen or St. John's wort (hypericum). *See* the Resource Guide (Hygieia).

Sitting with your feet elevated helps drainage of lymph in the groin and legs. Also, simply raising your arms for several minutes on a daily basis helps to stimulate flow of lymph under the arms.

The lymph fluid—up to three quarts daily—moves upward towards the chest. (This is why you want to brush upward during body brushing.) The lymph then drains into the bloodstream. Lymph in the head and neck drains down, toward the chest. Because the lymph depends on movement to encourage flow and has no pump (like the heart), we must help it. The natural aging process also impedes lymph flow. Exercise, muscle contraction, and a healthy, chemical-free diet encourages lymph flow. Lymphatic massage (light manual manipulation) also helps the flow to revitalize.

Foods to Help Remove Metabolic Waste

• Broccoli, oranges, carrots, spinach, and apples contain glucaric acid. Glucaric acid helps to eliminate harmful substances like pesticides.

• Consume foods that contain the strong anticancer substance *glutathione*. This potent antioxidant is protective to the liver, and helps to keep it function-ing smoothly so that toxins can't build up. Eat watermelon, asparagus, and parsley. Add asparagus to soups, steam it with leafy green vegetables, or blanch for a side dish or salad. Add parsley to vinaigrettes and salads, or consume it in fresh vegetable juice. Eat watermelon for breakfast in the summer. Milk thistle helps to increase glutathione levels.

• Vitamin C-rich foods help to cleanse the body. Foods that contain significant amounts of vitamin C also generally contain protective phytochem-icals that further protect the body. Supplemental vitamin C cannot offer this additional, profoundly important protection. The following foods are rich in vitamin C and many phytochemicals: red pepper, strawberries, oranges, cantaloupe, kiwi fruit, fresh, cooked broccoli, kale, cabbage, and Brussels sprouts.

> TIP: To preserve vitamin C, don't overcook vegetables. Steam until just tender, or if you boil, keep the water at a very gentle boil.

Things You Can Do Now to Improve Lymphatic Health

• **Consume foods in their most natural states.** Cleanse your lymph system several times a year by selecting two to three days when you eat only whole grains, raw vegetables, very lightly steamed vegetables and tofu, and fresh flaxseed oil.

• **Eliminate sugar.** Sugar can keep your lymphocytes from functioning effectively, perhaps because it prevents vitamin C from entering them, according to Alan H. Pressman, author of *The GSH Phenomenon: Nature's Most Powerful Antioxidant and Healing Agent*. Steve Rissman, N.D., of the Natural Health Clinic, Bastyr University, Seattle, told *Delicious!* magazine in October 1997 that "sugar interferes with the ability of white blood cells to get rid of bacteria."

• **Switch from table salt to unrefined, unheated mineral salt.** Heating salt, part of the process of refining table salt, encourages hardening of body tissues, including lymph glands. For more information on salt, *see* Chapter 18, "Secrets of a Healthy Kitchen."

• **Deep breathing** increases oxygen within the body, encouraging movement of lymph fluids. Breathe deeply, through the nose.

• **Explore acupuncture.** Studies indicate that it increases lymphatic cleansing.

• **Consider lymph drainage therapy.** Lymph drainage therapy is done by delicate manipulation of the lymphatic glands to reduce waste. (*See* the Resource Guide for information on seminars on lymphatic drainage therapy) Lymph drainage therapy has been practiced in Europe for decades. This gentle palpating of the lymph glands and system rejuvenates and strengthens our natural defenses.

• **Exercise:**
   Brisk walking can encourage stagnant lymph to move through the body.
   Rebound exercise has been found to be the most effective method of lymphatic circulation stimulation because the body is subjected to a change in velocity and direction twice, with each jump. This exercise is similar to the use of a trampoline, but has been found to be more efficient and safer. The gentle stimulation is very different from the jolting and jumping you see with a trampoline. (*See* the Resource Guide for information on the Health Circulator.)

Lymphatic Power Teas

• **Ginger tea** is a lymph gland cleanser. Combine 1/2 teaspoon freshly grated organic ginger with 6–8 ounces of boiling water. Cover and steep for 12 minutes. Strain and drink.

• **Lymphatic teas:** Combine red root and organic orange peel with a touch of ginger juice in filtered water. (One part herbal blend to five parts water.) Simmer for 15 minutes. Cover with a bamboo mat and steep for 10 minutes. Strain and add several drops of echinacea tincture.

For strengthening lymphatic circulation, cleavers and violet leaves can help to protect the breasts from potentially harmful substances by redirecting them away from the breasts to the liver (for elimination), according to the *Vegetarian Times* (July 1997). Place approximately ½–¾ teaspoon of each herb into a cup or mug. Add 4–6 ounces of boiling water. Cover with a bamboo mat or plate for 20 minutes; strain and drink. Other herbs that have general cleansing properties are nettles, dandelion root or leaf, and red root.

• **Red root extract:** Known as blood purifying and cleansing, it helps to discharge waste from the lymph. Extract of red root is recommended for lymphatic health: 25 drops, three times a day. (*See* the Resource Guide to order Herb Pharm's red root extract from NEED's Pharmacy.)

- **Echinacea:** A tincture of echinacea, rather than capsule form, is recommended, at a dose of 10–20 drops three times a day.
- **Silica Homeopathic** helps cleanse the lymph.
- **Bach's Crab Apple** is suggested for lymphatic drainage by Carolyn Heller West, knowledgeable nutritionist and Bach Flower Remedy expert. (*See* the Resource Guide.)

> TIP: Asparagus is a cleansing food for the lymphatic system.

Sauna Detoxification

Saunas help to release pesticides and other chemicals that accumulate in the body from foods and the environment. Lighten the burden of the lymphatic system by encouraging removal of these substances. If you don't have access to a sauna, try a steam bath or regular hot Epsom salt baths, to induce sweating. Heat strengthens immunity by killing pathogens and aiding the excretion of harmful substances like pesticides. (*See* the Resource Guide for information on ordering soft-heat saunas.)

> TIP: A hot cup of ginger tea effectively encourages sweating while bathing.

Breast Structure and Lymph Nodes

There are six to nine overlapping sections, called lobes, that make up each breast. Smaller lobules, containing dozens of milk-producing bulbs, make up each lobe. There are tiny, thin tubes called "ducts" that are found throughout each lobe, lobule and bulb, linking them together. Blood vessels and lymph vessels also make up breast tissue. The lymph vessels are connected to lymph nodes (small and bean-shaped) which are clustered together in the chest, under the arms, above the collarbone, and in many other parts of the body.

Does Wearing a Bra Impede Lymphatic Flow?

The Case for Bralessness
Can wearing a bra many hours a day increase women's risk of developing breast cancer? Sydney Ross Singer, Ph.D., and Soma Grismaijer interviewed 4,500 women for their book *Dressed to Kill: The Link Between Bras and*

Breast Cancer. They found that women who wore a bra for more than twelve hours a day had a nineteen times greater risk of developing breast cancer than women who wore a bras less than twelve hours a day. Women who never wore bras had the most protection. Based on statistical observations, the authors theorized that wearing a bra depletes and constricts lymphatic drainage in the breasts. Because the breasts are especially sensitive to the accumulation of fat-soluble toxins, owing to the fatty tissue that makes up the breast, perhaps not wearing a bra means that lymph flow in the breasts will be less restricted. Thus the removal of potentially harmful chemicals from breast tissue will be encouraged.

Questioning the Singer and Grismaijer Study

Adriane Fugh-Berman, M.D., a Washington, D.C.-based medical researcher who specializes in women's health and alternative medicine and the author of *Alternative Medicine: What Works* (Odonian Press), took issue with Singer and Grismaijer's theory. In a column in *Bottom Line* (March 1997), Dr. Fugh-Berman had some questions about how the study was conducted. Dr. Fugh-Berman felt no effort was made to ensure the women in the two groups were "matched" properly: that is, had similar family histories, were of similar ages, and had similar risks for breast cancer. She felt that these issues would have disqualified the study from being published in a reputable medical journal.

What to Think?

My conclusion is that, even though Singer and Grismaijer's study was not published in a medical journal and may have been conducted in a less-than-airtight way, perhaps there is still something we can learn from their book, *Dressed to Kill.* Certainly, in the meantime, some women may want to wear bras fewer hours in the day, and purchase bras that aren't constricting, until we have more information.

CHAPTER 14

The French Mediterranean Diet: Natural Food at Its Best

Enjoying Natural Foods: Marianne's Story

Working with women who want to improve their health by improving their diets is extremely rewarding. My greatest pleasure is being a catalyst for such positive change. Another pleasure is being able to dispel the myth that natural foods taste boring! Let me tell you about one of my clients, Marianne Hickey. Marianne's changes in diet and health are chronicled in detail in *Gary Null's Encyclopedia of Alternative Health* (Kensington).

Marianne had some chronic health problems when she initially consulted me. She was really upset about being on a variety of medications that did not seem to be helping her. In fact, as time went by, Marianne appeared to be getting worse instead of better. She was ready to try anything, including drastic changes in her diet. Marianne was empowered to change by her need to claim responsibility for her own health, and as a result, she explored natural foods cooking in depth. Because she was so struck by the discovery that she could positively influence her health by improving her diet, Marianne worked to build a repertoire of delicious, healthy recipes. Marianne's health steadily improved as the quality of her diet improved, and she has been off her medication for more than four years.

When I first met with Marianne, I told her (as I tell all my clients) that a truly healthy, natural foods diet utilizes the best of ingredients: lots of really fresh vegetables; robust flavors, such as lemon and garlic and herbs; beautiful, fresh fish; servings of whole grain (to replace French fries); and lots of salads. I pointed out to Marianne that natural foods cooking is exemplified by the delicious cuisines of the Mediterranean. The best chefs from the top restaurants in the world look to Mediterranean cuisine for inspiration. Beginning with the French Mediterranean, let us examine the aspects of these foods and food preparation techniques that are so protective of health.

A REPORT FROM SOUTHERN FRANCE

The French Riviera, redolent of lavender and thyme, is blessed with the most wonderfully healthy foods imaginable. It doesn't seem surprising that the people who live in such relaxed and beautiful surroundings are healthy. The rates of breast cancer and heart disease are much lower in the Mediterranean than they are in North America. An important reason for this may be diet. People living in the sixteen Mediterranean countries don't consume processed foods, partially hydrogenated cheese spreads, or other junk foods like most Americans. Instead, they frequent farmers' markets that offer the most extensive varieties of fresh, beautiful produce, herbs, fish, and whole grains. Healthy eating is simply a part of the Mediterranean way of life.

Weekly and even daily farmers' markets are commonplace in the region. In Cannes, on a 400-year-old stone floor, the Marche Forville is a riotously colorful, aromatic, and noisy display of regional foods: vegetables, fruits, mushrooms, honey, herbs, fresh goat's cheese, and even essential oils. Every square foot of this very large market is filled with display counters, stalls, and truck beds proffering the greatest variety of food to be found anywhere. The Marche Forville market is a living tribute to the proud heritage of the region's farmers and artisans.

The Widest Variety of Vegetables Imaginable: Marche Forville Farmers Market

Strolling through the long aisles and observing the strikingly beautiful flower displays, colorful produce, glistening olives, and aromatic fresh goat's cheese, I was struck anew by the health benefits of the Mediterranean diet. Stall after stall contained the most incredible dark leafed greens, including spinach, turnip, beet, and dandelion; bitter greens (some wild, and many with French names I could not readily translate into English); a variety of alliums, including garlic, green onions (with the big white root bulbs), chives (rich in vitamin A), shallots, leeks, scallions, and onions; daikon and red radishes; big, round orange squash and turnips; all sorts of potatoes; fennel (including wild, young, smaller types); a huge selection of asparagus; amazing amounts of fresh sardines (rich in protective fish oils); freshly pressed olive oil in brown or green glass; selenium-rich mushrooms (both cultivated and wild); unpasteurized, fresh chevre (goat's cheese), full of living, healthy enzymes, wrapped in chestnut leaves tied with raffia; and lots of antioxidant-rich herbs and peppers.

The Restaurants of Cannes

Classic Moroccan, Provençal, Vietnamese, Chinese, Italian—Cannes presents so many choices of cuisines! Whatever the ethnic influence, seafood predominates, as it does in the regional fare, which features seafood flavored with garlic, herbs, and olive oil. Meat is usually small amounts of chicken or lamb, from naturally raised animals. Salads are available in abundance. Lunch is often simply a large salad, perhaps salade Niçoise, with tuna and spinach. Salad is usually the first course at dinner as well; it typically includes dandelion greens (rich in minerals and cancer-fighting phytochemicals) and onions and/ or chives (which have strong anticancer, anticholesterol properties). Lunch or dinner's main course generally consists of poached, steamed, or stewed seafood accompanied by fresh vegetables. Olive oil is the oil of choice, and it is revealing that much food preparation is done without using heated oil. There seems to be a pervasive, unwritten rule that keeps sautéing to a minimum; when necessary, only olive oil or a small amount of butter is used. Although the French love bread and consume as much of it as Americans do, the rest of their diet includes plenty of fresh vegetables and fruits—much more than we eat!

A Table in the Kitchen

At La Palme d'Or, considered by many to be the best restaurant in Cannes, I had the unique experience of eating at the chef's table in the heart of the kitchen. For nearly four hours, I watched Chef Christian Willer and his staff prepare five-course, mouth-watering meals of imaginatively combined and presented foods. The defining moment of each course seemed to occur when the Chef personally anointed each dish with freshly pressed olive oil (bottled in opaque glass) before serving. Very little of our meal had sautéed ingredients.

La Palme D'or can boast an incredibly clean, healthy, and smoke-free kitchen. Not only was it a wonderful evening and a delicious repast, but it was more educational than any cooking class I have ever attended.

Even Fast Food in Cannes Boasts a Healthy Use of Oils

With the exception of McDonald's, which recently opened in Cannes, the French approach to fast food is unique, and it's anything but unhealthy. When residents don't have time to cook, they generally stop into an *épicerie*, or deli, that carries prepared food. Foods sold in these shops are made daily; typical items include a seafood salad (generally consisting of shrimp, calamari, scallops, and red pepper, and occasionally a little corn, with a light olive oil vinaigrette), or raw vegetable salads of beets and onions, grated carrots, red cabbage, and other fresh vegetables. Additional "fast foods"—bouillabaisse and risotto, resplendent with shrimp, clams, and squid; pizza with onions and anchovies; fresh sardines prepared in countless ways; the most appetizing seafood; and prepared vegetables (asparagus, green beans, artichokes, and fennel)—can be purchased fresh daily at the local *épicerie*.

Back to the USA: Junk Food and Fats

Flying out of Nice, one of my last images of the French Mediterranean was an airport worker, carrying a lunch tray back to her office. On her tray was a piece of roasted chicken breast and a large serving of bright green beans. This contrasted sharply with my initial image of New York City's Kennedy Airport—a long row of ugly steel vending machines offering corn chips, peanuts, crackers with cheese spread, and candy, all full of trans-fats and rancid, chemically altered oil.

The Mediterranean Gift of Combining Fresh Vegetables: Creative and Delicious

The French have a simple, natural way of combining fresh ingredients to create some of the most enjoyable foods in the world. The Mediterranean use of vegetables, seafood, and herbs results in truly healthy eating. The vine-ripened tomatoes must surely be the juiciest found anywhere in the world.

Consider, for example, the following combinations:

Salade Niçoise

- Spinach
- Green pepper strips
- Ripe tomatoes (Ripe produce has been shown in studies to contain much greater amounts of phytochemicals than produce picked before it's ripe.)
- Minced celery
- Olives
- Hard-boiled eggs
- Onions
- Tuna
- Vinaigrette: olive oil, red wine vinegar, lemon, and a touch of mustard

Salade Verte

- Mixed mesclun greens
- Minced parsley
- Sweet onion (The French Mediterraneans eat lots of raw onions—probably half a cup a day—which offer many health benefits.)
- Tomatoes
- Dressing: lots of lemon, garlic, and a drizzle of olive oil

Salade Compose

- Spinach
- Butter lettuce
- Tomatoes
- Marinated scallops (lightly broiled)
- Artichokes, surrounding the plate
- Garnish with very thin shavings of cheese
- Aioli dressing: Lots of raw garlic, touch of Dijon mustard, egg yolks, olive oil, lemon, and freshly ground black pepper

Simple Salads

- Grated raw carrot salad
- Thinly sliced beets, cooked until just soft and lightly drizzled with olive oil and lemon, simply seasoned with sea salt and ground pepper
- Thinly sliced, crisp cucumber salad
- Asparagus and green beans

Simple Side Vegetable Dish to Accompany Entrée

A melange of the following perfectly cooked vegetables (*legumes*, in French), with the lightest touch of olive oil or butter:

- Leeks
- Turnips
- Zucchini
- Beans
- Carrots

Green Bean Salad with Arugula

- A mixture of arugula, sweet onion, and juicy red tomatoes topped with bright, fresh greenbeans, cooked to crisp perfection
- Vinaigrette: Olive oil, red wine vinegar, touch of Dijon mustard

Salad of Lightly Cooked Shrimp in a Bed of Greens and Herbs

- Melange of greens
- Delicate mixture of fresh herbs, such as baby wild fennel leaves, marjoram, touch of tarragon
- Plum tomatoes that were lightly prepared by deseeding, peeling, and then marinating in a little olive oil, sea salt, herbs, and lemon
- Shrimp (slow cooking by braising in the oven, says Chef Christian Willer at La Palme d'Or, gives a much softer texture to the shrimp and also complements the freshness of the seafood)
- Vinaigrette: extra virgin olive oil and balsamic vinegar

Lycopene, a phytochemical in tomatoes, has been strongly linked to a reduced risk of certain types of cancer (breast, prostate, colon, and rectal). Lycopene is a more potent antioxidant than beta carotene and offers protection against free radicals.

Mediterranean Power Foods

Abundant research has shown that these foods—rich in phytonutrients, phytochemicals, essential fatty acids, and fiber—may lower the chance of developing breast cancer.

Vegetables

An impressive variety of fresh vegetables is consumed daily in the Mediterranean, in soups, salads, side dishes, stews, as crudités with dips (as opposed to the chips and prepackaged dips, containing trans-fats, that Americans consume), and garnishes. Mireille Johnston, author of *Cuisine of the Sun*, points out, "Some Niçois residents claim they know more than seventy ways to cook vegetables." Vegetables are also used to thicken sauces and stews, rather than richer thickeners that incorporate butter, flour, and cream.

> TIP: In place of heavy butter and cream, use puréed vegetables to thicken sauces as they do in the Mediterranean.

Alliums: onions, leeks, scallions, chives, and green onions. These extremely popular foods are eaten daily in the Mediterranean. A salad will frequently contain both onions and chives, which are especially rich in vitamin A. Active compounds found in alliums stimulate the production of enzymes that are responsible for neutralizing free radicals linked to cancer development. Research shows that the best way to consume these compounds without deactivating them is to eat them raw, and the French are happy to comply.

Artichokes. This vegetable's bitter taste stimulates and aids digestion by encouraging secretion of gastric juices. Artichokes are said to "tonify" the digestive process.

Asparagus. High in selenium, a breast cancer-protective phytonutrient that also cleanses the body of cholesterol, according to Paul Pitchford (author of *Healing with Whole Foods: Oriental Traditions and Modern Nutrition*), asparagus also helps to cleanse the lymphatic system and has bitter properties which are healing for the liver.

Green beans. Very popular and exceptionally delicious, green beans are a darker, vivid green in France. Green beans contain strong anticancer phytonutrients.

Beets. Grated, raw beets, a very popular salad and fast food in the south (available in all *épiceries*), strengthen both immune and liver health.

Bitter and spicy greens. Endive, frisée, and rocket (arugula) are very popular. These foods aid digestion and stimulate the liver.

> Raw chives, rich in vitamin A, are wonderful tossed with bright green, lightly blanched green beans, then drizzled with olive oil and lemon, or used as a garnish on poached or soft-boiled eggs.

Cabbage family: broccoli, cabbage, cauliflower, bok choy, collard greens, rutabaga, kale, daikon and salad radishes, mustard greens, turnips, and watercress. These immune-strengthening foods are part of daily French Mediterranean fare. They are known to prevent the initiation and growth of cancers. Some of the breast-protective phytonutrients contained in these foods are indoles, flavonoids, polyphenols, antioxidants, isothiocyanates, chlorophyll, lutein, and beta carotene.

Solanaceae vegetables. Plenty of tomatoes, eggplant, and peppers are eaten in southern France. These vegetables are rich in bioflavonoids, and may contain other phytonutrients that are also anticarcinogenic. Tomatoes, used in many Mediterranean dishes, are wonderful anticancer foods, and frequent consumption correlates strongly with lessened risk of cancer.

Spinach. A lot of carotene-rich spinach—raw and cooked—is consumed on the Riviera. Studies show women who consume the most spinach have the lowest rates of endometrial and cervical cancer. Spinach contains a large amount of lutein, and is three times richer in cancer-protective carotenes than even carrots. Spinach, along with other vegetables and fresh tuna, is often served in salad Niçoise.

TIP: Consuming carotene-rich foods with extra virgin olive oil or flax-seed oil (or any other fresh, unprocessed oil) helps to utilize the powerful benefits of carotenes because they are oil-soluble. Be sure to enjoy your salad Niçoise with plenty of vinaigrette made with health-giving fresh oils.

Potatoes. Since the Mediterraneans don't eat tofu or soybeans, it is interesting to note that their low rates of breast and other cancers may be attributed in part to their consumption of potatoes. Potatoes contain protease inhibitors that are just as effective as soybean protease inhibitors. Traditional French Mediterranean fare includes potatoes served either cold (in salade Niçoise, for example) or warm (as a side dish or in stews). Susun Weed points out in *Breast Cancer? Breast Health! The Wise Woman Way* that virtually every member of the potato family has, at some point in history, been regarded as a cure for cancer, even the poisonous ones (such as Belladonna atropa). Small amounts of potatoes can be consumed as part of a green vegetable-based diet, and *no*—French fries are not considered to be breast-protective.

Purslane. Another wild food, these delicate, vivid greens are eaten raw with salads. Don't cook purslane; it does not hold its shape or flavor when heated. This vegetable is an excellent source of omega-3 fatty acids, carotenes, glutathione, and antioxidants, all of which are powerfully cancer protective.

Umbelliferal vegetables: fennel, parsnips, winter squash, carrots, celery and celery leaves, and parsley. Epidemiological studies show these vegetables, rich in beta carotene and chlorophyll, may be effective against certain cancers. Celery leaves are often induded in salads and other dishes in the Mediterranean; they contain powerful anticancer agents that emulsify cancer-initiating chemicals and carry them out of the body. Polyphenols in carrots, celery, and parsley are foods that protect DNA against potential carcinogens.

Winter squash. Orange-fleshed pumpkin, butternut, and other hard-rind squash provide an abundance of cancer-protective antioxidants and carotenes.

Wild vegetables. Dandelions, wild chicory (also popular in Greece, known as horta), tiny wild asparagus, and field lettuce ("lamb's tongue") are particularly rich in minerals and phytochemicals that guard against cancer. Dandelions, eaten often in the Mediterranean, have been found to be especially beneficial for the breasts; this food can reverse cancerous changes and stop the promotion of oncogenes (genes that contribute to the development of cancer).

Fruit

Rutin is a powerful antioxidant that has been shown in animal studies to inhibit early stages of breast cancer. It is found in two popular French Mediterranean fruits, grapes and berries (as well as in broccoli).

Berries. Among members of the berry family, raspberries and strawberries contain rutin. Wild strawberries, strawberries, raspberries, blackberries, and other berries also contain catechins, antioxidants that prevent the initiation of cancers. Strawberries can actually prevent the formation of powerful, cancer-causing agents in the body.

Grapes. Cancer-protective ellagic acid (known to scavenge cancer causing agents), antioxidants, and trace minerals, such as breast-protective selenium, are found in grapes. Consumption of significant amounts of grapes is said to provide strong protection against recurrence of cancer and actually put primary tumors into remission. Dr. Gary D. Stoner at the Medical College of Ohio, Toledo, has found that ellagic acid works best when added to the system before exposure to cancerous chemicals. OPCs (oligomeric proanthocyanidins) are among the most protective antioxidants; they can be obtained from red grapes. Grape with seeds are widely available in the Mediterranean, and grape seeds are full of protective OPCs. Unfortunately, most grocery stores in the United States now offer seedless grapes almost exclusively. For more information on OPCs, *see* Chapter 9, "The Hidden Power of Plant Foods."

Red Grapes: The Folkloric "Grape Cure"

In 1928, South African naturopath Johanna Brandt came to the United States and published a book, *The Grape Cure*, which recommended a combination of fasting and consuming only grapes to heal cancer. The success of her extreme approach to healing cancer is only anecdotal.

OPCs extracted from grape seed have been found to benefit a variety of health problems, including breast cancer. For more on how OPCs benefit health, *see* Chapter 9, "The Hidden Power of Plant Foods."

Other fruits that contain anticancer phytochemicals include:

Apricots. Apricots' anticancer carotenes are particularly potent in the dried fruit.

Lemons. These tart fruits provide liver protection and contain flavonoids that are anticancer and immunosupportive.

Melons. The flavor of small, delicious, southern French melons are known throughout France; they contain cancer-protective phytonutrients (like vitamin C).

Orange peel. The peel is actually the most medicinal part of the orange, containing oils that help break down carcinogens. Orange peel is frequently used to flavor stews or as a light addition to marinades. *Science News* (May 1993) reported that the limonene in orange peel can prevent and reduce breast cancer. Susun Weed points out in *Breast Cancer? Breast Health! The Wise Woman Way* that traditional Chinese medicine has employed orange peel for its anticancer properties for hundreds of years.

> TIP: Use organic orange peels by mincing them into thin strips and mixing into salads, steeping in teas *(see* Chapter 16, "Power Teas"), or using in marinades.

Seasoning Herbs

Mediterranean meals (except breakfast) contain a wide variety of fresh herbs. In addition to providing no-calorie flavor to foods, herbs and spices help to suppress cancer growth by acting as neutralizers of free radicals. For more information on specific phytochemicals in these herbs and how they help to prevent breast cancer, *see* Chapter 10, "Herbs, Spices, and Mushrooms: Potent Enhancers of Flavor and Health."

Basil is used often in Mediterranean cooking, especially in combination with tomatoes.

Bay laurel, also known as "true bay," contains protective phytochemicals, and is frequently used in preparing stews and marinades.

Herbs de la Provence combines rosemary and thyme; this distinctive combination, always used in regional herbal blends, is particularly rich in protective, anticancer antioxidants.

Hot red and green peppers contain carotenoids, flavonoids, and Vitamin C. Vietnamese cuisine, which is popular in France and other countries on the Riviera, frequently utilizes hot peppers. Olive oil bottled with a generous amount of dried red peppers is used as a condiment for salads and vegetables.

Juniper berries (*genièure* in French) have long been used for healing and purification; even the fragrance was thought to help prevent disease. In *Aromatherapy, A Complete Guide to the Healing Art*, Kathi Keville and Mindy Green

point out that, until World War II, the French burned juniper berries in their
hospitals as an antiseptic. Used in many recipes to marinate foods, juniper
berries are high in vitamin C. Traditionally, they have been used as a diuretic,
to stimulate the flow of urine and to treat gout caused by high uric acid levels
(uric acid is secreted in urine). Gin was actually created by a Dutch pharmacist
by mistake. He was attempting to combine juniper berries with alcohol to
sell as a diuretic!

Nutmeg contains anticancer agents; it is always used freshly grated.

Rosemary, used in a variety of ways in Provence, has been shown in animal
studies to stop mammary tumors from developing.

Turmeric, used in the Moroccan couscous and stews which are very popular
throughout the French Mediterranean, contains potent anticancer phytonutrients.

Other Cancer-Protective Foods of the Mediterranean

Breast-Protective Fatty Acids. Mediterraneans consume a variety of foods
that are rich in beneficial fatty acids, such as sardines, tuna, salmon, olives
and olive oil, avocado, walnuts and walnut oil, and purslane. The basic
Mediterranean diet is high in substances that aid utilization of fatty acids—
such as antioxidant rich vegetables and herbs—and low in substances that
work against it, like saturated fats, sugar, trans-fats (margarine, hydrogenated
and partially hydrogenated oils), and fried foods. Therefore, metabolism of
beneficial fatty acids is optimized.

> A bonus that sardines offer for breast cancer prevention is that they
> are high in vitamin D. Research has shown that vitamin D is beneficial
> in preventing breast cancer.

Chickpeas. These legumes are frequently eaten in hummus, as well as in
Moroccan couscous restaurants; they are one of the richest sources of breast-
protective protease inhibitors.

Eggs. No one can deny that heart disease is virtually nonexistent throughout
the Mediterranean, or that eggs are regularly consumed. Although omelets
are popular in Provence, eggs are generally boiled (as in salad Niçoise) or
unheated (in mayonnaise) or heated gently (in crème Anglais). Nutritionally,
eggs are considered an almost perfect food, containing an incredible balance
of nutrients: vitamin A, breast-protective vitamin D, thiamin, lecithin, and
iron. The lecithin in eggs speeds the detoxification of fat-soluble chemicals
such as organochlorines. Additionally, the chances are good that eggs eaten
in the Mediterranean are organic.

Enzyme-rich salads and raw foods. Lunch in the French Mediterranean is often just a large fresh salad, featuring tomatoes, rocket (arugula), raw onions, radishes, tomatoes (with breast-protective lycopene), onions, boiled potatoes, green beans, and tuna, drizzled with fresh, unprocessed olive oil, and lemon—delicious! If lunch isn't just a large salad, then salad is luncheon's first course, followed by an entree course. Dinner generally follows the same pattern, beginning with salad, followed by the entree.

> Mediterraneans consume large amounts of raw foods, herbs, and garlic, which offer an abundance of beneficial enzymes.

Another favorite presentation of raw foods is as crudités (slices of raw vegetables, substituted for trans-fatty-acid-containing corn chips, crackers, or potato chips) with dips, for a healthy appetizer. The love of raw foods runs so deep in the French Mediterranean that a radish is often presented with stem and tiny leaf still attached. (In macrobiotics, the part of the stem that joins the radish—or turnip—is thought to contain the most healing benefits. Do the French know something intuitively?) Raw foods provide breast-protective enzymes and antioxidant vitamin C. Even though the French are known to eat smaller portions of food than we do, this is not true for the salads they love so much!

Fresh goat's cheese. Rich in naturally occurring enzymes and made from organic, unpasteurized milk, goat's cheese is a daily food in southern France. Fresh cheese does not contain the oxidized (aged) cholesterol found in aged cheese; oxidized cholesterol is the type that is so detrimental to health.

Garlic. The National Cancer Institute recognizes that garlic offers protection against cancer. Garlic has been shown in studies to prevent cancer at all stages (initiation, promotion, and recurrence). It contains allylsulfides and antioxidants as well as selenium and germanium. Remember, selenium is the breast-protective mineral that lowers the incidence of breast cancer. Garlic also contains isoflavones. (Because tofu is not popular in the French Mediterranean, it's important to note that women get breast-protective isoflavones from another food in their daily diet—garlic.) Garlic is often eaten raw, minced in small amounts into vinaigrettes.

Lentils. These legumes are extremely rich in phytochemicals and nutrients known to be breast-cancer-protective: genistein, lignans, and protease inhibitors. Many different types of lentils have shown breast-protective results. Lentils can repair damaged DNA, reverse cellular changes from effects of cancer, and repair damaged cells. Lentil soup is extremely popular throughout the Meditenranean.

Mushrooms. Many different types of wild mushrooms, gathered by expert foragers, are rich in anticancer phytochemicals and nutrients such as selenium, antioxidants, and lignans. Other compounds found in mushrooms are also anticarcinogenic, helping to enhance immune functioning and to slow the growth of tumors.

> ### Small Amounts of Lean Lamb Provide an Antioxidant
>
> Lipoic acid, an antioxidant nutrient, was first studied by Dr. Lester Packer at the University of Berkeley. In 1993, Dr. Packer found that lipoic acid can have a protective effect on our genes. There are only two food sources of lipoic acid: red meat and yeast.
>
> Because the French Mediterraneans eat small amounts of red meat, usually lamb, several times a week, they are regularly obtaining the benefits of lipoic acid. Remember, the Mediterranean diet is low in saturated fat, partly because the amount of beef or lamb (which is usually more available than beef) they eat is extremely small compared to the amount of meat consumed by Americans. Conjugated linoleic acid (CLA) is especially rich in lamb. This compound is thought to help protect against breast cancer. Even small amounts of meat can provide the important nutrients it contains; consuming large amounts of meat, however, with its high levels of saturated fat, is linked to illnesses like heart disease.

Mediterranean Consumption of Fats and Oils

The Paradigm: Breast and Heart Healthy

Traditional Mediterranean fare does not contain the dangerous trans-fats found in the junk foods we eat in North America. The diet consists of whole, natural, very fresh foods, primarily fish, vegetables, garlic, herbs, and olive oil.

What the Mediterraneans Are Not Eating

• Partially hydrogenated vegetable oils: Many restaurants in North America use this cheap oil for frying. A doughnut contains 5 grams of trans-fats.

• Shortening: Used in prepared foods, and recommended for cake and brownie mixes. Shortening contains 1 gram of trans-fats per tablespoon.

• Margarine: Still used in place of butter, margarine contains trans-fats.

• Packaged microwave munchies: Microwave popcorn contains almost 2 grams of trans-fats per four-cup serving.

• Snack foods: Corn chips, cheese puffs, and crackers may contain up to 6 grams of trans-fats. Trans-fats are added to these junk foods to give them "body."

• Candy: Most chocolate contains partially hydrogenated fat to give it shape, as well as to promote shelf life; therefore, it also contains trans-fats.

Many "cholesterol-free" foods are sources of hidden trans-fats. For heart health, do as the Mediterraneans do: Consume a diet of whole, unprocessed foods and oils. Trans-fats have the same harmful effects on heart health as do saturated fats, raising LDL (bad cholesterol) and lowering HDL (good cholesterol).

The Healthy Fat Mediterraneans Eat: Olive Oil

For 6,000 years, olive oil has been the oil of choice throughout the Mediterranean. Mediterranean people are slender, even though they consume up to four times the amount of olive oil as Americans. Olive oil helps to metabolize the fat-soluble vitamins A and D, which create lustrous, beautiful skin and hair.

Unfortunately, olive oil consumption may be dwindling in the French Mediterranean, as consumption of cheaper sunflower or grape seed oils increases. Young Mediterraneans are developing a taste for French fries and hamburgers, which can be found in newly opening fast food restaurants.

Olive oil's profile shows some of the reasons it is such a health-giving oil:

• Contains oleic acid (omega-9), a monounsaturated, nonessential stable fatty acid (MUFA).
• It is a relatively stable oil for sautéeing.
• Contains LA (omega-6).
• Contains "minor ingredients" (making up less than 2% of the oil) that offer important health benefits. These minor ingredients:
• Improve liver function and bile flow, important in processing unhealthy forms of estrogen into safer forms vital for breast cancer prevention.
• Improve gall bladder function.
• Improve our hearts and arteries.

Some of those "minor ingredients" are: phytosterols, which help to prevent cholesterol absorption from food; the heart-protective phytosterol precursor squalene; chlorophyll, which contains magnesium and other nutrients; vitamin

E, an antioxidant that is heart- and artery-protective; and beta carotene, also an antioxidant.

Since the 1950s, studies have shown the Mediterranean people's use of olive oil to be heart protective. Subsequent studies have determined the specific benefits of olive oil in maintaining heart health.

Olive Oil and Heart Health

Olive oil:

- Increases HDL, good cholesterol.
- Lowers blood pressure.
- Thins the blood, helping to prevent dangerous blood clots that can lodge in coronary arteries!
- Stimulates enzyme production in the pancreas.
- Helps liver function.
- Protects against the peroxidation of cholesterol (and fatty acids) and decreases cholesterol absorption from foods.

Death rates from heart disease in the Mediterranean are one-half to one-third lower than in Northern Europe or the United States. A study conducted in Lyon, France (The Lyon Diet Heart Study), found there was a 76 percent reduction in heart attacks in patients following the Mediterranean diet with olive oil, compared to those following the American Heart Association's diet, which is much lower in fat. This is of great significance for all women, since heart attacks claim more lives every year than breast cancer. In fact, women with a family history of breast cancer (or any hormone-sensitive cancer) may be hesitant about taking the artificial hormones generally recommended at menopause to prevent heart disease. It is important to note that prevention of heart attacks or strokes can also be accomplished by diet and lifestyle choices.

Olive Oil and Breast Cancer

Olive oil has been shown to help prevent breast cancer. While more studies need to be done to state unequivocally that consuming olive oil will prevent breast cancer, Dr. Antonia Trichopoulou of the Harvard School of Public Health wrote an editorial in the June 1995 issue of the journal *Cancer Causes and Control* noting that, since mid-1994, four important studies—one from Greece, one from Italy, and two from Spain—have demonstrated a beneficial effect of olive oil consumption on breast cancer risk. Dr. Trichopoulou also noted that vegetables are frequently consumed with olive oil in these countries, and pointed out that consuming large amounts of vegetables also plays a role in reducing cancer risk. "Nevertheless, the necessary caution should not overshadow the fact that the existing evidence converges in support of a protective role of olive oil against breast cancer," Dr. Trichopoulou concludes.

It's also been shown that women who consume olive oil at more than one meal a day have a much lower rate of breast cancer than women who use it less frequently. A study published in the *Journal of the National Cancer Institute* reported that breast cancer rates were 25% lower among Greek women who consumed olive oil more than once a day, according to researchers from the Harvard School of Public Health and from the University of Athens in Greece. (It's important to note that women in Greece consume a diet that's much higher in fat than American women's diet, but much of that fat is from olive oil.) These researchers also reported that the women who ate the most vegetables had a 48% lower cancer risk. Studies in Spain and Italy have resulted in similar findings.

A 1995 study of breast cancer in Greece found that consumption of olive oil, vegetables, and fruits strongly correlated with reduced breast cancer risk. Margarine intake, however, is associated with an increased risk of breast cancer. Epidemiological studies have found that olive oil offers protection against lung, ovarian, and colon cancers. Colorectal cancer rates are lower in the Mediterranean compared with most countries in the West. A 1998 study published in the *Archives of Internal Medicine* found that a diet containing olive oil can reduce a woman's breast cancer risk by as much as 50%.

The Mediterranean Essential Fatty Acid Profile

The type of fat consumed is important in preventing breast cancer. Excessive amounts of saturated fat and processed oils promote breast cancer. Unprocessed olive oil, omega-3-rich sardines, tuna, purslane, and walnuts—all foods that are all part of the Mediterranean diet—help to prevent breast cancer.

In the United States, high intake of processed, omega-6, junk fats and oils, margarine and trans-fats in packaged foods, and too-little consumption of omega-3-rich foods has given Americans a very unhealthy fatty acid profile. In fact, most women in North America are deficient in breast-protective omega-3 essential fatty acid.

The fatty acid profile of the Mediterranean people is much healthier than our own. Let us consider some of the differences:

• Lower intake of saturated fat. A diet low in saturated fat is linked to lower levels of breast cancer. Mediterraneans consume smaller portions of meat and eat it less frequently than we do. They also eat less dairy.

• Consumption of unprocessed, antioxidant-rich olive oil. Studies show consumption of unprocessed olive oil, together with a whole foods, vitamin-rich diet, to be breast protective.

• Greater consumption of omega-3-rich fish.

• Fatty fish contains protective oils, which numerous studies found to prevent breast cancer, heart disease, arthritis, and more.

• Greater consumption of purslane and walnuts, other omega-3-rich foods.

• Lower consumption of heated oil. Heated oil blocks the benefits of healing fats and oils and contains many toxic substances.

• Little or no consumption of trans-fatty acids, linked to cancer and heart disease.

High Consumption of Health-Protective Fish

The Mediterraneans eat at least twice as much fish as we do, and much of the fish they eat—such as sardines, cod, tuna, and salmon—is rich in breast-protective fish oils. (The salmon available in the Mediterranean is from Norway. It is far richer in beneficial fish oils than the farm-raised variety becoming popular in the United States.)

Mediterraneans also consume a rich condiment of sardines and anchovies, an age-old dish called pissolat. It's a home-made jelly of rich, flavorful fish fats, olive oil, and herbs.

Red Wine

In the Mediterranean, red wine has been linked to lower rates of heart disease and possibly cancer, largely due to the presence of polyphenols (which prevent cholesterol oxidation even better than vitamin E) and proanthocyandins or OPCs (powerful antioxidants). Other beneficial substances found in Mediterranean red wine include resveratrol, a substance in grape skins that can prevent blood clots and raise the difficult-to-increase HDL cholesterol, and an anticancer agent called caffeic acid (also found in grapes).

I suspect that Mediterranean red wine is generally healthier than what we drink in the United States. My personal experience is that drinking Mediterranean wine does not carry the penalty of headaches and hangover. Why? I have asked myself this question many times, and finally, I know. It doesn't contain added sulfites. In all wine, there is a small amount (less than 10 parts per million, abbreviated "ppm") of naturally occurring sulfites, but adding sulfites to control the fermentation process has become common practice in commercial wine making. The U.S. government permits adding another 350 ppm. The vast majority of wine consumed in the Mediterranean on an everyday basis comes from small vineyards, and is produced for local use only; hence there is no need for added sulfur. (Even certain wine vinegars contain sulfites, so check the labels.)

The relative purity of the locally produced Mediterranean wines should heighten the positive effects of beneficial phytochemicals (polyphenols and OPCs). Also, grapes grown in the region come from soil and water rich in minerals because of the presence of limestone.

Red wine contains 600 percent more polyphenols than white wine; this is why it may be more health promoting. A study in Israel comparing different types of wine demonstrated that all wines are definitely not created equal. Researchers from the Lipid Research Laboratory of Rambam Medical Center found that red wine drinkers had decreased oxidation of their LDL cholesterol (the bad cholesterol). Conversely, white wine drinkers showed a remarkable increase in the oxidation of LDL cholesterol. Oxidation creates cholesterol deposits inside arteries, thereby increasing the risk of heart disease.

Chèvre (Cheese Made from Goat's Milk)

Fresh, unaged cheese offers powerful health benefits. Chèvre, goat's milk cheese, is made from unheated raw milk, just as it comes from the animal— alive and vibrant with powerfully beneficial, living organisms and rich in enzymes. Enzymes are a powerful ally in preventing and healing breast cancer. The fresh cheese available throughout the Mediterranean is made from very high quality, organic, unpasteurized milk. These cheeses are not available here, because regulations require all cheese sold in the United States to be made only from pasteurized milk.

> During pasteurization, milk is heated above 100°F. While this kills contaminating organisms (like bacteria), it also kills enzymes and neutralizes much of milk's flavor.

Being a nondairy consumer for many years (partly because of my macrobiotic roots), I was initially hesitant to try chèvre. However, its wonderful, fresh fragrance spoke to me of vibrant green meadows, wild herbs, and dewy mornings. This food could be nothing but natural! Still, I hesitated before I brought the plump, chestnut-leafed morsel to my mouth. (The artisans who produce chèvre in Provence choose only green chestnut or grape leaves, tied in raffia, for wrapping. No plastic for them!) At first bite, I knew I was eating a nourishing natural food. The flavor of chèvre is hard to describe: strong and woodsy, nutty and fruity, really delicious.

While traditional cheese is produced throughout the Mediterranean, cheese production is not a commercial enterprise. In fact, it is rare to see a Provençal cheese for sale in the United States.

Chèvre and feta, unaged cheeses, do not present the health problems that aged cheese presents. Aged cheese contains oxidized
cholesterol, the type of cholesterol that can collect in the body and
lodge in coronary arteries. Aged foods containing animal products (or
fats) have decreased amounts of the antioxidant nutrients (vitamins C
and E, carotene, selenium, and sulfur) that protect our arteries.

Mineral-Rich Water

Mediterranean water contains high concentrations of minerals because
there is so much limestone in the region. Dramatic, rocky limestone cliffs
define the coastline throughout the Mediterranean.

Studies analyzing the drinking water in one hundred large cities throughout
the United States found four factors associated with a reduction in cancer
deaths of as much as 25%: moderately high levels of minerals, referred to as
"total dissolved solids" or TDS (the minerals measured by TDS include calcium, magnesium, copper, zinc, chromium, and selenium); particularly high
levels of two of these minerals, calcium and magnesium ("hard" water); an
alkaline pH (above 7.0); and water with 15 milligram per liter of the mineral
silica.

In the mid-to-late 1970s, studies found that people who drank water containing high levels of TDS had lower death rater from cancer, heart disease,
and other chronic illnesses. Conversely, such deaths were higher in cities with
water containing local amounts of TDS.

Look for water hardness of around 300 milligrams per liter and an alkaline
pH (above 7.0). Water in the United States requires a filtration system to
remove contaminants, but we must not remove the minerals if we want to
protect our health.

In researching bottled water from the United States, I was disappointed to
find that some companies offer water with low mineral content, low pH, and
low TDS concentration. "Mineral water" is not necessarily high in minerals.
Ask for the company's mineral, TDS, and hardness profile in writing. In the
Mediterranean, most people drink bottled water, but they still cook foods vith
tap water, which is very hard, mineral-rich water. Could the harder water
available in the Mediterranean be linked to lower rates of cancer and heart
disease? I think so!

The French Mediterranean Lifestyle at a Glance

• **Do Mediterranean children get a healthier start in life?** Parents don't hesitate to purée fresh vegetables, fruits, and other foods for their babies. Packaged baby foods are not as popular in the Mediterranean—or as available—as they are in the United States. Most mothers choose to breastfeed infants, instead of using formula. (The enzymes in breast milk build powerful immunities.) Because children aren't exposed to antibiotics and other chemicals in dairy foods (as they are in Northern America), childhood ear infections and sore throats aren't as typical. Also, a childhood operation we take for granted in our culture—tonsillectomy—is not regularly performed on Mediterranean children. Many nutritionists oppose removing tonsils, believing that they are necessary for a strong immune system.

> Mediterranean children aren't exposed to the constant hormonal assault of estrogen-laced meat and dairy that is part of everyday life in North America. Do these artificial hormones in our food supply distort the endocrine system? I think so, and believe that this is one of the reasons hormone-related cancers are significantly lower in the Mediterranean.

• **Mediterranean farmers don't pick produce prematurely for commercial purposes.** Vegetables and fruits are allowed to ripen on the vine, which adds both flavor and nutritional value. Powerful nutrients are obtained the last few days of ripening; for instance, cancer-preventative lycopene is richest in vine-ripened tomatoes.

• **Many Mediterranean foods are acidic.** This creates an alkalizing effect on the body, which in turn encourages better mineral absorption, as explained by Lendon Smith, M.D. Tomatoes, vinegar, lemon, eggplant, and fruits all have alkalizing effects. Another very significant factor is that the French Mediterranean diet is based on whole foods, without additives, preservatives, and sugar, all of which rob the body of vital minerals. For more information on acid/alkaline foods, *see* Marilyn Diamond and Dr. Burton Schnell's book *Fitonics*.

• **The lymphatic system is not underestimated.** Numerous centers for lymphatic drainage massage offer treatment to cleanse the lymphatic system. Many foods included regularly in the Mediterranean diet (like asparagus) have a naturally cleansing effect on the lymphatic system. Junk foods that clog the lymphatic system are not consumed. All of these factors help to prevent breast cancer.

• **Relaxing, low-stress lunches and dinners.** Meals in the Mediterranean are wonderful, calm experiences, without that hectic, "eat-on-the-run" feeling. Try to take more time to eat, in a calm environment, if possible.

• **Avoidance of plastics and other harmful artificial substances.** Microwaving in plastic, or microwaving at all, isn't done in the Mediterranean. Health food stores avoid plastic containers for oils, supplements, herbs, and other products. Opaque glass bottles are always used.

• **Minimal exposure to free radicals.** Substances that encourage the production of free radicals, such as medication and food additives, aren't as prevalent in the Mediterranean as they are in the United States. Mediterranean people turn to homeopathy, herbs, lymphatic drainage massage, and other natural forms of healing to restore health before they resort to medication. Foods are consumed fresh, so there is no need for preservatives and other chemicals.

• **Consumption of fewer calories, lower total body weight, and more active life style.** The French Mediterranean people are slender. Meal portions are much smaller, although salad size is definitely larger. Obviously, they burn more calories than they consume, which is believed by researchers to be linked to lower cancer risk.

• **Fiber-rich diet.** Rice, couscous, lentils, peas, salads, vegetables, and fresh fruits provide Mediterraneans with many sources of healthy fiber. The American Cancer Society, National Institutes of Health, and other organizations devoted to reducing (and eliminating) cancer recommend a diet high in fiber.

• **Limited intake of sugar.** Mediterranean people eat much less sugar than we do, which is vital in maintaining immune health. For example, sugar interferes with the transport of key antioxidants present in our body, primarily vitamin C. When candy is consumed in the Mediterranean, it is in small amounts. and quite infrequently, mostly by children at holidays. Desserts are generally much less sweet, and are also consumed in much smaller amounts. Fruit and cheese is as frequent a dessert choice as something sweet.

• **Less saturated fat.** The Mediterranean diet, with smaller portions of meat and dairy, focuses on vegetables, olive oil, fish, and fruit.

• **Organic food.** Restaurant chefs (and owners) personally know the farmer who sells them wheat, eggs, cheese, produce and other foods. Mediterranean farmers take a lot of pride in growing and producing foods that are as closely allied with nature as possible. Even in Paris, a movement toward the organic, earth element called the *terroirs* has been evolving since the 1970s.

• **Processed foods.** These foods just aren't consumed in the Mediterranean. Devotion to whole foods, unprocessed olive oil, fresh fish, nuts, and seeds ensures a diet with the broadest spectrum possible of breast-protective nutrients and EFAs.

• **Avoidance of charred foods.** Grilled steaks, barbequed ribs, and blackened fish aren't popular in the Mediterranean. Food preparation is creative, emphasizing lightness. In fact, browning over high heat and then roasting is not the current trend in French cooking. Instead, food is cooked over very low heat for hours, using methods like braising. Poaching, steaming and other very light cooking techniques are also employed. Jean Carper, author of *The Food Pharmacy* and *Food—Your Miracle Medicine*, points out that meat can be carcinogenic unless it is slow-cooked at low temperatures.

- **Avoidance of hormone-laced dairy and meat.** Animals aren't given hormones to increase meat and milk production, as they are in this culture. The Mediterranean cattle farmer would see no sense in that practice, because a need for more medication would soon follow. The animals' udders become infected from increased milk production, and antibiotics must then be used. These hormones and antibiotics directly affect our own endocrine systems.

- **Consumption of red grapes and wine, rich in protective OPCs.** While it is true sulfite-free red wine isn't as abundant here as it is in the Mediterranean, the same OPCs (oligomeric proanthocyanidins) are obtainable from the red grapes and seeds.

- **Sun-filled lifestyle.** Don't underestimate the power of the sun. Vitamin D, from the sun, helps to prevent breast cancer. Vitamin D is an antioxidant that helps inhibit the initiation of breast cancer. In fact, people who habitually use sunscreen have very low levels of Vitamin D (*see* Chapter 20, "Personal Care Guide").

TIP: A little natural light, on arms and legs for twenty minutes a day with no sunblock, may be beneficial. Caution: Be sure it's early morning or late afternoon sunlight.

Fresh, Unprocessed Foods Common Throughout the Mediterranean Countries

Tomatoes, onions, olive oil, a wide variety of vegetables (many consumed raw), lamb, chicken, goat, chickpeas and other dried peas and beans, garlic, herbs, and antioxidant-rich spices are used throughout all the Mediterranean countries.

Garnishing herbs, however, can vary from country to country. In Italy, use of fresh basil is common; in Greece, wild thyme and oregano are frequently utilized. Fresh mint, parsley, and dill are used often in Middle Eastern cooking.

The Middle East

The Middle East could be called the "home of olive oil." Middle Eastern cooking employs lots of olives and olive oil, vegetables (raw and cooked), scallions, onions, tomatoes, garlic, cracked wheat (bulgur), barley, fish (such as sardines and others), fresh herbs at every meal (parsley, dill, mint), liberal use of lemon juice, sesame seeds and sesame paste (tahini), tomatoes, fava beans, and chick peas. Consider the following dish, which is actually eaten at breakfast: Cooked fava beans are mixed with raw garlic, salt, red pepper and lemon juice, and garnished with chopped parsley, green onion, and paprika. Lots of unheated olive oil is drizzled on this and most dishes before eating.

Paprika is an antioxidant, parsley is a source of breast-protective glutathione, and green onions and garlic contain anticancer phytochemicals. What protective foods to start the day with, especially compared to what Americans eat!

Morocco

Fresh coriander is common in Moroccan cooking, and northwest African spices such as turmeric, cinnamon, cumin and ginger are frequently used. Moroccan cuisine also utilizes a wide variety of fruits. A typical cooking technique is slow stewing over a long period of time. A clay pot cooking technique called "tajin" is also used; it features mixtures of meat and grain combined with onions and tomatoes. An example of a typical Moroccan slow-cooked dish combines the following foods "tajin" style: lean, boneless lamb, cut into cubes, 5 fresh tomatoes, several cups of cooked chickpeas, garlic, onions, carrots, olive oil, and turmeric.

Italy

In southern Italy, a wide variety of vegetables is consumed, especially leafy greens, zucchini, beans, mushrooms, tomatoes, bell pepper, and onions. Fish, shellfish, anchovies, and chicken are combined with dried beans, garlic (liberally used), olive oil, parsley, pine nuts, basil, hot red pepper, and red pepper flakes.

Consider the following Italian dish: green beans cooked briefly in rapidly boiling salted water, seasoned with chopped garlic, olive oil, chopped parsley, chopped tomatoes, and a touch of balsamic vinegar. Adjust seasonings to taste.

Greece

Olive oil is consumed in abundant amounts by women in Greece. In fact, 42 percent of the calories that they consume is from fat—primarily olive oil. Furthermore, as Dimitrios Trichopoulous, M.D., reported at the Seventh European Nutrition Conference, Greek women have "substantially lower mortality from breast cancer than women in the U.S. who consume 35% of their calories from fat"—a finding that raises serious questions about the low-fat diet. The source of fat in American women's diets is not olive oil, but "other foods, mostly meat," according to Dr. Trichopoulous. Greece is known for delicious, fresh salads of lettuce, tomatoes, scallions, cucumber, grape leaves stuffed with rice, olives, green pepper, and feta cheese, seasoned with garlic, olive oil, lemon, dried oregano, ground pepper, and salt.

Spain

A typical Spanish condiment is ground nuts, olive oil, and garlic used as a sauce. Olive oil, onions, and bell pepper are frequently used, and dishes are often flavored with saffron and garlic.

Summary

The Mediterranean people consume a diet rich in protective fats from olive oil, sardines, and tuna, as well as plant sources of omega-3 (avocado, purslane, and walnuts). In fact, Mediterranean people consume a diet much higher in fat than people in the United States, yet they have lower rates of cancer and heart disease. Researchers suspect that other aspects of the Mediterranean diet—such as the consumption of greater amounts of fresh vegetables and cooking herbs as well as lower consumption of satured fats—have protective benefits. The correlation of trans-fats in the diet with increased risk of breast cancer has led some researchers to hypothesize that a diet low in trans-fats may also have protective effects against breast cancer.

CHAPTER 15

Alcohol, Coffee, and Sugar

The evidence linking alcohol consumption and breast cancer is much stronger than any suggesting a connection with dietary fat.
— *Tufts University Diet and Nutrition Letter,* December 1996

M ost women take morning coffee and an evening glass of wine for granted. What do these substances do to our immune systems? Do they play a part in contributing to breast cancer?

Although it's distressing to think that these sources of pleasure and relaxation that play a part in many of our lives are most likely damaging to women's health, consider the facts presented in this chapter seriously, and also consider the possibility of reducing or eliminating these stimulants from your diet.

Alcohol

Did you know that more studies show a correlation between alcohol consumption and breast cancer than correlate fat consumption and breast cancer? One study of women taking Premarin showed a fourfold rise in blood estrogen levels for several hours following only two alcoholic drinks, Christiane Northrup, M.D., reported in the *Health Wisdom for Women Newsletter.*

The American Institute for Cancer Research's brochure on breast cancer recommends that alcohol be consumed in moderation, if at all. *Even in moderate amounts, consumption of alcohol is linked to greater risks of developing breast cancer.* A study published in the *New England Journal of Medicine* in 1987 found a 40-60 percent increase in breast cancer with only moderate drinking. In 1990, *The Lancet* published a study finding that the greater the consumption of alcohol, the higher the risk for breast cancer. The Food Network's *In Food Today* website announced the results of a Harvard study finding that, in women undergoing estrogen therapy, consuming one drink containing vodka increased hormone levels by more than 300 percent (December 5, 1996). These researchers concluded that alcohol might affect the way estrogen is broken down in the body, but noted that more research is needed to be certain that there is a possible link between alcohol consumption and the risk of breast cancer.

Researchers at the Seventh European Nutrition Conference (May 24-28, 1995, in Vienna) reported that "drinking during the early years of a woman's life might enhance breast carcinogenesis." They also pointed out that "further investigations need to focus on assessment of alcohol use, and other potentially confounding nutritional characteristics, at varying points in a woman's life."

> TIP: Alcohol is thought to have a more profound effect on increasing the risk of breast cancer when consumed during the teenage years.

Although two important studies showed no association between alcohol consumption and breast cancer (one conducted in Southern France, the other in Northern Italy), I feel that there is enough evidence for women to acknowledge a possible association between alcohol consumption and breast cancer.

We know that alcohol adversely affects the liver, which helps to break down and metabolize estrogen; alcohol may, therefore, have an adverse effect on the liver's ability to process estrogen. We also know that alcohol depletes important immunoprotective nutrients like magnesium and zinc, and promotes the production of free radicals. Furthermore, alcohol is harmful to the digestive system. It is important for digestion and elimination to work efficiently so that excess estrogen may be removed from the body.

> If an occasional glass of wine is difficult to give up, insist on organic wine. Combine sparkling mineral water with white wine, reducing the amount of wine you consume.

Coffee

Chemicals like methylxanthines in coffee and decaffeinated coffee have been linked to cancer, as have the roasted hydrocarbons, which are especially high in darker coffees, like French roast. Eliminating coffee may slow the growth of malignant breast lumps.

Caffeine is known to cause reproductive system problems. During pregnancy, coffee can contribute to miscarriage and low birth-rate babies. Fibrocystic breast disease and symptoms of PMS are worsened by caffeine. It also aggravates hormonal fluctuations and other symptoms of menopause, like hot flashes.

Methylxanthine-rich substances include decaffeinated coffee, chocolate, and many over-the-counter medications such as diet pills, aspirin, and a widely used medication for symptoms of PMS and menstrual relief. Methylxanthine has been linked to cancer.

Doctors advise patients to eliminate coffee for a variety of health conditions. Some of the health problems worsened by coffee are:

- Anxiety and nervousness
- Chronic fatigue syndrome and other auto-immune disorders
- Hypoglycemia
- Heart palpitations
- Insomnia (it's amazing how deep sleep becomes when you eliminate coffee)
- Liver disease
- Gallstones
- Kidney, bladder disease, and kidney stones
- Migraines
- Osteoporosis
- Urinary tract infections

Coffee can create other deleterious internal conditions.

Blood sugar swings, leading to more coffee consumption. Caffeine forces the liver to release glycogen into the bloodsteam, increasing blood sugar levels. The pancreas responds to the sudden rise in blood sugar by releasing insulin, the hormone which causes excess carbohydrates to be stored as fat. Within the span of an hour or two, the result is a sharp drop in blood sugar, resulting in hypoglycemia (low blood sugar), cravings set in for a sweet, starchy snack like cookies or a doughnut and another cup of coffee, and the whole cycle starts again.

Acid imbalance. There are more than 208 acids in coffee that contribute to many different health problems resulting from overacidity, including arthritic and rheumatic conditions. Optimal health requires an alkaline pH balance in the body—the opposite of the acidic condition encouraged by coffee. Caffeine breaks down into the by-product uric acid, which the body excretes through the kidneys. An excess of uric acid taxes the kidneys and can cause kidney stones and gout. Additionally, men need to be concerned about coffee consumption aggravating prostate conditions. Many people experience a burning sensation in their stomachs after drinking coffee because coffee increases the secretion of stomach acid.

Essential mineral depletion. Coffee inhibits the absorption of some nutrients and causes urinary excretion of calcium, magnesium, potassium, iron, and trace minerals, all essential elements for good health. Women need to be concerned about osteoporosis as they enter menopause, and studies show that women who drink coffee have an increased incidence of osteoporosis compared to non-coffee drinkers.

Exhausted adrenal glands. Caffeine is a central nervous system stimulant. It causes the adrenal glands to secrete adrenaline, the hormone the body depends upon in emergencies to elevate the heart rate and increase respiration and blood pressure for a rapid "flight-or-fight" response. When you overuse stimulants, the adrenals become exhausted. If your caffeine sensitivity has diminished, or you are one of those people who can drink three shots of espresso and go to sleep, guess what? Your adrenals have given up responding. This means that you have less resistance to stress, which leaves you vulnerable to health hazards such as environmental pollutants and disease pathogens.

As we age, the adrenals become more important as the producers of essential youth and sex hormones. Many people in their forties find that they cannot tolerate the same coffee consumption as they could in their twenties or thirties. The adrenals can be considered the storage center for the vital force. They require nourishment for optimal health.

Natural grain coffee provides a delicious alternative to coffee. (*See* Teecchino in the Resource Guide.)

Finally, coffee raises homocysteine's level in the body. Homocysteine is a compound that is naturally produced from the amino acid methionine. Research shows that if homocysteine levels become too high, heart attack, stroke, and osteoporosis can result. Be sure to consume adequate B12, folic acid, and B6 if you are a coffee drinker.

Espresso and French Coffee Press Raise Harmful LDL Cholesterol

Tufts University's *Health and Nutrition Newsletter* reported in January 1998 that a study conducted in the Netherlands found coffee made without filters, in a coffee press called a cafetière (or plunger pot), can raise harmful LDL cholesterol as much as 14%. Cafestrol and kahweol, compounds that raise cholesterol, are removed by the filters used in the drip method of coffee preparation. These compounds are also present in espresso.

Sugar

In 1983, an article in the journal *Medical Hypothesis* drew a correlation between the intake of sugar and an increase in breast cancer; several subsequent studies have also found high sugar intake to be a strong risk factor for breast cancer. Otto Warburg, twice winner of the Nobel Prize in Medicine, has commented, "The prime cause of cancer is the replacement of oxygen in normal cells by a fermentation of sugar." Highly refined sugar is so detrimental to immunity, a single taste can lower resistance for up to six hours.

A can of soda contains about 10 teaspoons of sugar. Look for Reed's Premium Ginger Ale in health food stores. Reed's is gently sweetened with honey and flavored naturally with ginger. Another natural soda is one you can make yourself by combining one part each of kukicha tea, apple juice, and sparkling mineral water.

Consuming sugar robs the body of minerals. Enzymes, which are so important in the digestive process, depend upon minerals. When enzyme supplies diminish because we have eaten sugar, the other food we've consumed is not digested. Instead, the undigested food gets into the bloodstream. The immune system then has to work overtime to help cleanse the bloodstream of substances from fermenting, undigested food. Years of being overburdened from cleansing the bloodstream may cause the immune system to become vulnerable to invaders like viruses, bacteria, and cancer cells. Sugar can also cause triglycerides to rise and may upset the endocrine system. It interferes with the absorption of calcium/magnesium. In addition, sugar can cause urinary tract infections.

Dr. Weston Price, a dentist who studied the nutrition and dental health of native people throughout the world in the 1930s, discovered that sugar cane does not cause teeth to decay like refined sugar does. Dr. Price found that native people who ate sugar cane frequently, even daily, had perfect jaw aligment and no cavities. Succinat is the sweetener that is most similar to sugar cane. Because regular use of any type of sweetener can raise glucose in the body—which encourages tumor growth—sweets should be eaten infrequently, perhaps once or twice a week. If you have young children, consider using Succinat, especially for baking.

TIP: Saccharin is considered a cancer-causing substance; switch to stevia instead. Stevia, an herb that has been consumed for centuries in South America and for decades as a government-approved sweetener in Japan, China, and Korea, is a calorie-free, all-natural alternative to artificial, "calorie-free" sweeteners.

When you crave sweetness, select natural desserts. Baked apples, soy milk puddings, or oatmeal cookies can satisfy any sweet tooth. Make them at home and use an unrefined, natural sweetener like maple syrup, honey, or Succinat with a very light touch, or buy them from a natural bakery that uses healthy ingredients, including sweeteners. Make sure that baked goods are not made with canola or other processed oils. Butter is the healthiest choice for baking—and the most delicious!

To reduce sugar cravings, make sure you:

• Eat bitter foods such as escarole, watercress, frisée, endive, dandelion, and broccoli rabe on a regular basis.

• Ingest adequate protein intake at every meal, balanced by generous servings of vegetables.

• Reduce amounts of breads and pasta to help eliminate cravings for more carbohydrates which helps to reduce cravings for donuts, cookies, cakes, and other sweets.

• Eliminate coffee.

• Take Epsom salt baths to restore levels of magnesium.

• Exercise.

• Supplement with chlorella, a source of protein (and minerals) helpful in stabilizing blood sugar.

Products such as diet cola, mints, gum, and ice cream made with artificial sweeteners, as well as artificial sweeteners for coffee or tea, have been associated with headaches, dizziness, diarrhea and other stomach upsets, mood swings, dry eyes, loss of memory, and depression. Americans currently spend more than $250 million a year on the artificial sugar substitutes Equal and Sweet and Low.

CHAPTER 16

Power Teas

In eighth-century China, people began making healing drinks of "leaves of a bush," as described much later by visiting Hollanders. Tea began as medicine, and we can enjoy using it that way today, as both a soothing beverage and a healing medicine.

Teas contain active, nourishing agents that can help heal and may actually help to prevent disease. Disease-fighting catechins are found in ordinary green, oolong or black teas. Even mild herbal teas like lemon balm or nettles are rich in nutrients such as bioflavonoids, carotenes, minerals, and vitamins. Mild, herbal teas are the safest form of enjoying herbs and can provide many benefits with no side effects. Herbalist and author Susun Weed describes nourishing herbal teas such as red clover, lemon balm, nettles, alfalfa, and chamomile as "nourishing foods, just as leafy greens, garlic, and carrots are."

The quality of the teas you brew will only be as good as the raw materials or packaged product you select. Christopher Hobbs, author and herbalist, reminds us to "choose products that contain organically grown herbs."

I usually recommend that people begin exploring herbal teas by purchasing organic packaged teas and following the brewing instructions with care.

The teas I have recommended as Power Teas are *gently* nourishing. Herbs can be potent, and using some of them requires the help of an herbalist or other professional. None of those types of herbs is recommended here.

Teas can be wonderful tools in improving our health. They can calm, soothe, revitalize, cleanse, and in some cases, even offer potent protection against breast and other cancers. This chapter includes my favorite teas that I rely on—my "power teas."

TIP: For information on specific teas for ailments, compresses, and tea baths, read Marie Nadine Antol's *How to Prepare and Use Teas to Maximize Your Health (see* the Bibliography in the Resource Guide).

Herbal Teas: Rich Sources of Vitamins and Minerals

Phytosterols in herbs balance hormones and are a rich source of vitamins and minerals. In fact, the vitamins and minerals in herbs are assimilated more efficiently than those from supplements.

Phytosterols are plant hormones that provide hormonal building blocks, allowing the body to produce both the amount and combination of hormones needed. It is not necessary to know the exact amount to consume. Phytosterols also support the liver. Some of my favorite phytosterol rich herbs are red clover, dandelion, nettle, and sage.

Nettles. I am drinking a fortifying cup of nettles tea as I write this. It is pleasantly bitter, and very satisfying. Nettles is one of the most potent sources of calcium and other minerals, and is nourishing and cleansing. It contains silicon, boron, magnesium, and potassium, as well as chlorophyll, carotenes, vitamin C, vitamin D, vitamin B complex, and flavonoids. Nettles is excellent for the adrenal and endocrine glands.

Dandelion. This powerful tea is useful in protecting, cleansing, and regenerating the liver. I love dandelion root tea in the winter, and the lighter, leaf tea during the spring and summer. Modern research has confirmed that traditional use of dandelion is especially effective for preventing and treating breast and other cancers. Dandelion's roots and leaves are rich in minerals. For a liver cleanse, combine 1 part dandelion roots and leaves with 10 parts water. Simmer for 20 minutes, steep for 10, and drink 1 cup two to five times a day. Dandelion root concentrate can be added to a cup of hot water or tea to promote liver health (*see* the Resource Guide).

Red clover. This tea is rich in anticancer genistein, especially protective for breast and other cancers. It also helps the lymphatic system cleanse the body and bloodstream of toxins.

Flor-essence. Available in health food stores (*see* Resource Guide), this tea contains red clover, burdock root, and other cleansing herbs.

Lemon balm. A relaxing, nighttime tea, lemon balm strengthens the liver, is a source of abundant antioxidants, and helps relieve headaches.

Sage. Great for alleviating hot flashes, sage also helps depression, nervousness, mood swings, and headaches. It is excellent for women going through menopause. Women report that sage tea at night is effective at relieving night sweats. Make sage tea and drink throughout the day. Also helpful in strengthening the liver, sage is rich in minerals and antioxidants.

Chamomile. Known as a wonderfully relaxing herb, chamomile is also antibacterial, antiseptic, and has antinausea properties. It also has antinflammatory properties, so it may be beneficial for people suffering from arthritis or rheumatism. What I like best about chamomile is that it provides a calming energy in the day, so if I'm under stress, I can drink chamomile tea without becoming sleepy. At night, however, chamomile tea imparts that "ready for a good night's sleep" feeling, especially when you drink a cup while in a lavender bath.

Peppermint. This tea has been used since Ancient Egyptian times as a digestive, and for good reason. It is extremely effective at relieving digestive problems ranging from indigestion to stomach cramps from mild food poisoning. Always have peppermint tea on hand in your own kitchen.

TIP: Power teas that are effective for bloating and to reduce gas are fennel, anise, caraway, coriander, chamomile, and peppermint.

Green. When discussing breast health, green tea belongs in a special category all by itself. I try to drink one cup of green tea each day because of the extensive research showing how this potent beverage stops the initiation and growth of breast cancer. Green tea has been found to be the most protective against breast (and other) cancers, followed by oolong and then black tea. Green tea protects DNA from cell damage and helps to rebuild already-damaged DNA. Having powerful anticancer properties, it inhibits tumor promotion and proliferation by reducing the adhesion ability of the tumor cell surface. Green tea is especially effective in preventing and treating esophageal, lung, stomach, and skin cancers. It is rich in polyphenols and epigallorachin gallate (EGCG), chemicals that can neutralize the free radicals associated with cancer. Green tea is also a rich source of antioxidants, and can be measured in the blood up to eight hours after it is consumed.

TIP: Green tea contains caffeine, so be careful not to drink too much of it during the day, or at all in the evening.

Kukicha. This calcium-rich Japanese tea, which is very popular in macrobiotics, contains more calcium per cup than milk. Kukicha tea is made from the twigs of the plant, as opposed to the leaves. Because most of the caffeine in tea is found in the leaves, kukicha ("twig tea") is relatively low in caffeine.

Be sure to purchase only organic kukicha tea, because many pesticides are used in the farming of teas in Japan, and throughout the world.

Lotus root. Valued in Asian folk medicine as a tonic for the lungs, it can be helpful in cleansing the lungs when there are respiratory problems of any kind. (*See* the Resource Guide.)

Ume extract. Unripe Japanese ume plums are pressed carefully to extract the juice, which is then cooked for about a day to concentrate it. Ume concentrate is salt-free, and can absorb and neutralize several hundred times its weight in acid. It also possesses antioxidant properties. Ume extract is wonderful to have on hand for headaches, nausea, or constipation.

Ume was first produced on a commercial basis in Japan in the mid-1920s. At that time, the Japanese Army and Navy officially used it as an antiseptic to guard against food poisoning, dysentery, and other illnesses. Ume extract is effective for both constipation and diarrhea. It increases or decreases bacterial action when necessary to reestablish the proper balance and restore normal bowel movement. It has both the capacity to suppress breeding of bacteria in the small intestine that leads to diarrhea, and to promote bacterial growth to aid bowel movements. Simply add ¼ teaspoon of ume plum extract to 1 full cup of tea (I recommend kukicha tea). Stir and drink.

> If you like sweet teas and are used to artificial sweeteners, stevia contains no calories and is a much healthier choice. Be careful, because this dark green leaf from Paraguay is twenty-five times sweeter than sugar. Use only ⅛ teaspoon of stevia per cup or glass of tea. Amazingly, stevia can be used by people with hypoglycemia. If you use a chemical, calorie-free sweetener, make the switch to natural stevia. The Japanese have researched stevia's safety and effectiveness, and have been using it since the 1970s (*see* the Resource Guide).

Tips For Brewing Power Teas

To use the *infusion* method, place 1-2 teaspoons of dried, cut leaves and/ or flowers (double this amount if using freshly picked herbs) in a cup. Add 1 cup of boiling water, and stir. Cover and steep for 8-10 minutes; for a stronger, medicinal effect, steep for 15-20 minutes. Strain and drink.

Glass teapots are recommended for superior teamaking. They aren't easy to find, but Natural Lifestyle mail order (*see* the Resource Guide) offers a functional, handled, nontoxic glass teapot that is flame resistant and dish-washer safe. A removable glass infuser allows for convenient, strain-free preparation of loose teas. You need a diffuser for electric stoves, but you can use directly on a gas stove.

An enticing option often recommended by herbalists is to mince ½ tsp of organic orange peel and add it to the tea while steeping (be sure to cover the tea). Citrus peels provide a bitterness that is healing for the liver, and contain enzymes and phytonutrients that aid in the detoxification of carcinogens. Limone, the phytochemical in orange peel, has been found to be a potent breast protector. You may want to boost your calcium intake by saving (clean) organic egg shells and using them in the water you boil to make tea.

A final suggestion: I regularly add Swedish bitters to a cup of hot kukicha or other herbal tea to get the liver and digestive system going. Swedish bitters are a combination of cleansing herbs and aloe, in liquid form, available in the health food store. (*See* the Resource Guide.)

CHAPTER 17

Mammography: Foods and Supplements That Offer Protection

Your breast health plan should be built on the foundation of prevention, including nutrition, exercise, relaxation, and frequent breast self-examination. The importance of breast self-exams cannot be underestimated; most women find their own breast cancers through self-examination. For information on self-exam and how a breast sensor pad can help you better examine your own breasts, *see* the Personal Care Guide.

Visits to the gynecologist for thorough, breast exams are also very important if a woman is at higher risk for breast cancer. The decision about when or how often to have a mammogram is one that every woman must make with her physician, based upon her family history and age. The *Women's Health Advocate Newsletter* recommends regular mammograms in women age 50 and older, citing the statistic that mammograms can reduce breast cancer deaths in this age group by up to 30 percent.

In 1997, *Women's Health Advocate Newsletter* reported the findings of three national health organizations that reviewed current data regarding mammography for women in their forties. Here are the health agencies' conclusions:

• The National Institutes of Health concluded that there is no scientific basis for women in their forties to have routine mammography.

• The American Cancer Society recommends that women in their forties have mammograms as frequently as once a year, an increase in its past recommendation of once every one to two years.

• The National Cancer Institute recommends women at "high risk" seek medical advice about beginning mammograms as early as their thirties. For women in their forties at "average risk," a mammogram every one to two years is suggested.

Getting a Good Mammogram

If you need to have a mammogram, be certain the technician is qualified. Make sure that the person reading the films is a certified radiologist, and is experienced at interpreting mammogram X-rays. Ask whether the equipment has been certified by the American College of Radiology, as well as by the Food and Drug Administration, as mandated by the Mammography Quality Standards Act of 1992. The clinic's certificate—which is white, with a blue stripe—should be displayed in plain view. It indicates that the facility receives an annual inspection insuring that the facility meets legal requirements: i.e., the equipment is safe and is inspected annually, and the personnel's continuing education is up-to-date. (*See* the Resource Guide for information on the American College of Radiology.) Ask the radiologist to have your prior mammogram available to note personal breast patterns, in case a change develops. It is important for you to keep your mammograms, especially if you change facilities or move. In addition, the accuracy of mammograms is questionable if performed during the last half of the menstrual cycle. Breasts are more sensitive during this time, and technicians hesitate to compress the breast fully (which insures a better X-ray image). Women are more than twice as likely to have a false negative reading during the last half of the menstrual cycle, according to a report in *The Globe and Mail* (August 1997).

> TIP: Find a clinic specializing in mammography where you can actually receive your results that same day.

Breast Ultrasound Gaining in Use

Dixie Mills, M.D., an expert in breast care from the "Women to Women" clinic in Yarmouth, Maine, reports that more and more centers are becoming familiar with *breast ultrasound*. She predicts that this method of diagnosis is going to be extremely popular in the future. Dr. Mills compares the current state of breast ultrasound to the early years of black and white television, which evolved into color—in other words, the technology will become even more beneficial as time goes by. Dr. Mills utilizes breast ultrasound to complement mammography if a woman's breasts are dense on mammography, or if there is a question about a mammogram, like a suspicious or tender area.

Using first-generation breast ultrasound technology, it is difficult to image the whole breast. It is also difficult to compare images; one facility's machine may be slightly different from another's. Breast ultrasound is also dependent upon technique. The angle at which the ultrasound probe is held may vary from technician to technician.

How does it work? Sound waves are bounced off breast tissues in order to locate dense tissue. Cancer tissue is denser than normal tissue. Ultrasound can be used to identify solid lumps that require further evaluation. Solid masses with thin, sharp, smooth margins are often benign; those with jagged edges or irregular shapes might be malignant.

An early cancer screening test that detects malignancies up to nineteen months before clinical diagnosis is possible, the **AMAS test** measures an antibody that is present in people who have cancer of any cell type in any location. This antibody, called the "antimalignin antibody," is detected by a simple blood test and is highly associated with the presence of cancer cells. The AMAS test is an important diagnostic option for people from families with a high cancer incidence, or for individuals who've previously had cancer. (For information on the AMAS test, *see* Resource Guide.)

If you need to have a breast biopsy, try to find a doctor who knows about the new needle specifically used for biopsies that helps to prevent scarring. Nationwide, about 500 hospitals are now using this new needle for biopsies.

Power Foods and Supplements That Offer Protection

For strengthening DNA against radiation, eat a lot of cooked, carotene-rich foods such as orange winter squash, sweet potatoes, pumpkin, dark leafy greens, and dandelion greens. Carotenes will protect your DNA from radiation, and also provide lots of anticancer protection. The darker and richer the oranges and greens in the vegetables, the more antioxidant-rich carotenes they contain. Although carotenes become more protective when cooked, pink grapefruit and cantaloupe also possess carotene power. In addition, load up on the following:

Astragalus can help to strengthen the immune system. Use this herb for protection the week of your mammogram. Immunitea, from UniTea Herbs (*see* the Resource Guide) is a mixed blend herbal tea containing astragalus. Another way to use astragalus is to purchase it from the health food store and use it in soups. (*See* the Recipes.) Interestingly, astragalus is currently under investigation as an adjunct to cancer therapy. A 1990 study conducted at the M.D. Anderson Cancer Center in Houston found an extract of astragalus to increase the body's ability to kill cancer cells tenfold (*Women's Health Advocate Newsletter*, December 1996).

A week before a mammogram, grate fresh *ginger* on vegetables and drink tea to begin benefiting from ginger's antimutagenic and antioxidant properties. For convenience, ginger supplements are available (*see* the Resource Guide).

Paul Schulick, author of *Ginger: Common Spice and Wonder Drug,* recommends that women make a tea from *red clover, burdock,* and grated fresh *ginger root,* to drink before and after mammography. Simmer herbs in water for 20 minutes. Strain, and add 2-3 drops of organic tangerine essential oil.

Chlorella can be used (at least 1 teaspoon daily of powdered chlorella mixed in 6 ounces of water or juice) the week before, and several weeks after, the mammogram. A 1996 study published in *Radiation and Environmental Biophysics* reported that natural beta-carotene supplements, derived from algae, are effective in protecting against free radical damage produced by exposure to radiation. Algae offer more protection from radiation than synthetic beta carotene.

Siberian ginseng has been shown by studies conducted in Russia to have radioprotective effects. It has also been found to be helpful for women with breast cancer. (*See* the Resource Guide for Siberian ginseng tea.)

An *organic apple,* consumed with the peel, is rich in pectin, thought to help to draw out harmful chemicals like radioactive substances from the body.

Tofu, soybeans and *miso* contain protease inhibitors which guard against radiation. These protease inhibitors are destroyed if cooked at very high temperatures, so steam tofu and roast soybeans instead of pressure-cooking them. It is also important to add miso just as a soup or sauce is finishing cooking, so that the miso doesn't boil.

Sodium alginate, a substance in some sea vegetables, helps to protect against radiation. For convenience, explore sea vegetable supplements (*see* the Resource Guide).

Grape seed extract is one of the most protective antioxidants. Take 100 milligrams of OPCs (*oligomeric proanthocyanidins*), per day for two days before the mammogram, and 100 milligrams a day for several days afterward. (*See* the Resource Guide.)

N-acetyl-cysteine (known as NAC) is an antioxidant that can protect cells and DNA from radiation, and also helps to boost the body's production of L-glutathione, an antioxidant. Robert Haas, M.S., reports in *Permanent Remissions* that a typical dose of NAC is 500 milligrams.

> TIP: Try this delicious Kombu condiment. Lightly wipe kombu with a damp cloth. Soak in filtered water (to cover), until soft. Cut into small pieces about ½ inch thick (prepare about ⅓ cup). Bring kombu, ⅔ cup water, and ¼ cup tamari soy sauce to a boil. Reduce flame and cook gently until kombu is soft. Grate fresh ginger root over cooked kombu and consume a few pieces with lunch and dinner. Store in a covered bowl in the refrigerator for up to 1 week.

Miso contains dipisolinic acid, which helps to reduce the harmful effects of radiation. Include it daily in soup, or pureed in a little water to sauté vegetables.

Buckwheat contains glucoside rutin, a phytochemical that helps to protect against radiation. Rutin is a flavonoid with powerful antioxidant properties that plays a key role in gene repair, by activating the repair enzymes in DNA. Rutin is related to quercitin, another flavonoid with antioxidant benefits. Foods that contain these flavonoids are buckwheat berries, grapes, and broccoli.

Burdock root helps to eliminate radioactive isotopes from your body. Burdock root tincture is available as a supplement. (*See* the Resource Guide.)

Eggs and *flaxseed oil* are sources of lecithin, also offering protection against radiation.

Apples and *sunflower seeds* contain pectin, a type of fiber that helps the body to eliminate radiation.

Lentils help to protect DNA.

Lentil Miso Soup

4-inch piece of
   kombu
1 medium onion
2 medium carrots
1 small turnip
1 cup green lentils
2 bay leaves
2 tbsp minced
   parsley
6 cups filtered water
3 tbsp barley miso
¾ cup cubed tofu
minced chives

Wipe kombu with a damp cloth and reconstitute in a small amount of water. Cut into ½-inch squares. Peel onion and scrub vegetables with a vegetable brush, cutting them into bite-size pieces. Wash lentils, and place in soup pot together with vegetables, kombu, bay leaves, parsley, and water. Slowly bring to a boil. Reduce flame and simmer for 45 minutes to 1 hour. Puree the miso into a little soup broth in a small bowl. Slowly add to the soup, continuing to cook over low heat for 20 minutes more. Add cubed tofu. Garnish with chives.

Lentils contain genistein, an inhibitor of estrogen-sensitive cancers. Con-

suming lentils provides dual benefits for women interested in breast health—
they protect DNA, and help to prevent the formation of breast and uterine cancer.

> TIP: If you work at a computer and are concerned about the cumula-
> tive effects of radiation, special shields are available that help to
> minimize the risks. (Refer to the Resource Guide for radiation shields
> for computer monitors.)

Sample menus using foods that protect against radiation:

Breakfast: Soft-boiled egg, lightly drizzled with flaxseed oil, with canta-
            loupe or pink grapefruit.
Lunch: Miso soup with shiitake mushrooms, kombu, and carrots.
Snack: Apple and sunflower seeds.
Dinner: Soba noodles in broth with burdock condiment, and steamed
            butternut or buttercup squash.

Soba Noodles in Broth

6 dried shiitake mushrooms
5-inch strip of kombu, wiped lightly
5 cups filtered water
3 minced scallions
4½ tbsp tamari
4 cups cooked and drained soba noodles
⅓ bunch cleaned and chopped watercress
1-2 tsp fresh grated ginger

Rinse shiitakes. Reconstitute mushrooms and kombu in water for 15 minutes. Remove the tough stems, and slice mushrooms. (You can use the stems
in vegetable broths. Bring water, tamari, mushrooms (including stems), and
kombu to a boil over medium-high heat. Reduce heat and simmer for 20
minutes. Add the scallions and ginger and cook for another 2-3 minutes.
Adjust seasoning by adding more tamari, if necessary. Place noodles in four
bowls, with watercress. Ladle hot broth and mushrooms over each serving.

> TIP: One of my favorite soba noodle recipes is simply to cook them
> according to the instructions on the packet, and while they're cooking,
> make a quick vinaigrette from minced garlic, a few pinches of sea

salt, some minced rosemary, and a light drizzle of extra virgin olive oil. Add just a touch of wine vinegar. Before the noodles are done, add a few asparagus spears to the hot water, and finish cooking. Drain soba and asparagus. Mix the vinaigrette throughout. Season with cayenne pepper. Look for Eden's 40 percent Soba, made with wheat and buckwheat flour. I especially like this soba, because it is a thin noodle.

Burdock Condiment Helps to Protect

The easieset and the tastiest way to prepare burdock is to scrub the burdock root with a vegetable brush, leaving the skin on, since it is rich in nutrients. Cut the burdock into matchsticks and place in a small pot or pan with ½ organic apple juice and ½ organic shoyu or soy sauce. Bring to a boil, reduce heat, cover, and cook over medium heat for 20 minutes. Let cool and eat as a condiment with fish, rice, noodles, or tofu. If you are too busy to make burdock root condiment, you can simply cut the burdock root into matchsticks and toss it into soups. Easier still, purchase Eden's delicious Tekka miso vegetable condiment containing burdock root, available in the macrobiotic section in health food stores. Use Tekka on brown rice. (*See* the Resource Guide.)

TIP: Burdock seed extract is available in tonic form, and can be added to tea or water as a protective supplement. (*See* the Resource Guide.)

A Soothing Bath and Chest Rub
to Shield Against Radiation

For added protection against the effects of radiation, try a baking soda and sea salt bath. Simply add a handful of each to your bath. Finish with cold water. Some women have used a combination of St. John's wort oil and calendula oil as a chest rub before mammography to protect tissue and encourage repair. Just mix a little in the palm of your hand, 1 part St. John's Wort oil to 2 parts calendula oil. Calendula is a healing oil that is great for the skin and helps to enhance the effects of the St. John's Wort, traditionally used to treat minor burns and encourage tissue repair.

Mammography Follow-up?

Women's Health Advocate reported in August 1997 that scintimammography (sometimes called mikaluma or sestamibi) has been formally approved as a follow-up for mammography. When an initial mammogram isn't able to provide a clear image (such as when the breasts are too dense, as they can be in women in their forties), a woman is injected with a radioactive tracer. The radiologist then uses a camera to image the breast so that the areas of tissue that took up more of the tracer can be observed in detail. The suspect areas will stand out from the surrounding breast tissue, because they will appear darker.

Mammography can be a lifesaver. Indiscriminate use of X-rays, however, can be harmful; their effects are cumulative. Decline unnecessary X-rays, such as during routine visits to the dentist, when they aren't specifically indicated to diagnose a problem.

The Center for Medical Consumers offers an informative pamphlet, "Mammography Screening: A Decision-Making Guide." *(See* the Resource Guide.)

CHAPTER 18

Secrets of a Healthy Kitchen

Before I discovered that old macrobiotic book in the basement of my Manhattan apartment, food preparation was simply a matter of convenience. It was one-stop shopping for me—everything I needed could be found at the local grocery store.

When I later discovered just how much of an impact fresh, organic vegetables, herbs and freshly pressed oils had on my health and sense of well-being, I realized that extra time devoted to food was profoundly well spent.

You, too, will notice many rewards from investing just a little more time in caring for yourself by preparing life-giving, fresh, beautiful foods—improved sleep and energy; fewer headaches and hormonal problems; and many others specific to you. Before I improved my diet, for instance, I was beginning to experience serious arthritic pain from a bone injury I suffered when I was twenty-two. I had fractured my femur, an injury that left me with an eight-inch metal plate in my leg. After making dietary changes like those outlined in *Total Breast Health*, my pain diminished significantly. As long as I practice prevention—exercising daily (including gentle stretching); not abusing my condition (by carrying heavy items or standing all day, for instance); and consuming a diet free from processed foods like white sugar, white flour, white rice, soda, and food additives—I feel very well.

Each of us must take responsibility for our own health and find ways to nourish ourselves. Maintaining an exercise program, getting enough sleep, and selecting and preparing high-quality, fresh foods will help to safeguard health. As you increasingly feel (and look) better, the old ways will disappear from thought. Every meal, every exercise session, every day presents an opportunity to create health.

Don't worry if you are distracted from healthier habits by holidays or travel. Such events and activities may feel disruptive, but allow yourself to enjoy these experiences for what they offer. Interacting with family and friends, sharing a holiday meal or a birthday celebration, also provides nourishment. Just choose the best food available at these activities, and enjoy.

After enjoying a family visit or holiday, I really look forward to returning to my own routine of exercise, lightly prepared foods with a variety of vegetables, and leisurely walks on my favorite beautiful street. This routine makes me feel too good—my body feels both slender and limber from regular exercise, my mind is calm, my sleep deep—to imagine giving it up.

I'd like to share some selected questions from clients over the years and my suggestions to them about convenience, preparing basics (like brown rice), and other general information to make healthy meal preparation easier to incorporate into your routine. I hope these ideas will encourage you to spend more time in your own kitchen. Most women are busy with so many activities, they find it hard to focus on protecting their health. We've become all too accustomed to take-out and restaurant food. Getting back into the kitchen may seem inconvenient initially, but there are no magic bullets that provide instant health. It's necessary to spend time selecting and preparing the freshest, highest-quality foods to create health and prevent (or heal) breast cancer and other illnesses.

I promise that this time will be well spent. The benefits you experience will reward you for all your effort. It's too alluring to feel and look better! Protecting the most beautiful gift we are given—a healthy life—is a profound and wonderful responsibility.

Sometimes I pick up a frozen dinner from the health food store. Is this a good idea? If you don't recommend frozen foods, can you recommend some healthy foods that are convenient to prepare when I'm pressed for time?

One of the interesting things I learned from my study of macrobiotics is Oriental face reading. When you observe a person's face carefully, you can learn a lot—even about the freshness of his or her diet. If a person is eating very fresh vegetables, bright green leafy ones in salads, and other freshly prepared foods, including freshly pressed oils, it shows on his or her face. Are the eyes clear and bright? Is the skin soft and clear? Does the hair shine and look full? Are the facial features calm, reflecting a healthy central nervous system? When deli food—or frozen food—is consumed on a regular basis, the diet lacks the vitality and energy that fresh foods provide. A 1997 study showed that freshly prepared Brussels sprouts, cooked until just tender and eaten right away, contain more protective phytochemicals and nutrients than Brussels sprouts that were cooked longer and consumed later. Recent studies also indicate that it is best to cut vegetables right before eating to preserve optimal nutrients. The key is freshness, which is fundamental to protecting health.

Eat at home for greater antioxidant consumption. *The American Journal of Public Health* published results from a 1997 study of the cancer-preventative carotenoids that found people who eat at home consume greater amounts of carotenoids (like lycopene and beta-carotene).

Time-Saving Tips:

• Stopping at the deli: I strongly recommend that you only use prepared foods from either the best natural foods store or the best gourmet foods establishment in your area. This will ensure the purchase of deli foods with fresh, quality ingredients. Select from among poached salmon, tofu salad, roasted skinless white meat chicken, or sliced, preservative-free, all-natural turkey breast. To complement prepared foods, prepare a simple salad and a cooked green leafy vegetable or a cooked orange vegetable. Drizzle flaxseed oil or Udo's Choice Perfected Oil Blend on your salad or cooked vegetable, add a fresh herb, and you've got a relatively convenient, breast-protective meal.

• Stopping at the health food store: This option gives you access to organic produce, so you can pick up fresh herbs and vegetables. Think color and variety.

Chives, a source of potent breast-protective allyl sulfides, can be minced into your salad, or tossed with lightly steamed kale, right before serving. *Carrots* (especially if they're organic) are a deliciously sweet, powerful antioxidant containing carotenes, which are made even more protective when cooked. Cut carrots into julienne strips, or grate, for fast cooking. *Dark leafy greens* contain indispensable chlorophyll, folic acid, vitamin K (for bones), and a variety of breast-friendly phytonutrients. Boil water, put a steamer basket in the pot, fill it with grated carrots and fresh kale or collard greens, and steam them briefly. Finish the dish with minced chives, a splash of delicious ume plum vinegar (look for the Eden brand), and a drizzle of oil.

It's easy to put together a quick salad of *raw spinach* (a source of cancer-preventative glutathione and protective vitamin E) and thinly sliced *red peppers* (which contain nine times the beta carotene of green peppers and twice the vitamin C), with *mild onion* and *grapefruit* segments (which contain terpenes, protective enzymes that help to excrete certain carcinogens). Drizzle olive oil and lemon juice over your salad—tangy, fresh, and delicious!

Quick Dinner with Deli Protein

3–3½ ounces of protein (choose between prepared salmon, tofu salad, organic chicken or turkey breast, and other prepared proteins)
Cooked greens and carrots, with minced chives

Spinach salad with peppers, onion, and grapefruit segments
Protective fats: flaxseed and olive oil, and if you selected salmon
as your protein source, breast- and heart-protective oils.

• A well-stocked kitchen and pantry provide inspiration to create health-ier, time-saving meals. Keep flaxseed oil, Udo's Choice Perfected Oil Blend, and olive oil, soy sauce, umeboshi vinegar, mirin, shallots, garlic, and fresh ginger on hand. For days when you are really rushed, make sure you have a good selection of canned salmon, tuna, and sardines. My favorite low-sodium pink salmon and solid white albacore tuna packed in spring water are from the Crown Prince company (*see* the Resource Guide). Crown Prince tuna has no hydrolyzed vegetable protein or vegetable broth, additives containing naturally high levels of MSG that are found in almost all canned tuna. Also look for Crown Prince natural sardines and anchovies.

Keep organic tomato products on hand for easy meal-making. I especially like Eden's delicious organic spaghetti sauce in glass. Crushed tomatoes, diced tomatoes, and lightly seasoned tomato sauce are convenient pantry staples.

Dana Farber Cancer Institute researchers reported in March 1997 that processed tomato products help to reduce cancer risk. Research also shows that tomatoes offer significant protection against breast cancer because they contain the phytochemical lycopene.

Quick Scallops in Tomato Sauce with Basil and Olive Oil

Put about 2 cups of Eden's organic tomato sauce in a broiler-proof dish. Clean 2 cups of fresh scallops purchased that day. *Select beige, slightly pink, or orange scallops to avoid "processed" ones that have been dipped in a chemical solution to keep them looking fresher longer.* Drain seafood and add to tomato sauce, along with several cloves of finely minced garlic and minced fresh marjoram. Place under a preheated broiler for about 10 minutes. Remove from broiler and garnish with natural black olives, minced basil, and a drizzle of extra virgin olive oil. Serve with steamed broccoli rabe.

Other Time-Saving Suggestions

Poach fish or chicken breasts. Simply rinse fish or chicken and add water to cover, along with a little onion, carrot, bay leaf, celery, pepper corns (a serrano chili, for the brave!), garlic, and fresh herbs (marjoram, rosemary, and oregano). Add salt, and place over medium heat. Bring to a gentle boil, and cook until just tender. Remove from the broth right away, or it will continue to cook. Make extra poached fish or chicken for lunch or dinner the following day.

Quinoa. A quick-cooking, high-protein grain (which contains greater amounts of the B vitamins than rice) can be prepared in just 15–20 minutes.

Make a salad for dinner. Combine salad ingredients, season with sea salt and ground pepper, dress with your favorite vinaigrette, and top with cooked shrimp, poached chicken, tofu, or organic feta cheese.

Tempeh. Rich in protective isoflavones and phytosterols, tempeh cooks quickly in a braising liquid of mirin, soy sauce, and water with sliced garlic or shallots. Slice tempeh thinly for quicker cooking. Let cool, mash with your favorite minced vegetables, mellow light miso, lemon, and tahini for a quick and healthy protein source.

Poached eggs on baked potato or blanched spinach. Try this very easy, delicious supper. Scientists are finally acknowledging that eggs are nutritious. Dr. Krauss, the chairman of the American Heart Association's nutrition board, stated, "Even for people at high risk of heart disease, eggs are low on the list of worries." Put an organic Idaho potato in the oven, and bake for 1 hour. Take a relaxing bath. By the time your bath is over, you can poach an egg, take the potato out of the oven, make a quick, simple salad, and enjoy a nutritious, light meal.

Why do you recommend baking a potato in the oven instead of using a microwave? Microwaving is so fast!

My husband Thomas, who has a degree in mechanical engineering, has always questioned the safety of microwave ovens, so we've needed no convincing in our decision not to have one in our home. Here are some of our concerns:

• Microwave radiation, the energy source for heating foods in a microwave oven, may be a concern. Make sure the seals are tight on your microwave oven so that the radiation can't leak.

• Foods can absorb harmful chemicals from the containers in which they are microwaved—especially if the containers are plastic. It's not a good idea to warm a baby's formula or food in plastic containers in the microwave. We don't yet know the long-term effects of this practice.

• Foods sometimes cook unevenly in microwave ovens, which means harmful bacteria may multiply.

• Approximately 60 percent of the energy that microwave ovens use isn't used to cook or heat food, and so is wasted.

TIP: Look for a convenient, counter-top convection oven to use in place of a microwave. Convection ovens use air-driven heat to cook up to 30 percent faster (using 30 percent less energy) than regular ovens. Harmony ovens (Italian-made convection ovens) are available by mail-order. *(See* the Resource Guide.)

I'd like to include more healthy oils in my diet, but I've been on a low-fat diet for years. How can I get used to the taste of unrefined oils?

It's easy to become accustomed to the taste of freshly pressed, unrefined oils. Remind yourself that essential fats will not make you fat, in fact, the right kind and amount of fat will help to prevent overeating by fighting food (especially sugar) cravings, and increase the metabolic rate to help burn calories. Essential fatty acids (EFAs) help to prevent the overconsumption of calories that turn to fat in the body. Healthy fats also provide more energy to burn calories during exercise, and they help to promote prettier skin and hair, which makes people feel like taking better care of themselves. Including EFAs in your diet will provide a number of health-promoting bonuses.

• Immune system enhancement: EFAs improve functioning of the T-suppressor lymphocytes that defend the body from invaders.

• Cancer prevention: EFAs inhibit some types of cancer cell growth.

• Heart disease prevention: EFAs help to lower blood cholesterol and triglyceride levels, and regulate blood pressure.

• Diabetes control: EFAs promote more efficient insulin utilization.

• PMS: EFAs can alleviate 90 percent of PMS tensions and discomforts.

I began by using flaxseed and extra virgin olive oil. Combine, in a suribachi (*see* the Recipes), a little olive or flaxseed oil (or a little of each) with a clove of minced garlic and some minced fresh rosemary or basil. Add a bit of lemon or wine vinegar, some freshly ground pepper, and a little sea salt, and you've created a healthy, flavorful salad dressing. Another delicious use of flaxseed oil is to drizzle it on soft-boiled or poached eggs. The breast-protective antioxidant carotenoids in the egg yolk are made more potent by the addition of the flaxseed oil. Drizzle extra virgin olive oil lightly on minestrone soup, seafood cooked with tomatoes and garlic, or fresh salads and vegetables. Soon you will be used to the flavor and silky texture of fresh oils. Select other oils to experiment with, like pumpkin and sunflower seed, and walnut. The recipes and suggestions throughout this book will give you many ideas on delicious ways to incorporate health-giving oils in your diet.

Are oils that have been "expeller-pressed" healthy?

"Expeller-pressed" is a confusing term. It describes a process that results in clear oils, but how much pressure is used to produce the oils? If the pressure is high, it can result in the oil being exposed to a very wide range of temperatures, which is damaging to the delicate oil.

How do I select a good-quality oil if the "expeller-pressed" label is misleading?

Look for an oil that is deep golden in color to assure that it hasn't been refined, deodorized, or bleached. Select oils that are labeled "certified organic," free from pesticides and herbicides. These harmful substances are oil-soluble, which makes them even more dangerous. Oils should also be labeled "unrefined." Make sure you buy oils bottled in glass (to avoid potential health problems associated with unhealthy and ecologically unfriendly plastic), complete with a pressing date. Dark glass bottles help to protect the oils from damaging effects of light. I recommend Flora oils. My favorites are flaxseed, Udo's Choice Perfected Oil Blend, sunflower, walnut, almond, and pumpkin seed oils. (*See* the Resource Guide.)

> *Spectrum* magazine reported in its March-April 1997 issue that "Britain's Ministry of Agriculture, Fisheries, and Food found traces of plasticizers in every food sample taken since 1993. High levels were found in vegetable oils."

Studies show that olive oil is heart healthy and helps to prevent breast cancer, especially if complemented by a diet rich in vegetables and salads.

Dimitrios Trichopoulos, M.D., of the Harvard School of Public Health, notes that, "Studies showing olive oil is protective were done with extra virgin olive oil, not light olive oil," which comes from subsequent pressings of the olive. (Extra virgin olive oil is derived from the first pressing of the olives.) It's also important to note that "light" olive oil is *not* lower in either calories or fat.

The benefits to health will be greatest if you select an excellent-quality olive oil. Ask questions, and sample olive oils. Many health food and gourmet stores offer consumers extra virgin olive oil tastings. What should you look for in a good oil? "Nutty, grassy, buttery [taste] . . . like green apples," Nancy Harmon Jenkins, author of *The Mediterranean Diet Cookbook*, told *Self* magazine (September 1997). What to avoid? An oil that is "greasy, muddy, or musty." "You shouldn't buy it," Jenkins cautioned.

Olive oil can be stored for up to one year in a tightly closed container in a cool, dark place. Olive oil's cancer-protective qualities are enhanced by seasoning herbs, which contain antioxidants, so combine extra virgin olive oil frequently with rosemary, basil, and other herbs.

I don't have breast cancer, and even though I have greatly reduced my use of heated oils, I occasionally want to sauté. What are the safest oils for sautéing, and the safest method?

Sautéing is kept to a minimum in our home, purely as a preventive measure. When I do sauté—about two or three times a month—I use one of the following sources of fat:

• Butter is the safest, stablest fat for heating because it sautés at a lower temperature than oils. Butter heats to about 300 degrees; oils need more heat, around 360–420 degrees. It is amazing how little butter is needed for sautéing. Recently, I gently sautéed sliced mushrooms in a tiny amount of organic butter, with minced lemon grass and garlic, which I later added to rice.

• The two stablest oils for sautéing are sesame and extra virgin olive oils. (Avoid "roasted" or "toasted" sesame oil, because it has already been heated.) These two oils are safest for heating because they have a higher smoking point than other oils. When oil turns to smoke, it undergoes chemical changes that create carcinogenic substances. (For more information on the dangers of heating oils, refer to Chapter 1.)

TIP: Extra virgin olive oil is made from good quality, ripe olives, pressed without the use of heat, and is unrefined.

Suggested method for heating olive and sesame oils: Put a little water in the pan—approximately 1–2 tablespoons of water to 1 tablespoon of oil. The water not only acts as a buffer between the heat source and the food, but decreases the amount of oil needed.

Another method I often use is water-sautéing, without using any oil at all. You can easily "brown" a medium to large onion in about 2 tablespoons of water, stirring occasionally to prevent sticking.

I have trouble digesting beans. Any suggestions?

Spices and herbs help with the digestion of beans, and create a more flavorful dish. In her *Natural Health* article, "Better Beans with Spices," Leslie Cerier pointed out that certain herbs and spices contain volatile oils that reduce flatulence and relax stomach muscles, including ginger, cinnamon, thyme, cayenne, cardamom, coriander, and dill. Garbanzo, pinto, and black beans may protect against breast cancer, according to Jean Carper's *Food, Your Miracle Medicine*. Carper reported findings from a study conducted by Dr. Leonard Cohen at the American Health Foundation (in New York City) in which Hispanic women who ate ¾ cup of beans six days a week were found to have a lowered rate of breast cancer.

Tips on cooking beans: Soak beans in unsalted water that covers them by several inches. Discard soaking water and cook with fresh water. Use a deep, heavy pot, and place a 1–2-inch piece of kombu sea vegetable (a 1 inch piece per cup of beans) in the bottom of the pan. Boil the beans for about 12 minutes on high heat. Kombu contains glutamic acid, which helps to make the beans more digestible. Chewing beans thoroughly also aids the digestive process. Don't add salty or acidic ingredients like tomatoes or vinegar during cooking, or the beans will not break down easily. Onions and garlic can be added to beans while cooking.

What types of fruit are the healthiest?

I eat a lot of grapefruit because I like its sour, astringent taste in the morning. I feel that it stimulates the liver. Flavonoids in grapefruit (as well as its noringenin, and hesperitin in oranges) have been found to be especially effective at protecting against breast cancer. They aid the body in detoxifying carcinogens, and also help to guard against tumors. Interestingly enough, when you eat citrus fruits, the flavonoids work in unison with soy isoflavones to help prevent cancer, as Jeffrey S. Bland, Ph.D., reported in *Delicious!* magazine in September 1997.

Vogue magazine reported in November 1997 that a Rutgers University study found that, "ounce for ounce, kiwis offer the widest range of vitamins and minerals" of the twenty-seven common fruits analyzed. Kiwi fruit is used in traditional Chinese medicine to treat breast cancer. Raspberries and strawberries have cancer-blocking substances, and grapes with the seeds have potent antioxidant properties. Apples contain pectin, which has been found to help prevent tumors (buy organic, so you can eat the skin for more fiber). Figs have been found to contain breast-protective phytochemicals, and are high in enzymes. Watermelon, also high in enzymes, is another healthy choice. Pomegranates contain protective ellagic acid and other nutrients, and are a rich source of phytoestrogens. Pomegranate seeds mixed with organic plain yogurt is one of my favorite yogurt-fruit combinations.

> TIP: Avoid flavored yogurt; the flavorings have an adverse effect on yogurts living cultures. Flavor yogurt with plain fruit instead.

How should I select salt?

Table salt from the grocery store is not a healthy choice, because it:

- Is heated at high temperature. Normally, pure mineral salt contains calcium. However, when heated, the calcium is damaged and cannot be used by the body.

• Contains anticaking substances for "pourability"; these substances interfere with salt's ability to dissolve in your body.
• Contains sugar, which is added to stabilize the iodine.
Mineral salt is a rich replacement for table salt. Be sure mineral salt is not
white in color, which indicates that it has been refined. Look for light beige,
off-white, or pink mineral salt.

Mineral salt:

• Has been used in traditional medicine for centuries. For example, in
Ayurvedics, mineral salt is used to restore energy.
• Can counteract poisoning from poor-quality foods.
• Can actually soften some inflamed or hardened areas of the body, such
as hardened lymph nodes, hardening of the arteries, calcium deposits in joints,
and muscle inflammation.
• Can create bowel action.

> TIP: Avoid overuse of salt—especially a problem with processed
> foods—because it can block calcium absorption. Restaurant food
> is often over-salted.

Why is brown rice so much healthier to eat than white rice?

Brown rice contains more fiber than white rice, which becomes "white"
when the kernel is stripped of the brown bran layer that surrounds it. Each
cooked cup of brown rice yields approximately 3.2 grams of fiber, and white
rice only approximately 0.6 grams. The recommended daily intake of fiber
is 20–35 grams. According to Los Angeles dietitian Martin Yadrick, R.D.,
"Brown rice contains insoluble fiber, which is especially important because
it helps digestion and has been linked to lower incidence of bowel cancer
and other digestive disorders." Fiber may also help to avoid overeating,
because high-fiber foods make you feel fuller than low-fiber foods. Brown
rice also contains slightly more protein, calcium, potassium, and vitamin
E than white rice. Brown rice and other whole grains contain lignans,
phenolic acids, phytosterols, vitamin E, B vitamins, chromium, magnesium,
and fiber.

Pressure-Cooked Rice

Pressure cooking brown rice is both easy and delicious. I am convinced
that pressure-cooked whole grains not only taste better but are more digestible.

Pressure cooking, which uses high-temperature steam, decreases cooking time, enhances flavor, and preserves foods' nutrients. I like the Innova pressure cooker (*see* Resource Guide). If you don't pressure-cook brown rice, use a heavy, stainless steel pot, with a heavy, tight-fitting lid.

Pressure-Cooked Scallion Rice with Chestnuts

2 cups short grain brown rice
¾ cup of dried chestnuts
3 cups filtered water
3 pinches sea salt
2 minced scallions

Rinse rice in a bowl of cold water. Repeat until water is clear. Soak chestnuts overnight. Rice can also be soaked overnight, which helps to create a "lighter," more digestible rice, and is especially delicious when pressure-cooked. Soaking rice and other grain also helps to reduce phyates. (For more on phyates and phytic acid in fiber-rich foods, *see* Chapter 7, "Soybeans Protect Against Breast Cancer.")

Place rice and chestnuts in the pressure cooker. Add water and sea salt. Engage the pressure cooker lid, following the manufacturer's directions. (Innova's pressure cooker is 100 percent safe; it does not open until all the pressure inside is released.) Bring the cooker up to full pressure over medium-high heat. Once pressure is "up," turn down the heat to medium-low. You can also use a "flame tamer" under the pot (*see* the Resource Guide), which helps to produce a lower temperature. Cook the rice for about 20 minutes, then turn the heat down to low and cook for 30 minutes. You will hear a hissing sound from the pressure cooker, indicating that the cooker is working properly, while the rice is cooking.

Turn off the flame, remove from heat, and allow the pressure to dissipate naturally. The indicator button will drop when the pressure has released. At this point, remove the lid. I like to use a wooden paddle to remove the rice. Place the hot rice and chestnuts into a bowl, mincing scallions while they cool. Add scallions to the rice and chestnuts, and cover the dish with a bamboo sushi mat to keep it warm (bamboo mats are available at Oriental food markets). I prefer bamboo mats to cover cooked foods; a lid can capture enough heat to overcook food.

Facts About Chestnuts

Chestnuts are consumed regularly by some of the longest-lived peoples in the world, including the Hunzas of Pakistan, Soviet Georgians, and Abkhasians. They have also been a staple for thousands of years in the diets of Europeans and Asians.

I like to use dried chestnuts, because they need no roasting or peeling and are ready to use—but not ready to eat! They require soaking and cooking before eating.

- Chestnuts are sweet, tender, and flavorful.
- They contain 190 calories per cup.
- They are at home in sweet or savory dishes.
- Chestnuts should be soaked at least 4 hours before cooking.

Why shouldn't I use nonstick cookware?

The two healthiest types of cookware are stainless steel and enamel-covered. I strongly advise against using nonstick cookware, because the chemicals used to create the no-stick surface may raise unhealthy levels of estrogen by creating xenoestrogens. Aluminum, too, is not a healthy choice for cookware; high levels of aluminum have been found in people with Alzheimer's disease. I also advise against using iron cookware. A 1991 study showed that excess iron is present in breast cancer, and iron skillets and other cookware are definitely a source for iron.

What type of flour do you recommend for baking?

I recommend purchasing whole grain flours, cornmeal, oats, and other flours from companies that are aware of the possibility of spoilage. When grains are ground into flour, the fragile fats they contain spoil easily. Flour should be stored in the refrigerator section of the health food store. The most whole foods benefits are gained from flours that are ground from fresh grains and refrigerated to prevent spoiling. Home grain and flour mills are available through Miracle Exclusives (*see* the Resource Guide).

TIP: Don't purchase unrefrigerated whole grain flours or wheat germ.

How can I increase the fiber in my diet?

It's great that you've decided to add more fiber to your diet. Most Americans, in fact, need to double their fiber intake to obtain the recommended daily amount of 20–35 grams, which is easy to do when eating whole foods.

Seven Secrets for Increasing Fiber

• Use the whole vegetable. For instance, radish leaves make a great addition to salads.

• Purchase organic produce and a vegetable brush. Scrub the skins of fruits and vegetables, and eat the whole food. Don't discard peels.

• Consume more vegetables and fruits. Peas, corn, carrots, and broccoli are especially good sources of fiber.

• Eat more whole grains and eliminate or reduce carbohydrates in the form of bread, rolls, and pasta.

• Ingest flaxseeds on a daily basis. Grinding, and then soaking, increases bulk and aids metabolism. After the flaxseed is softened (2–8 hours of soaking, depending on your digestive system), you can add it to health shakes, juice, or water.

• Consume small amounts of beans to add fiber; balance them with herbs and spices to aid in digestion.

• Snack on raisins to boost your fiber intake. (For more information on fiber, *see* Chapter 11, "Food, Hormones, and Breast Cancer: What's the Connection?")

TIP: Be certain to drink plenty of water to increase fiber's bulk and speed its intestinal transit.

How can I select a good water filter?

More people than ever before are realizing that chlorine and other harmful chemicals in water (like pesticides) weaken our immune systems and contribute to cancer. Current research indicates that chlorinated water plays a significant role in breast, colon, and rectal cancers. We need to think about the water we shower in, as well as the water we drink.

Chlorinated shower water releases chloroform, a toxic gas created when chlorine (from the chlorination process) interacts with the natural organic matter in tap water. Fifty percent of the pollution from water is absorbed through the skin. Your body absorbs more chlorine from a 15-minute shower in chlorinated water than it does from drinking eight glasses of the same water.

I recommend purchasing a point-of-use drinking water filter and a shower filter (*see* the Resource Guide).

The health reasons for drinking water are many. Water keeps cells and bodily systems working. It absorbs shock in joints, muscles, and bones, and helps to disperse nutrients, vitamins, and minerals throughout the body. When you drink sufficient water, your skin glows, and your glands and hormones operate more efficiently. Water helps the liver to break down more fat.

Bottled water can be a breeding ground for bacteria. A single bacterium can multiply into 30,000 germs in just twelve hours. Be aware that warm weather—when people often carry bottles of water with them— encourages bacterial growth. The bottle's spout is a specific area in which bacteria multiply. Furthermore, states obviously cannot monitor each bottle of water to ensure that standards are consistent. I have also noticed some bottled water marked with an expiration date, which is puzzling. Water should not "expire." Another concern is the plastic bottles in which water is generally packaged. There is such a strong smell (and often, taste) of plastic that it makes me wonder if the plastic leeches into the water. It is possible, and Dr. Andrew Weil expressed his concern about this prospect in *Natural Health* magazine (January–February 1997).

Water Filter Secrets

Look for a filter that is certified by the National Sanitation Foundation. NSF is the organization that the Environmental Protection Agency depends upon to regulate the water filter business. You need to be sure your water filter is certified in two categories:

Health effects. This is the most difficult to find. It includes protection from contaminants such as pesticides, trihalomethanes, lead, and volatile organic chemicals (VOCs). Ask about the range of chemicals, pesticides, microbes (such as infectious agents like cryptosporidium and giardia) and other contaminants that the unit is certified to remove, and make sure it has NSF certification.

Aesthetic effects. Most units are certified by NSF for aesthetic effects, meaning "taste and smell" (removal of the smell of chlorine, for instance).

Combinations of pesticides can be especially lethal. Pesticides used in farming and on lawns end up in ground water, and then in our tap water. Research has found that combinations of pesticides have the ability to imitate estrogen; excessive estrogen contributes to breast, uterine, and prostate cancer.

How can I include a greater variety of vegetables in my diet? There is such emphasis placed on consuming at least five different vegetables daily, and I find this difficult to do.

It's extremely important to consume a variety of vegetables. Jane E. Brody reported in her *New York Times* "Personal Health" column (May 7, 1997) that women who eat the most vegetables have a 54 percent lower risk of developing breast cancer. The message from researchers is that we have to put health before convenience. People may think that they are ingesting adequate phytochemicals from supplements containing isolated plant chemicals. However, according to the co-chair of the World Cancer Research Fund expert panel on diet and cancer, Dr. John D. Potter (who also heads the Cancer Prevention Research program at the Fred Hutchinson Cancer Research Center in Seattle), the "chemical composition of the compounds may be altered" from so much processing that they "ultimately yield few health benefits for the consumer." Supplements just can't provide the protection that vegetables offer in terms of preventing cancer and other illnesses.

Eight Secrets For Including a Greater Variety of Vegetables in Your Diet

1. *Purchase smaller quantities of vegetables.* Buy one yellow squash, a cup of sugar snap beans, one small turnip, and a single leek. You can then select three or four different vegetables to steam for dinner. Place the denser, more fibrous vegetables (sliced turnips, squash) in the bottom of the steamer basket. When the steaming is almost completed, add the lighter, more delicate vegetables (sugar snap beans, leek). Steam for another 3–4 minutes until all vegetables are just tender.

2. *Salads provide a great opportunity to eat a variety of vegetables and fruit.* Remember to purchase small amounts of vegetables so you can continue to change which vegetable is consumed. Instead of buying a pound of cucumbers, for instance, but a single cucumber, a few Jerusalem artichokes, and a red pepper.

Jerusalem artichoke is actually a sunflower with edible tubers; they are sometimes called "sunchokes." They can be eaten raw in salads, steamed, roasted, boiled, or diced into soups. Next time you make chicken or tuna salad, replace celery with minced Jerusalem artichoke.

3. *Think color, and be willing to experiment.* Try new vegetables, like Easter egg radishes (which are purple, light red, white, or dark red), or magenta broccoli. If you buy green cabbage one week, select purple the following week. A meal should ideally reflect a variety of colors to assure that you are obtaining the broadest spectrum of phytochemicals, vitamins, and minerals. For example, to accompany salmon, select:

Yellow	Corn
Green	Broccoli
Red	Red pepper
White	Onions
Orange	Blood orange segments
Dark green	Arugula

A sample menu would be:

Salmon
Steamed broccoli
Corn on the cob
Salad of arugula, roasted red pepper, blood orange segments, and
     sliced Vidalia onion.

This menu includes six different vegetables (and fruit) in one meal. If you have already consumed ½ grapefruit (for breakfast or dessert), and a salad with three vegetables for lunch (along with your protein, like chicken or tofu), you are meeting the recommendation of eating ten different vegetables each day, and well on your way to reducing your breast cancer risk by 50%, as current studies report.

TIP: Be experimental. Purchase yellow and orange tomatoes in the summer from farmers' markets, instead of just red ones.

---

4. *Evaluate your favorite recipes.* Consider ways to reduce their meat portions, and replace meat with more vegetables and grains. As the American Institute for Cancer Research suggests in its brochure, "Feast on fruits and vegetables." Turn your chicken and shrimp with vegetables dish into a vegetable dish with chicken and shrimp.

TIP: Don't overcook vegetables, and be aware that leftover vegetables are not as protective as freshly cooked ones. A 1995 study from the Department of Gastroenterology and Food Research Institute in the Netherlands found that freshly cooked vegetables are the most powerful detoxifiers of carcinogens.

---

5. *Don't underestimate the protection that a variety of fresh cooking herbs can offer.* Get in the habit of buying fresh herbs on a regular basis. Some of the most readily available fresh herbs include rosemary, dill, basil, parsley, cilantro, tarragon, sage, and mint.

Make easy vinaigrettes with freshly minced herbs as often as possible. Use a suribachi with a wooden pestle. This is a traditional Japanese method for making dressings and condiments. A tip I learned in Jordan is to begin vinaigrettes by blending minced garlic with salt before adding olive oil and lemon. Try it, and you'll discover how quick, easy, and effective it is to blend a delicious vinaigrette. Simply blend several pinches of sea salt with several cloves of minced garlic in a suribachi. After the garlic and salt are blended, slowly add flaxseed or olive oil, and lemon juice. You can then add a touch of wine vinegar, and 2 teaspoons of your favorite minced herb. I love rosemary or mint, but I try to use a variety of fresh herbs in daily cooking because of their protective qualities.

6. *Purchase a zester, a handy little lemon and orange peel grater.* Use grated, *organic* citrus peel in rice, over fish, or on salads. Citrus peels contain potent breast-protective phytochemicals.

TIP: A sharp, pointed end on your knife makes it easier to mince shallots or garlic.

---

7. *Use the whole vegetable.* Don't throw away tangy radish leaves, for instance. Radish, turnip, and beet leaves make healthy additions to salads or steamed vegetables.

8. *Add diced root vegetables to soups, as thickening agents, or to stews.* Use a convenient immersion blender right in the pot to puree. You will have fewer bowls to clean and a greater variety of vegetables. Immersion blenders, available at gourmet stores, are also convenient in making soy or yogurt shakes.

What if I am too busy to cook? How do I get enough soy?

A diet rich in soy foods offers breast cancer protection. In fact, in a 1997 study, David T. Zara, Ph.D. (California Public Health Foundation, Berkeley), reported that the soy isoflavonoid genistein is better than other flavonoids, even quercetin, for breast cancer prevention. Genistein inhibits cell growth and is a strong estrogen antagonist. These two factors suggest that soy may also offer protection against the growth of malignant human prostate cells, indicating that men can receive the same benefits from soy as women. Soy is also heart protective. In 1995, the *New England Journal of Medicine* reported an analysis of thirty-eight controlled studies showing that soy helps to reduce both bad cholesterol (by 12.9%) and triglycerides (by 10.5%). Supplement with soy for both breast and heart protection.

The following soy products can offer convenient supplementation on days when you are too busy to cook:

- Iso-Gen tablets from Bio-Nutritional Formulas.
- Harmonizer soy nutrients combined in tablets with herbs to help women avoid discomfort associated with hormonal fluctuations like PMS or menopause.

(Iso-Gen may be taken by men and women; Harmonizer is formulated specifically for women.)

TIP: A soy shake can be a quick breakfast. I like to combine Edensoy with strawberries and 1 tablespoon of flaxseed oil—easy and healthy! Soy milk contains half the calories and fat but nearly as much protein as whole milk.

I really love the richness of dairy foods. Could you tell me which foods are the healthiest to select, or do I really need to avoid them all?

If you are concerned about preventing breast cancer, you should know that bovine growth hormone, a potent stimulator of cell growth in both cows and humans, has been found to have cancer-promoting effects on breast cells. Recombinant bovine growth hormone (rBGH), the type usually administered to cows, also promotes cancerous changes in colon cells.

Why was rBGH approved for use by the Food and Drug Administration? Perhaps because injection of rBGH causes cows to produce 20 percent more milk than they had previously produced. As a growth hormone, rBGH stimulates the pituitary to produce a substance called insulin-like growth factor (abbreviated "IGF-1"). IGF-1 is transported throughout the body to all cells, affecting their "growth, division, and differentiation, particularly in children, and has been increasingly linked by modern research to human cancer development and growth," Samuel S. Epstein reported in the *International Journal of Health Services in 1996.* An additional concern for consumers is that cows "treated" with rBGH appear to develop mastitis regularly, and are then treated with antibiotics (another problem). Milk contaminated with rBGH has been found to contain pus from mastitis. When the FDA approved the use and sale of rBGH in November 1994, it also banned the labeling of milk to show it contained this substance.

On the eve of the second anniversary of the FDA's approval of rBGH in 1996, the Cancer Prevention Coalition and Food and Water released a new study suggesting that rBGH increases risks of breast and colon cancers in humans.

I recommend that women avoid all milk that is not organic and hormone-free. Fats of all kinds—milk fat, saturated fat, vegetable oils, and trans-fats—are powerful components of either health or disease. All cells are affected by fats and oils. It pays to be selective.

Another alternative is to switch to goat milk products. Goat's milk is gentler on the digestive system than cow's milk. Many people who are allergic to cow's milk have found that the fat and protein in goat's milk is more easily absorbed. A recent study indicated that, of 300 infants with milk allergies, 270 of them could easily digest goat's milk and became symptom-free. It has a sweet and slightly hazelnut-like flavor, and can be enjoyed either as a drink or as a replacement for cow's milk in recipes. Goat's milk contains a nutritional profile similar to that of cow's milk in terms of its calcium, phosphate, and vitamins A and B.

Mediterranean Salad Dressing

(MAKES 1¼ CUPS DRESSING)
Recipe courtesy of Meyerberg.

½ cup Meyerberg Goat Milk
¼ cup feta cheese, crumbled
3 tbsp olive oil
2 tbsp fresh lemon juice
2 tbsp Italian parsley, chopped
2 cloves garlic, minced
1 tbsp fresh oregano, minced
2 tsp anchovy paste
1 tsp dry mustard
¼ tsp salt
freshly ground pepper to taste

In a blender or food processor fitted with a steel blade, process all of the salad dressing ingredients together until blended. Dressing is thick and creamy. Refrigerate until ready to use.

Note: This recipe originally did not contain minced, fresh oregano. I substituted fresh oregano for a prepared condiment, to add the nutritional boost of phytosterols and the flavor of fresh herbs. Breast-healthy herbs can be substituted for other ingredients in many recipes.

Yogurt Contains Nutrients That Protect the Breasts

The newest fatty acid "star," conjugated linoleic acid (known by nutritionists as CLA), is a little-known fatty acid found in dairy products that may help to protect against breast cancer. Substances called cytokines, which are secreted by immune system cells, may be affected by CLA. Animal research shows that CLA builds muscle, protects against cancer, increases immune response, and can actually reduce the risk of heart disease. CLA can help stop damage caused by free radicals. Human studies of CLA have not yet begun. (Lamb and beef are also rich in CLA.)

In a *New York Times* "Personal Health" column in May 1997, Jane E. Brody discussed a study in the Netherlands that found frequent consumption of "fermented dairy products (yogurt, cheese, buttermilk)" appeared to result in "a 77 percent reduction in breast cancer risk." Calcium-D-glucarate (CDG) acts as a modulator of excess estrogen, and helps to prevent it from being absorbed into the body. Yogurt is a source of CDG; just 3 tablespoons a day provides enough CDG for breast health.

Yogurt also contains "friendly cultures," lactobacillus and acidophilus. Yogurt helps to strengthen the digestive system by creating a healthy environment. The protective bacteria found in yogurt interfere with the cancer-promoting effects of viruses and bacteria. Yogurt also contains tumor-suppressing agents. Yogurt is especially recommended for people at high risk of developing cancer because it is efficient in blocking the cellular changes that can lead to cancer. Numerous studies have shown that the more yogurt a woman eats, the lower her risk of developing breast cancer. If yogurt is consumed before puberty, it decreases breast cancer risk by half.

TIP: A recent study reported that the friendly flora in the gut helps women to benefit from soy isoflavones. Be sure you consume yogurt. (My favorite is goat's milk.)

Secrets for Healthy Dairy Selection

• Select only organic milk, cheese, yogurt, or cottage cheese from naturally raised animals that have not been given hormones, antibiotics, or other chemicals.

• Focus on organic, plain yogurt, a source of calcium D-glucarate (CDG) and conjugated linoleic acid (CLA).

• Select nonaged cheese. Choose from among fresh cheeses, including goat's milk, organic feta, ricotta, cottage cheese, or mozzarella.

Why is sauerkraut often recommended for health?
Sauerkraut, as well as yogurt, contains living cultures called lactic acid bacteria. These living cultures greatly strengthen immune function. The incidence of cancer is much lower in countries that consume large amounts of lactic acid–fermented foods, including Russia, China, Bulgaria, and Romania. Naturally pickled vegetables have also been a part of Far Eastern cuisine for centuries.

> During fermentation, the carbohydrates in vegetables decompose and form lactic acid. Lactic acid in turn activates gastric juices, thereby stimulating the breakdown of food in the bowel.

Ten Secrets of Sauerkraut's Healing Properties

• It is rich in acetylcholine, a substance that is calming to the central nervous system. Acetylcholine can produce a more restful mind and sleep pattern.
• It activates the pancreas, an important gland that is part of the endocrine system.
• It is rich in choline. Choline, like acetylcholine, plays a role in the nervous system, helping in the transmission of nerve impulses. Choline is also extremely important to liver and kidney function.
• The lactic acid in sauerkraut helps in enzyme production, which provides protection against cancer.
• Sauerkraut helps to cleanse the large intestines and regenerate the blood. It has been used for centuries for its ability to heal infectious intestinal diseases.

Foods rich in lactic acid include (be sure all sources are organic):
• Sauerkraut.
• Pickled daikon radish (from the macrobiotic section of the health food store).
• Natural yogurt with acidophilus.
• Miso (Add pureed miso at the end of cooking. Do not boil miso, as this destroys the lactic acid bacteria.).
• Kim chee pickles.

TIP: Select only organic, naturally made sauerkraut from the health food store. Sauerkraut from the refrigerator section is my first choice, because it's likely to contain more lactic acid bacteria. Be aware that pickled vegetables from the delicatessen and grocery store are *not* the same as naturally fermented, chemical-free sauerkraut. In fact, pickled foods are not recommended by the American Cancer Society.

Smoked and Cured Meats

Nitrites are used to preserve and flavor cured meats, and chemical nitrite salts are used as curing agents in making sausages and other cured meats. The American Cancer Society does not recommend consumption of foods that contain nitrites because they encourage the formation of N-nitroso compounds, which are linked to cancer in animal studies. Population studies have also linked nitrites and cured meats to esophageal and stomach cancers in humans. Nitrites (or nitrates) are not permitted in baby food, nor do federal standards permit hydrogenated vegetable oils, shortening, or trans-fatty acids in baby foods. What is unhealthy for babies and toddlers is also unhealthy for adults!

CHAPTER 19

Summary

Getting Sidetracked by Nutritional Theories

When I began the research for this book, a diet emphasizing precise amounts of protein, carbohydrates, and fat was popular. As I conclude *Total Breast Health,* eating according to blood type is trendy.

When I first became interested in health and nutrition as a teenager, a diet high in protein and saturated fat was common. My parents' generation, for whom steak and rich desserts epitomized the good life, became extremely concerned about having high cholesterol levels, and many of them took (and are still taking) cholesterol-lowering drugs.

The theory that high blood cholesterol levels contribute significantly to heart disease has been widely accepted for the last thirty years, despite the fact that most people who have heart attacks have normal cholesterol levels. Has this field of research been influenced by manufacturers of anti-cholesterol drugs, as the *New England Journal of Medicine* questioned in April 1996?

For the last thirty years, Dr. Kilmer McCully, a Harvard-educated physician and researcher, pursued another avenue toward understanding heart disease, one that focuses on prevention and nutrition, not drugs. In 1997, Dr. McCully finally received validation of his theory that a substance called "homocysteine" is a major contributor to heart disease. Homocysteine is a metabolite of the essential amino acid methionine; it builds up in the blood and harms blood vessels as a result of consuming excessive animal protein like milk, meat, and eggs. If the diet contains enough nutrients like vitamins B6 and B12 and folic acid, the body is able to metabolize homocysteine before it can damage blood vessels. If the diet is poor—like the highly refined and processed diet most people in Northern America consume—it's very difficult to obtain the important nutrients that prevent arteries and blood vessels from clogging, and help to prevent heart disease and other illnesses.

According to Dr. McCully's theory, many (if not most) cases of heart disease can be prevented by taking the simple, inexpensive steps of adjusting our diets to contain less animal protein and making sure we consume adequate amounts of B vitamins to prevent the buildup of homocysteine.

How can we determine what is sensible in the field of nutrition amid all the confusion? I often remind women I counsel that commonsense, traditional cultures that rely on a plant-based diet have the lowest rates of cancer and heart disease. The Asian and Mediterranean diets emphasize vegetables and fruit, grain, beans, and small portions of fish or meat and, in Asia, protective soy foods.

The Oldways Preservation and Trust in Cambridge, Massachusetts, is a nonprofit organization made up of culinary professionals from all over the world, national and international public health officials, and progressive research organizations interested in improving nutrition. The focus of Oldways is not calorie counting or trendy theories, but study of traditional, health-giving foods. Oldways President K. Dunn Grifford believes that, above all, food should be enjoyable. In the research Oldways sponsors, a healthy population within a specific geographical area is studied. Over a two-year period, fifteen or twenty advisors analyze information that applies to this population and develop a type of "blueprint," composite diet that retains flexibility.

I suspect that Dr. McCully's theory about heart disease and homocysteine has met with strong opposition because there is no money in it. The B vitamins that prevent the buildup of homocysteine are widely available. Sadly, there has never been a lot of money in the prevention of disease.

We can, however, use the resources available to us to create a health-promoting and illness-preventative lifestyle. Consider, for instance how our grandparents and great-grandparents lived and ate before the rates of cancer and heart disease skyrocketed. They were more physically active; they didn't spend hours in front of a television set. It took more physical effort to wash clothing and clean house; they got exercise from performing this work rather than from going to the gym, as people do now. Stress was lower; there was no mass media reporting up-to-the-minute news about natural disasters, death, and political conflict. Today, many people watch the news while eating a fast-food dinner from the neighborhood pizza restaurant. What is this kind of stress and nutrient-deficient food doing to our immune systems?

Earlier in the twentieth century, a typical dinner gathered the family together, and communication was encouraged, partly because there was no distracting TV. A meal most likely included a vegetable-based stew, with a small amount of meat or a piece of fish. Real butter was spread on bread, not margarine. If cheese was consumed, it was made from animals raised naturally, without antibiotics or hormones. In fact, all animal protein, eggs and dairy were free of hormones, antibiotics, and other chemicals. Heavy-duty pesticides were not applied to produce. Fruits and vegetables were grown locally and consumed in season. Foods were not processed, and did not contain chemicals like aspartame and saccharin, or artificial colorings like FDC and Red #3.

People also did not consume refined vegetable oils made with trans-fatty acids to promote shelf life, then deodorized and chemically treated. Chips, snack foods, cookies, and other baked goods were not made from hydrogenated and partially hydrogenated fats containing health-destructive trans-fatty acids.

People Are More Deficient in Essential Fatty Acids Than Any Other Nutrient

It should not be a surprise that the rates of both cancer and heart disease have greatly increased in our century. For decades, people believed that margarine was better than butter because it didn't raise cholesterol, not knowing it was filled with health-destroying trans-fatty acids. We eat a preponderance of fast and fried foods. Oils heated at high temperatures are loaded with dangerous by-products that have unknown long-term effects on our healths and contain some trans-fats. Heated oils also prevent essential fatty acids from being absorbed. *People are now more deficient in essential fatty acids than any other nutrient.*

We cannot absorb the protective essential fatty acids (EFAs) when the proportion of heated fat and trans-fats eaten are so much greater than healthy fats that the EFAs are displaced. In a 1997 study performed by researchers at the University of North Carolina at Chapel Hill, trans-fats were found to increase the risk of breast cancer. Given what we now know about trans-fats, that is most likely because, in part, people are so deficient in essential fatty acids.

The effect of a given increase in trans-fats may depend upon the amount of unsaturated fat competing with it for binding sites. Women with the lowest levels of polyunsaturated fat had a 3.6-fold greater amount of trans-fats. In other words, trans-fats *displace* other, healthier fatty acids, such as those found in flaxseed and fatty-rich fish, or in nuts and seeds.

Trans-fats have an adverse effect on protective enzymes in the body that potentially have antiinflammatory effects.

Transfats are associated with chromosome breakage.

It was known as long ago as 1975 that fried foods, margarine, and shortening were linked to a significant increase in breast cancer risk. Roland L. Phillips noted in *Cancer Research* in 1975 that "the association with fried potatoes and fried foods in general raises the possibility that carcinogens may be produced by excessive heating of fat during frying."

I wrote this book because I was inspired to create a collection of recipes using unheated, fresh, life-giving oils. Along the way, I investigated the body of research on the topic of fats and oils (as well as soy foods, vegetables, cooking herbs, and other nutrient-dense, protective foods) to understand better the powerful effect they have on our health. I am neither a scientist nor a physician. I have written this book for women like myself who are interested in nutrition and want to understand which foods protect our breasts, and our health.

I hope the recipes in Part Three illustrate that it is possible to prepare food that tastes delicious without heating oil, help women reduce the frequency at which they fry foods, and encourage experimentation with their own healthy versions of light cooking techniques. *Bon appetit!*

PART THREE

Recipes

The recipes I have selected for *Total Breast Health* are a sampling of the many dishes I have created over the years as a result of my love of beautiful, life-giving foods, influenced and flavored by travel overseas. I have drawn from many cultures in recommending these breast-healthy foods. Olive oil from the Mediterranean; flax seed oil from Northern Europe; and soy foods from Japan have been found to protect our breasts.

Food should delight and refresh us. The wonderful, fresh cuisines of both the Mediterranean and Japan demonstrate that health and flavor not only can exist side-by-side, but also enhance each other. The freshest, ripest tomato is the most flavorful and the healthiest tomato we could eat.

The following recipes incorporate foods that have been found to protect our breasts, as well as to support liver health. The liver is essential to breast health, as we've learned, because it metabolizes hormones and fats.

The recipes in *Total Breast Health* provide the bonus of helping to prevent colon and prostate cancer, which, like breast cancer, are hormone-sensitive cancers. The heart is also protected by these foods. Making the healthier choices I've recommended and including these wonderful foods in your diet will protect you and your family in many ways. Enjoy!

A note on soy products: Select organic misos, tamari, and shoyu from companies that use naturally grown soybeans. Shoyu contains soybeans, whole wheat, and sea salt. Tamari is wheat-free, and is made from soybeans and sea salt. (*See* Resource Guide.)

Power Foods for
Breast Health

Vegetables	Select from the widest variety of the freshest produce available. There is much that science has yet to discover regarding phytonutrients. More research will undoubtedly discover many more protective phytochemicals that haven't yet been identified. To safeguard health, selecting a variety of vegetables (and fruits) ensures that we are consuming the widest spectrum of protective phytochemicals.
Cabbage family	Savoy cabbage, Brussels sprouts, cabbage, broccoli, cauliflower, rutabagas, turnips, daikon radish, horseradish, radish, watercress.
Orange, red, and yellow vegetables	Carrots, squash (kabocha, buttercup, delicata, spaghetti, butternut, hubbard, longneck) yams.
Dark, leafy greens	Kale, savoy cabbage, bok choy, collards, mustard, turnip greens, green leaf and romaine lettuce.
Bitter greens	Dandelion, watercress, broccoli rabe, endive, escarole.
Raw greens and vegetables for salads	Radish, tomato, onion, celery, romaine lettuce, grated raw spinach, beets, broccoli sprouts, purslane, cucumber, dandelion leaves.
Wild greens	Nettles, lamb quarters, watercress, dandelion, purslane.
Fruit	Grapes with seeds, raspberries, strawberries, tangerines, grapefruit (especially pink), kiwi, watermelon, figs, pineapple, apricots, apples.
Glutathione-rich foods	Asparagus, parsley, spinach, watermelon, purslane.
Fresh cooking herbs	Rosemary, mint, lemon grass, basil, parsley, sage, marjoram, and other fresh herbs. Note: Utilize herbs such as marjoram, mint, and basil with bibb lettuce and other salad greens in raw vegetable salads.
Protective alliums	Garlic, chives, leeks, onions, spring onions, shallots, scallions. Note: These foods contain

	protective protective compounds that also help in glutathione production.
Peppers	Hot red and green peppers, especially potent when combined with garlic.
Grains	Brown rice, millet, corn, quinoa, bulgur, buckwheat (including soba noodles), oats.
Legumes	Lentils, chickpeas, white and black soybeans, mung beans, and other dried beans.
Soy foods	Tempeh, miso, shoyu and tamari, natto, tofu, and soy milk.
Sea vegetables	Wakame, kombu, hijiki, arame, and other sea vegetables.
Mushrooms	Shiitakes, reishi, maitake.
Spices	Turmeric, ginger root, celery seed, cumin, paprika, nutmeg, caraway, cayenne, saffron
Lemon and orange peel	Note: It is especially important to purchase organic oranges and lemons when using the peel.
Seeds and nuts	Flaxseeds, milk thistle, sesame, pumpkin, sunflower seeds; brazil nuts, almonds, walnuts, chestnuts, hazelnuts.
Freshly pressed oils	Flaxseed oil, extra virgin olive oil, walnut, pumpkin, sunflower, hazelnut, sesame, and almond oils.
Fatty-rich fish	Tuna, rainbow trout, salmon, eel, sardines, herring, mackerel.
Meat	Lamb, turkey.
Dairy foods	Unflavored yogurt, goat's milk and cheese.

More Easy Lunch Ideas

• Blanched broccoli, udon, soba, or yam noodles served on a bed of chopped dandelion greens and thinly sliced tofu. Garnish with lemon, umeboshi vinegar, scallions, minced garlic, and flaxseed oil.

• Fresh, raw vegetables such as radishes, cucumber, daikon, carrots, and lettuce served with a dollop of humus. Garnish with a splash of lemon and extra virgin olive oil.

Total Breast Health's Seven-Day Menu Plan

Every person is different, so proportions should be flexible. This menu plan is similar to traditional diets of the Mediterranean and Asia, where plant foods are the basis for a healthy diet.

Approximately 50% of total calories from   vegetables, fruits, whole grains, beans, and other sources.

Approximately 25–35% from   good-quality protein like fish, skinless lean turkey or chicken, lamb, beef, soy foods like tempeh or tofu, yogurt, eggs, or goat's cheese.

Approximately 15–20% from   protective fats such as fresh, unprocessed organic flaxseed oil, extra virgin olive oil, avocado, nuts, and seeds.

Breakfast
½ Red Grapefruit and Blueberries
Huevos Rancheros (with water sautéed onion, garlic, and pepper), and a Poached Egg
Soy Sausage
Green or Kukicha Tea

Midmorning
Fresh Vegetable Juice Combo with Ground Flaxseeds

Lunch
Corn and Fennel Miso Soup
Tofu Côte d'Azur in Radiccio
Steamed Savoy Cabbage with Mint Vinaigrette

Dinner
Mixed Spinach and Avocado Salad with Orange Peel
Quick Scallops in Tomato Sauce
Basmati Rice with Mushrooms and Onions
Apricot
Lemon Balm Tea

Breakfast	Midmorning	Lunch	Dinner
Watermelon Slice Steel Cut Oats with Sesame Seeds Soft-Boiled Egg Green or Kukicha Tea	Pomegranate and Yogurt with Ground Flaxseeds	Miso Soup Spicy Sardine Pita Pocket Fennel Salad Dandelion Tea	Wakame Salad Soybean Casserole with Chicken Broccoli and Leek Coulis Grated Beets with Vinaigrette of Extra Virgin Olive Oil, Garlic, Lemon, and Fresh Rosemary Brown Rice
Kiwi Fruit Muesli with Ground Flaxseeds and Soy Milk Green or Kukicha Tea	Fresh Vegetable Juice Combo with Chlorella	Quinoa Salad with Carrot Miso Dressing Tempeh Salad Nettles Tea	Grapes and Goat's Cheese Basic Miso Soup Hijiki and Arugula Salad Roman Pot Chilean Sea Bass Tri-Colore Vegetables with Marjoram Vinaigrette Mock Coffee Flan with Raspberry Sauce
½ Red Grapefruit Scrambled Tofu Small piece of Goat's Cheese Green or Kukicha Tea	Fresh Vegetable Juice Combo with Ground Flaxseeds	Basic Miso Soup with Asparagus Spicy Shrimp Salad with Basil Dandelion Salad Red Root Tea	Buttercup Squash Dip with Raw Vegetable Crudités Spicy Savoy Cabbage and Tomato Salad Yosenabe with Tempeh and Fish Brown Rice and Black Soy Beans Hot Co-Co Mocha

Breakfast
Bimbim Babb drizzled with Flaxseed Oil and garnished with Minced Scallions
Grapes
Green or Kukicha Tea

Midmorning
Soy Milk Shake with Raspberries and Ground Flaxseeds

Lunch
Hatfield High-Enzyme Salad
Quick Humus
Nettles Tea

Dinner
Miso Soup with Shiitake Mushrooms
Butter Lettuce and Tomato Salad with Horseradish Dressing
Tuna with Coriander and Onions
Mediterranean Potato Salad
Baked Apple

Tangerine
Goat's Milk Yogurt with Ground Flaxseeds
Almonds
Green or Kukicha Tea

Fresh Vegetable Juice Combo with Ginger

Wild Yam Soba with Herbs and Lemon
Blanched Mixed Greens and Tofu
Grated Carrots drizzled with Extra Virgin Olive Oil
Chamomile Tea

Basic Miso Soup with Carrots
Easy Middle Eastern Cabbage Salad
Moroccan Garbanzo Stew with Lamb
Barley and Shiitake Salad
Cantaloupe and Goat's Cheese
Dandelion Tea

Yogurt and Fresh Strawberry Shake with Ground Flaxseeds

Dried Apricots
Walnuts

Salad of Seasonal, Fresh, Raw Vegetables with Mediterranean Salad Dressing
Tempeh Sandwich Spread on One Slice of Whole Wheat Toast
Steamed Asparagus
Lemon Balm Tea

Mung Bean Soup with Ribbon Pasta
Baye Salad with Chicory and Tahini Parsley Dressing
Dilled Salmon in Miso-Lemon Sauce over leeks
Quinoa
Brussels Sprouts Piquant
Almond Amazake Pudding
Nettles Tea

- Salmon or albacore tuna (rich source of omega-3s) on a bed of escarole, Bibb lettuce, tomato, and vidalia onion with lemon and umeboshi vinegar.
- Thinly sliced chicken or turkey paillard atop a salad dressed with Dijon mustard, lemon juice, and olive/flaxseed oil vinaigrette.

BREAKFAST

Scrambled Tofu

(SERVES 1–2)

❦ A 1996 study published in *Nutrition and Cancer* reported that nor-ingenin from grapefruit works with soy isoflavones to protect against breast cancer. Have a half-a-grapefruit as your first course, followed by scrambled tofu.

½ lb tofu
½ cup finely chopped onions
⅓ tsp turmeric
½ tsp sea salt
2 tbsp filtered water
1–2 tsp flax oil

In a small skillet, heat water over high flame. Water sauté onions for about 10 minutes until almost brown. Stir frequently and season lightly with sea salt. Add a little more water and crumble tofu into pan. Continue to water sauté. Season with turmeric and cook over medium heat for 5 more minutes. Remove from flame, lightly garnish with a drizzle of fresh flax oil and serve.

Comment: Turmeric has been used in traditional medicine for the treatment of cancer for centuries. In modern time, it has been widely researched and found to be liver protective, and a stronger anti-oxidant than Vitamin C.

Research shows genistein, a compound in soy, blocks the growth of cancerous cells. Mark Messina, Ph.D., a genistein researcher in Port Townsend, WA, has found that just half a cup of tofu a day can reduce breast cancer risk between 20% and 50% (*Nutrition & Cancer*, vol. 26, 1996). Consider tofu for a breakfast choice.

Breast-Protective Power Foods: Tofu, onions, turmeric, and flax oil.

Korean-Style Rice and Eggs Bimbim Babb

(SERVES 1)

❧   *This typical Korean breakfast breakfast has a good combination of protein, egg; complex carbohydrate, brown rice; and protective fat, flax seed oil. If you like spicy food, you'll love Bimbim Babb.*

1 or 2 poached eggs
1 cup of cooked brown rice
2 tbsp flax oil
1 finely minced scallion
3 pinches of cayenne pepper
3 pinches of sea salt

Top brown rice with poached eggs. Garnish with minced scallions, and a drizzle of flax seed oil. Season with salt and cayenne pepper. Spicy kim chee pickles are the usual accompaniment to this Korean breakfast.

> TIP: Look for eggs from hens that have been fed flaxseeds. Ask about these eggs from your local health food store.

Breast-Protective Power Foods: Brown rice, flax oil, scallions, cayenne pepper.

Steel Cut Oats

(SERVES 2)

❧   *Sesame seeds are rich sources of essential fatty acids. Enjoy them over a hot bowl of oat cereal.*

1 cup rinsed organic steel cut oats
½ cup organic sesame seeds
1–2 tbsp honey
Pinch sea salt
2 cups filtered water

Rinse sesame or sunflower seeds. Bring water to a rolling boil, salt, and steel cut oats. Simmer over medium heat for 5–6 minutes. Stir and turn down. Cook gently for several minutes more. Take off heat and cover with a bamboo mat. Oats will continue to steam in the covered pot. Five minutes later, stir, and serve with your choice of sesame or sunflower seeds and honey.

TIP: Be sure all sources of dairy are organic.

Additional Breakfast Suggestions:

- Eggs, either soft boiled or poached with a teaspoon of flax oil.
- Unflavored yogurt, served with grapes. Consume seeds for additional source of OPCs.
- Fruit salad with kiwi, grapes, and watermelon, with yogurt or cottage cheese.
- Museli with soy or goat's milk.
- Goat's milk yogurt with fruit salad.
- Goat's cheese, almonds, and fruit.
- Soy sausage, oven roasted or based in water with the pan covered.

TIP: Be aware that most granola is made with oils that probably are not fresh or even natural. Choose museli instead.

Breast-Protective Power Foods: Oats, sesame seeds.

APPETIZERS

Quick Humus

(Serves 3–4)

❧ *A Lebanese "mazah" is the prototype for mezas served in Israel, Jordan and Turkey. They are the most wonderful experience in dining—that is, if you love the freshest vegetables, herbs, and extra virgin olive oil available. At the center of a table, a platter holds an endless variety of seasonal vegetables—a small head of beautiful, vibrant lettuce; cucumbers; scallions; watercress; incredibly flavorful tomatoes; green pepper; celery; and beautiful, garden-fresh mint. Around this abun-*

dance of vegetables are colorful, small, unmatched plates with pickles; tabbouleh; fresh tahini; parsley sauce; different kinds of hot fish; nuts; olives; cheese; shish kabob; stuffed grape leaves; green bean salads; foul (garlicy beans in tomato sauce); humus, and freshly baked pita. Humus is always served on the mazah table, drizzled with olive oil, and garnished with minced parsley.

    1 15-ounce can organic garbanzo beans
    1 tsp organic unroasted sesame tahini
    1 tbsp extra virgin olive oil
    1–2 cloves of garlic
    1 lemon
    1 tsp of light miso such as chick pea or
        mellow white
    3 tbsp minced parsley

Blend all ingredients. Delicious in pita with sliced onion, lettuce, and parsley.

Breast-Protective Power Foods: Garbanzo beans, tahini, extra virgin olive oil, miso, garlic, parsley.

Buttercup Squash Dip

❦   *This is a delicious, savory squash dip that goes well with crudité vegetables. It is full of unexpected sweet and savory flavors. Use very fresh basil, and combine ingredients right before serving.*

    4 cups cooked buttercup or hokaido squash
    2 tbsp sweet white or mellow white miso
    2 tbsp unroasted sesame tahini
    3 small red onions
    6 cloves of minced garlic
    2 tbsp mixed extra virgin olive oil and flaxseed oil
    filtered water
    2 tbsp minced basil

Peel squash and cut into chunks. Put in the blender. Dilute miso in water, and dilute tahini in a little water. Combine all ingredients except basil in the blender. Purée. Add the minced basil and mix through gently.

Serve with a colorful array of bright seasonal raw vegetables, such as red pepper strips, carrot sticks, celery sticks, radishes, summer squash, and so on.

Breast-Protective Power Foods: Squash, basil, miso, tahini, extra virgin olive oil, onions, garlic.

Tofu Côte d'Azur

(SERVES 3–4)

❦ *Fresh rosemary, red pepper, olives, and garlic are evocative of the aromatic, southern French coastline. Delicious tofu makes a wonderful background for these strong, savory flavors. A colorful way to present this flavorful dish is to put the tofu into "radicchio cups" surrounded by julienne carrot strips—color, flavor, and texture!*

> 1 small red pepper
> 2–3 heads Roasted Garlic (*see* page 260)
> 1 lb soft tofu
> ½ tsp extra virgin olive oil
> ½ tsp salt
> juice from ½ lemon
> 2 tbsp finely minced onion
> 1 tsp finely minced fresh rosemary
> 2 tsp chickpea miso
> 3 olives, pitted and chopped

Preheat broiler. Rinse pepper and remove seeds, and cut in half. Roast the red pepper on a piece of foil, turning a few times, for approximately 8–10 minutes until skin is charred. Let cool. Meanwhile, remove roasted garlic from the individual cloves by squeezing out, into a blender. Peel, seed, and chop cooled red pepper. Set aside. Combine tofu, extra virgin olive oil, salt, lemon juice, onion, rosemary, and miso with garlic in the blender. Puree for several seconds. Add the red pepper and olives. Blend for another minute. Adjust seasoning and serve.

TIP: To store an opened package of tofu, put it in a bowl and cover with water. Change the water every two days.

Breast-Protective Power Foods: Tofu, red pepper, garlic, rosemary, miso, onion, extra virgin olive oil.

Easy White Bean and Roasted Garlic Dip

❦ *Also evocative of southern France is aromatic cooked garlic. If you love the taste of roasted garlic, try this delicious white bean dip, equally wonderful with freshly cooked or, if you are short on time, organic canned beans.*

> 1 15-ounce can organic Great White Northern beans
> 2–3 heads of roasted garlic (*see* Roasted Garlic, below)
> ⅓ cup extra virgin olive oil
> several pinches of sea salt

Remove garlic from skin. Drain beans and puree all ingredients together in a blender and serve with raw vegetable strips, or as a spread on bread.

Roasted Garlic

YIELD: ABOUT 30 CLOVES OF GARLIC, OR ¼ OF A CUP.

> 2 heads garlic
> 2 tsp filtered water
> 1 tsp extra virgin olive oil
> ⅓ tsp sea salt
> freshly ground pepper

Smash the heads of garlic lightly to loosen. In a small casserole with a lid, put filtered water and garlic. Drizzle with the olive oil and lightly season with salt and pepper. Cover the dish with the lid and roast until soft at 375° for approximately one hour.

Let garlic cool down before handling. The garlic will peel by squeezing at one end. Cut off the very top of the head of the garlic with a sharp knife so that you can squeeze the softened, roasted garlic out.

Comment: If you don't have a casserole the right size, you can roast the garlic on a sheet of aluminum foil. Simply wrap tightly before cooking. You might also want to investigate the clay garlic roasters, available through a catalog. (*See* the Resource Guide.)

Breast-Protective Power Foods: Beans, garlic, extra virgin olive oil.

Red Lentil Dip with Cumin

(SERVES 6–8)

❦ *Roasted garlic also combines easily with red lentils, a quick-cooking dried bean. Red lentil dip can be served surrounded by refreshing slices of fennel and juicy black olives. Serve on a bright yellow plate, garnished with parsley, and you have a colorful and delicious appetizer.*

1 three-inch piece kombu
6 cups filtered water
1 lb dried red lentils
3 tsp extra virgin olive oil
1 tsp flaxseed oil
1 head roasted garlic
5 tsp fresh lemon juice
1½ tsp cumin
1 tbsp mellow miso
1 tsp sea salt
⅛ tsp cayenne pepper or to taste
4 tbsp minced parsley

Wipe kombu sea vegetable lightly with a clean cloth. Soak in water until soft. Drain kombu. Put lentils and kombu with water in a saucepan. Bring to a boil. Reduce to simmer. Stirring occasionally, cook until lentils are soft, about 30 minutes. Drain and place lentils in a blender with oils and puree a minute or two. Add remaining ingredients, *except* for parsley. Garnish with parsley and serve with crackers or pita, or stuff in celery.

CAUTION: **Be careful not to get cayenne pepper on hands or in eyes, where it can burn.**

Breast-Protective Power Foods: Lentils, kombu, garlic, extra virgin olive oil, flaxseed oil, cumin, miso, cayenne pepper.

Vegetarian Stuffed Grape Leaves

(SERVES 8)

❦   *When you make this dish with freshly picked mint, and use the sweetest mild onion available, the flavors are wonderful. A drizzle of extra virgin olive oil completes this delicious appetizer.*

    1 lb tender large grape leaves
    3 cups uncooked rice
    ½ cup finely chopped onions
    ⅓ cup finely chopped mint
    ¾ cup chopped parsley
    1 cup diced tomatoes
    ½ cup extra virgin olive oil
    ½ cup lemon juice
    4 tsp sea salt
    ½ tsp pepper

Dip grape leaves in boiling water. Separate and stuff with the following mixture: wash rice and mix with the rest of the ingredients (except for grape leaves). Put rolls, formed into the shape of fingers in a deep pan and cover with water and 1 tsp of sea salt. Cover and cook for 1½ hours or until the rice and leaves are well done. Serve at room temperature.

Grape leaves are rich in protective antioxidants.

Breast-Protective Power Foods: Grape leaves, onions, mint, parsley, tomato, extra virgin olive oil.

SOUP

Basic Miso Soup

(SERVES 2)

    1 small onion
    1 small carrot

2 cups water
2 oz tofu
2-inch piece wakame sea vegetable
generous grating of fresh ginger
minced scallions for garnish

Slice onion into strips. Scrub the carrot and cut into thin half-moons. Bring water to a boil and add carrots and onions. Cook for 5 minutes in a covered pot. Cut tofu into 1-inch cubes. Reconstitute wakame by soaking in a small amount of water for 5 minutes. When reconstituted, discard hard rib and chop into bite-sized pieces. Add tofu and wakame. Turn heat down to low. Simmer 5–8 minutes. Puree miso in a little bowl using some broth from soup. Add pureed miso to the pot and simmer on low for 2 minutes. Garnish soup with a generous squeeze of freshly grated ginger juice (peel and grate ginger root; squeeze juice from grated root, using hands) and minced scallions.

Breast-Protective Power Foods: Sea vegetables, tofu, miso, carrots, onion, ginger, scallions.

Miso Soup with Shiitake Mushrooms

(SERVES 2)

❦ *Include shiitake mushrooms as often as possible, both for the wonderful flavor they impart to soups and stews, and also for their many immune-enhancing benefits.*

2 cups filtered water
2 dried donko shiitake mushrooms
½-inch dried wakame or kombu sea vegetable
2 cups filtered water
½ cup sliced daikon
2 tsp barley miso
minced scallions for garnish
grated ginger juice (optional)

Soak shiitake mushrooms for 15 minutes until soft, and slice. Discard the hard stem. Soak the sea vegetable until reconstituted and chop into small pieces. Add the daikon, mushrooms and sea vegetable to a pot with the water.

Boil for about 15 minutes. Turn down and cook gently. Meanwhile, puree the miso in a small bowl using some of the cooking soup broth, and add miso-broth mixture back into the pot. Simmer for 4 minutes very gently, taking care not to actively boil. Garnish with scallions, ginger (optional) and serve.

Breast-Protective Power Foods: Shiitake mushrooms, sea vegetables, miso, daikon, scallions, ginger.

Corn and Fennel Miso Soup

(SERVES 4)

❦ *Corn and umeboshi plums are incredible together. Nothing is more American than corn, or more Japanese than umeboshi plums. A little umeboshi paste on a fresh ear of corn makes a great combination. The salty-sour flavor of umeboshi complements the crisp, fresh sweetness of summer corn. Umeboshi plum vinegar brings a great flavor to this corn soup.*

> 3 large ears of corn
> 4 cups filtered water or vegetable stock
> 2 cups filtered water
> 1–1½ cups finely minced fennel
> ¼ cup dulse sea vegetable
> ½–¾ tsp umeboshi vinegar
> 5–6 pinches white pepper
> ¾ tsp barley miso per cup of water

Remove corn from cobs. Place cobs in vegetable stock or filtered water. Bring to a boil and cook gently in a covered pot for 20 minutes. Discard cobs. Add an additional 2 cups of filtered water. Bring to a boil. Add fennel and simmer for 3 minutes. Add corn and dulse and continue to cook gently for 6 minutes. Add umeboshi vinegar and pepper. Puree miso in broth liquid, and add. Taste, adjust seasonings.

TIP: Umeboshi vinegar can be added as a final flavor enhancer to many dishes; use a light touch, though, because it is salty. I especially love the way steamed cabbage tastes drizzled with umeboshi vinegar.

Breast-Protective Power Foods: Corn, sea vegetables, miso, fennel.

Mung Bean Soup with Ribbon Pasta

(SERVES 6–8)

🐞   *Celery seed contains polyacetylenes and phithalides, two anticancer phyto-chemicals. The combination of mung beans and pasta was introduced to me by my friend, Lucianna Maiorano, from Milan. Lucianna first introduced me to how sophisticated natural foods can be, and inspired me with her wonderful cooking.*

> 1 3-inch strip kombu
> 3½ cup each diced carrots and onions
> ⅔ cup rinsed mung beans
> 4 quarts filtered water
> 6 bay leaves
> ⅔ tsp sea salt
> ground pepper
> 1 tsp celery seeds
> 3 tbsp organic shoyu or tamari sauce
> 2 cups ribbon pasta
> extra virgin olive oil

Wipe kombu lightly with clean damp cloth. In a small bowl, cover with a little water and soak until soft, for about 10–15 minutes. Put carrots and onions in a soup pot with 3 tbsp of water. Sauté over medium/high heat for 3–4 minutes. Add ⅛ tsp of salt and continue to sauté for another couple of minutes until vegetables are tender. Add beans, kombu and water. Bring to a boil, skimming the foam that accumulates at the surface until it stops forming. Reduce heat. Add bay leaves and cook for an hour and a half. Add salt and freshly ground pepper to taste. Continue to cook for 2 more hours, stirring occasionally. Add celery seeds during last 10 minutes of cooking.

Cook noodles and drain. Add shoyu and pasta to soup. Adjust seasonings, remove bay leaves and serve. Drizzle oil over soup right before serving.

Breast-Protective Power Foods: Mung beans, carrots, onions, celery seed, soy sauce, extra virgin olive oil.

Cream of Broccoli Soup with Soy

❦ *This spicy cream of broccoli soup is a dairy free version of an old favorite. The addition of Jalapeno peppers (and 1 tbsp pepper corns to the stock) give this delicious soup an unexpected dimension.*

    1 onion
    3 shallots
    2 tbsp filtered water
    2–3 tbsp sea salt
    1 small leek
    6 cups vegetable stock
    1 handful of parsley (whole on stems)
    1⅓ lb bunch broccoli, cleaned and cut into large chunks
    2 cups soy milk
    3 tbsp extra virgin olive oil
    2 tbsp flaxseed oil

Chop the onion and shallots and sauté in water in a medium-sized soup pot until soft, approximately 20 minutes. The last 5 minutes add ⅛ tsp of salt.

Clean and chop the leek. Add the vegetable stock and the leek to the pot with the onion and shallots. Bring to a soft boil, turn down, add the parsley and broccoli, and cook for 20 minutes, covered slightly.

Remove the parsley and discard. Take out most of the larger chunks of broccoli with a large spoon (with holes in the spoon for draining) and put into a blender. Puree for 3 minutes.

Add the pureed broccoli back to the pot with the rest of ingredients, and the soy milk. Bring to a soft boil, turn down, add salt to taste, and cook for 10 minutes on low. Right before serving, add the oils.

Breast-Protective Power Foods: Broccoli, soy milk, shallots, leek, olive oil, flaxseed oil, parsley.

Easy Vegetable Stock

❦ *Inspired by* **The Greens Cook Book** *by Deborah Madison with Edward Espe Brown (Bantam, 1987).*

❦ *Making vegetable stock is easy. Simply scrub vegetables, cut into small chunks (about ½-inch square), add filtered water, herbs, garlic and bay leaves, and* cook for 30–40 minutes. Use about 7 cups of vegetables to 8 cups of water. This will yield about 6 cups of stock. Create your own combination of vegetables to complement the soup you are creating.

Simple Tips for Vegetable Stock

Options:
- ¼ cup of lentils to 8 cups of water adds a hearty taste to vegetable stocks.
- Always use plenty of parsley.
- To extract garlic in stocks, simply cut *unpeeled* cloves in half and add to stock.
- Leeks and onions are important in all stocks.
- Use a couple of large bay leaves to deepen flavor.
- Use tough, outer leaves of lettuce that you ordinarily may discard for stock.
- Dried or fresh mushrooms impart deep flavor.
- Figure on a teaspoon of salt to 8 cups of stock depending on taste.
- Use less salt if you also plan to use miso or soy.
- Use hulls from shelled peas in stock.

Vegetable Stock

1 leek
½ hot Italian pepper
1 corn cob
1 white onion
1–2 stalks of celery
1 carrot
1 tbsp pepper corns
2 chopped jalapeño peppers (Do not handle without wearing gloves—can burn eyes.)
3 scallions
4–6 cloves unpeeled garlic
2 sprigs rosemary
2 bay leaves
8 cups filtered water

Scrub vegetables. Cut in half or thirds. Cut garlic cloves in half. Put all vegetables, garlic, rosemary, and bay leaves in a large pot with water. Bring to a boil and cook over medium/high for 30 minutes. Strain out vegetables and use for soup or stews.

Breast-Protective Power Foods: Leek, pepper, corn, onion, celery, carrot, garlic, scallions, rosemary, bay leaves.

Sweet and Sour Red Lentil Soup with Saffron

(Serves 6)

❦   *This soup was inspired by a trip to Istanbul. Turkey has been a sort of melting pot of several influences: Middle Eastern, European, and Asian. I enjoyed the tradition of many different appetizer dishes, similar to the incredible mazahs in Jordan.*

> ½ tsp filtered water
> 2½ tbsp extra virgin olive oil
> 4–5 cloves garlic
> sea salt
> 2 ripe fresh tomatoes
> ½ cup diced onion
> 1½ tsp diced fresh hot red
>   pepper
> ½ cup red lentils
> 6 cups vegetable stock
> 5 sprigs of parsley
> ¾ tsp dried coriander
> juice from ½ lemon
> 1 tsp umeboshi vinegar
> 1 packet of saffron (at least
>   5 grams)

In a medium-sized soup pot, add water and ½ tsp of olive oil. Coat the bottom of the pot evenly with this mixture. Mince garlic. Add garlic and onions to pot, and sauté on medium/low gently for 10 minutes. Add a couple pinches of salt. In a small pot, bring 4 cups of water to a rolling boil. With tongs, briefly submerge each tomato, one at a time. Let them cool. Remove skin and seeds. Cut tomatoes into small chunks and add to pot with garlic and onions. Add dried red pepper. Continue to sauté on medium/low for about 8 minutes. Add ¾ cup rinsed lentils, the vegetable stock, and parsley to pot. Bring to a low boil. Add coriander. Stir and turn down to medium/low. Cook for about 5 minutes. Turn down to low and cook for 25 minutes, covered. Stir gently a couple of times. Add saffron, ½ tsp salt, lemon juice, and umeboshi vinegar. Stir and serve. Drizzle oil over soup before serving.

Breast-Protective Power Foods: Tomatoes, lentils, garlic, onions, saffron, red pepper, extra virgin olive oil, yogurt.

SALADS

Mixed Spinach and Avocado Salad with Orange Peel

(SERVES 2)

🍃 *A powerful, anticancer substance called D-Limonene is found in citrus peels. Citrus peels are also rich sources of flavonoids and antioxidants. As always, try to select only organic fruits and vegetables. With citrus peel, however, it is of particular importance. Toxins and dyes may be in the peel if the fruit is not organic. Raw spinach is a source of glutathione, which is an enzyme with antioxidant properties. Glutathione is an important anticancer ally.*

2 cups spinach leaves
1 cup red leaf lettuce
12 cherry tomatoes
3 radishes
⅓ cup sliced cucumber
½ cup sliced mild onion
1 avocado
2 tbsp finely minced orange peel

Clean and drain greens. Dry and put in a large salad bowl. Cut tomatoes in half and add to greens. Clean and dry radishes, then slice. Combine radishes, cucumbers, and onion to the salad. Peel avocado, cut into chunks, and add to the salad ingredients. Before final tossing, add the minced orange peel.

Comment: Frequently, when I'm too busy to mix a dressing, I drizzle fresh lemon juice, umeboshi vinegar, and flax seed or olive oil on my salads. It's a tasty and fresh option.

Breast-Protective Power Foods: Spinach, tomatoes, avocado, cucumber, onion, radishes, orange peel.

Easy Middle Eastern Cabbage Salad

(SERVES 6)

2 tsp sea salt
1 clove minced garlic
½ cup lemon juice
2 tbsp extra virgin olive oil
1 lb shredded cabbage

Pound salt and garlic in a suribachi or small bowl. Add lemon juice and olive oil. Add to cabbage and toss through.

Comment: Blood orange juice is a delicious element in salad dressings. Simply combine with extra virgin olive oil and a dash of umeboshi vinegar to complete. Blood orange vinaigrette combines well with many different types of salad greens, especially the bitter ones like arugula.

Breast-Protective Power Foods: Cabbage, garlic, lemon juice, extra virgin olive oil.

Fennel Salad

❦ *Enjoy the faint sweetness and crisp texture of the delicate licorice, anise-like flavor of fennel. When selecting fennel, choose the roundest ones available, called "the female" in Italy. (They are more tender than the flatter "male.") During the Middle Ages in Italy, especially in Florence, the flowers of the fennel were frequently eaten.*

1 large fennel bulb
½ cup extra virgin olive oil
juice from ½ lemon

1 tsp sea salt
freshly ground pepper to taste

Cut the tops off the fennel and discard bruised outer leaves. Cut the bulb in half lengthwise and slice into very thin strips. Toss with remaining ingredients and serve.

Breast-Protective Power Foods: Fennel, extra virgin olive oil, lemon juice.

Butter Lettuce and Tomato Salad with Horseradish Dressing

(SERVES 2–3)

❦   *Do you want strong nails and more lustrous hair? Try including horseradish in your diet. It's high in silica, which is great for hair and nails. Horseradish has also been found to contain breast-protective phytochemicals.*

2–3 cups butter lettuce, rinsed and dried
1–2 ripe tomatoes
1 tbsp horseradish, peeled and grated
¾ cup filtered water
1–2 umeboshi plums
2 tbsp cold extra virgin olive oil
1 tbsp fresh ginger, grated

Arrange the lettuce and tomato on a pretty plate. Combine the rest of the ingredients, including water, in a blender or suribachi and serve over the salad.

> TIP: Ginger and silica are antifungal, effective in combating yeast associated problems.

Breast-Protective Power Foods: Tomatoes, horseradish, extra virgin olive oil, ginger.

Mixed Green Salad and Garlic Parsley Dressing

❦   *Some traditional cultures believe that parsley (rich in calcium and magnesium) helps to purify the blood. Parsley contains many breast-protective nutrients, including glutathione, an important anticancer ally.*

Mixed Green Salad

arugula
Bibb lettuce
Boston lettuce

Combine equal quantities of each, cleaned and torn into pieces.

Garlic and Parsley Dressing

½ bunch parsley, cleaned and chopped
juice of 2 lemons
1 tbsp Colman's dry mustard
2 tbsp extra virgin olive oil
2 cloves garlic, peeled and minced
3 tbsp water

Purée in blender. Serve over salad.

Comment: Arugula is a cruciferous vegetable. Its spicy, bitter bite is also thought to help stimulate the liver.

Breast-Protective Power Foods: Arugula, parsley, lemon juice, extra virgin olive oil, garlic.

Pressed Salad with Miso Tarragon Dressing

❦   *Pressed salads are a refreshing accompaniment to seafood, as well as other dishes. They add creativity to any menu by encouraging the use of fresh vegetables, herbs, or grated citrus peel.*

Salad

½ head Chinese cabbage
1 stalk celery, washed and finely minced
6 radishes, washed and thinly sliced
1 scallion, washed and finely minced

Dressing

1 tsp sea salt
1 tbsp white miso
2 tbsp lemon juice
few drops of natural shoyu or tamari
    sauce
1 tsp minced tarragon
1 tbsp flaxseed oil

Wash and slice cabbage, mix vegetables together with salt, and spread over large plate. Place another plate over the dish with salad, and use a heavy book or sack of flour to weight down. Press for 1 hour. Remove the vegetables from the plate and squeeze out excess liquid with your hands. Put vegetables in a salad bowl. Mix together the miso, lemon, and shoyu, and tarragon together in a small bowl. Toss through the salad mixture. Drizzle a little oil over the salad and serve.

> TIP: Grate a little organic lemon or orange peel on top for added zest and breast protective phytochemicals.

Breast-Protective Power Foods: Chinese cabbage, celery, radishes, scallions, miso, lemon juice, shoyu, flaxseed oil, tarragon.

Pressed Salad with Sauerkraut

raw vegetables, such as:
¾ cup romaine lettuce
1 cucumber
½ stalk celery
3 radishes
1 small onion
⅓ tsp sea salt, or to taste

½ cup drained
   sauerkraut
lemon juice
flaxseed oil

Wash, dry, and slice vegetables. Place them in a large bowl.

Sprinkle sea salt throughout vegetables to mix well. Add sauerkraut. Mix well. Place a small plate on top of the vegetables and place a weight on top of the plate. (It can be a heavy jar or a stone, etc.) Leave it on for 45 minutes. Taste the salad. If it is too salty, you can rinse it before serving. If it needs a little more salt, adjust and serve. Dress with lemon juice and flaxseed oil.

TIP: After pressing salad, toss with soba noodles and flavor with lemon juice, umeboshi vinegar, and flax seed oil. Delicious!

Breast-Protective Power Foods: Cucumber, celery, radishes, onions, and unheated sauerkraut.

Pressed Cabbage and Grated Carrot Salad

(SERVES 4)

❦   *Indoles, found in cabbage family plants (including radishes), nourish cancer-fighting enzymes. In laboratory tests, indoles lowered breast cancer rates in mice 450 percent.*

Dr. Jon Michnovicz, from the Institute of Hormone Research in New York City, has found that cabbage is scientifically proven to balance levels of estrogen, thus helping to prevent the development of breast cancer.

¾ cup grated carrots
½–¾ cup thinly sliced radishes
⅓ cup chopped dandelion
   greens
1 thinly sliced purple cabbage
⅓ cup sliced scallions
½ tsp sea salt
2–3 tsp umeboshi vinegar

juice of ⅓ lemon
4 tsp flaxseed oil

Wash vegetables. Scrub unpeeled carrots and radishes with natural scrubber, available in local health food stores. Chop vegetables. Place mixed vegetables on a large plate. Spread out around plate. Mix salt and umeboshi vinegar uniformly throughout the vegetables. Place another plate of the same size on top of the vegetables. Place a rock or other weight on top of second plate to press vegetables. Press until liquid extraction occurs, at least 10 minutes, or according to taste.

Remove vegetables from plate. Drain liquid. Garnish with lemon juice and flaxseed oil.

Comment: Pressing vegetables is another way to enjoy enzyme-rich raw foods. This method of food preparation is used in Japan, to lightly pickle raw foods, which makes them more digestible.

Breast-Protective Power Foods: Dandelion greens, purple cabbage, carrots, radishes, scallions, lemon juice, flaxseed oil.

Salad of Mixed Greens with Goat Cheese and Olives

❦ *Goat's cheese is a fresh, flavorful cheese, popular throughout the Mediterranean. I love the combined flavors of olives, bitter greens, and goat's cheese. Watercress is a cruciferous vegetable, with powerful breast-protective phytochemicals.*

About 10 ounces of mixed greens: mizuna, mustards, frisee, purslane, endive, radicchio, tatsoi, escarole, dandelion, watercress, loose-leaf or butterhead lettuces.

5 oz natural goat cheese
6–8 Greek pitted olives

Dressing

1 scallion, whole, cleaned and chopped
1 tsp minced garlic
6 tsp freshly squeezed lemon or grapefruit juice
1 tbsp rice vinegar
6 tbsp water

2 tbsp extra virgin olive oil
2 tbsp flax oil
2 tbsp grainy natural mustard
salt
ground pepper
1 tsp freshly minced oregano

In a food processor (or suribachi) combine scallion, garlic, juice, and vinegar until all ingredients are blended. Add remaining ingredients and continue to blend or puree. Taste, adjust salt or pepper.

Place cleaned and dried greens in a mixing bowl. Toss with dressing. Add crumbled cheese and olives. Toss through and serve.

Note: Be careful to dry salad greens well so that they will hold the dressing.

Breast-Protective Power Foods: Mustard, dandelion, endive, watercress, escarole, scallion, garlic, lemon and grapefruit juice, extra virgin olive oil, fresh oregano.

Spicy Savoy Cabbage and Tomato Salad

(SERVES 4–6)

❦ *This is a departure from the usual salads we eat in the West. Koreans are used to combining cayenne pepper with raw vegetables to create delicious and spicy salads. Try this appetizing and refreshing version of a typical Korean salad.*

Savoy cabbage is the richest source for indole-rich cancer protective phytochemicals, even more so than regular cabbage. The anti-oxidant properties of cayenne pepper also offer protective benefits.

4 cups firmly packed savoy cabbage, shredded
1 cup sliced tomatoes
1 cup firmly packed and thinly sliced vidalia onion
   (or similar mild onion)
¼ tsp cayenne pepper
2 tbsp Braggs Liquid Aminos
juice from ½ large lemon

Combine ingredients and marinate for 30 minutes to 1 hour.

Comment: Spicy dishes are particularly balancing during warmer weather.

Breast-Protective Power Foods: Savoy cabbage, tomatoes, onions, cayenne pepper, Braggs Liquid Aminos, lemon juice.

Baye Salad with Chicory and Tahini Dressing

❦ *Talented natural foods chef Myrna Baye, known for her extraordinary soups and other culinary creations, devised this delicious recipe.*

Salad

Equal parts of chicory, watercress, and daikon
  radish. Treat daikon like a carrot—dice, grate, or
  julienne.

Dressing

½ cup filtered water
2 tbsp unroasted sesame tahini
1 tbsp lemon juice
2 tsp umeboshi paste
1 handful of minced parsley
2 tsp finely minced mild onion

Rinse greens. Scrub daikon with a natural bristle vegetable brush. Slice daikon into julienne strips, or grate. Dry vegetables and place in a salad bowl. Combine dressing ingredients in a food processor or blender and serve over salad.

Breast-Protective Power Foods: Watercress, daikon radish, tahini, parsley, onion.

Hatfield High-Enzyme Salad

(SERVES 4)

❦ *Pamela Hatfield is a gifted designer with a rich sense of color, pattern, and texture. Her intuition about design elements is matched by her ability to cook, especially the delicious salads and vegetables she loves so much and prepares so creatively.*

> 4 cups firmly packed kale
> 1 cup firmly packed, very thinly sliced savoy
>   (or regular) cabbage
> 1 cup *very* thinly sliced purple onion
> 2 tbsp Braggs Liquid Aminos
> juice of ½ lemon
> 2 tsps flaxseed oil

Rinse kale and shred into large bite-size pieces. Rinse all vegetables and dry. Combine in a large bowl, and add Braggs and lemon juice. All you need to do is marinate ingredients for about 1½ hours, turning every 15 minutes or so, to mix vegetables through marinade.

Drizzle oil before serving, and toss throughout.

Breast-Protective Power Foods: Kale, savoy cabbage, purple onion, Braggs Liquid Aminos, flaxseed oil.

SEA VEGETABLE SALADS

Hijiki and other sea vegetables are rich sources of iodine, calcium, and other minerals nourishing to the endocrine system. Sea vegetables are used in recipes throughout this book.

Hijiki and Arugula Salad with Sweet and Sour Dressing

(Serves 4)

> ½ cup hijiki
> ¼ cup carrot slivers
> 1½ cups loosely packed arugula, cleaned and dried
> filtered water

Dressing

> ⅓ cup mirin
> ⅓ tsp minced garlic or 1 tsp ginger juice

3 tbsp organic sunflower seed oil
⅓ cup Braggs Liquid Aminos or shoyu
½ cup lemon juice

Bring 4 cups of water to a boil. Add the hijiki. Cook for 10 minutes, boiling gently. Before the last minute of cooking, add the carrots and continue to cook for another minute. Take off heat. Drain, set aside. Heat mirin in a small pot until it just reaches a boil. Reduce heat and cook for 1 minute. Take off heat immediately and put into small bowl. In a suribachi or food processor puree garlic with the rest of the ingredients. After carrots and hijiki cool, toss into arugula. Add a little of the dressing and serve.

Breast-Protective Power Foods: Hijiki, carrots, arugula, sunflower seed oil, Braggs Liquid Aminos or shoyu, lemon juice, garlic.

Myrna's Arame Salad

(SERVES 6)

1 package of arame
organic apple juice
1 large grated carrot
1 small grated daikon
grated fresh ginger to taste
pinch of sea salt or 1 tbsp of tamari sauce
2–3 tbsp lightly toasted sesame seeds

Soak rinsed arame in apple juice to cover for 15–20 minutes. Grate carrot and daikon. Drain arame. Heat about ¼ cup of apple juice and add arame, carrot, and daikon. Steam for several minutes. Add fresh ginger and salt (or tamari). Remove from heat and add sesame seeds.

Breast-Protective Power Foods: Arame, carrot, daikon, ginger, tamari sauce, sesame seeds.

Wakame Salad

(SERVES 2)

❦ *Daikon radish, a large spicy, white radish (Korean Daikon is rounder, Japanese is longer) is a great part of macrobiotic healing. Daikon is known to be a powerful anticancer food, containing protease inhibitors and vitamins C and D. Part of the cabbage family of vegetables, the daikon is used in Japanese and Chinese healing for cancer. Isothiocyanates, a phytochemical in the daikon and other radishes, offer special protection for DNA in breast tissues.*

¾ cup thinly sliced daikon radish
¾ cup thinly sliced cucumber
¾ cup shredded Chinese cabbage
3 strips of wakame sea vegetable
sea salt
1½ tbsp mirin
1½ tbsp shoyu or tamari sauce
2½ tbsp lemon juice
1 minced scallion

Place radish, cucumber, and cabbage on a plate with about ¾ tsp of sea salt. Soak wakame in filtered water for 10–15 minutes. When reconstituted, remove inner rib. Boil gently for 8 minutes. Let cool and drain. Heat together in a small pot for 1 minute the mirin and soy sauce. Put in a small bowl and combine with lemon juice. Cut wakame into bite-sized pieces and combine with vegetables. Pour dressing over vegetables and sprinkle finely minced scallions to garnish and serve.

Breast-Protective Power Foods: Daikon radish, cucumber, Chinese cabbage, shoyu, lemon juice, scallion.

VINAIGRETTES

Sunflower Vinaigrette

(Serves 6)

⅓ cup mirin
½–1 tsp minced garlic or 2 tsp ginger juice or minced shallots
3 tbsp organic sunflower seed oil
⅓ to ½ cup Braggs Liquid Aminos or natural shoyu
½ cup lemon juice

Heat mirin in a small pot until it just reaches a boil. Reduce heat and cook for 1 minute. Take off heat immediately and put into small bowl. In a suribachi or food processor, puree garlic with the rest of the ingredients.

Optional: For a thicker dressing, add up to 1–2 tbsp chickpeas or mellow white miso. Any finely minced fresh herb, such as cilantro or rosemary, works very well with this basic mixture. Create your own favorites, by using walnut, pumpkin, flaxseed, or olive oil.

Note: Sunflower seeds contain genistein.

> TIP: Lemon vinaigrette with sunflower seed oil can be tossed through a simple salad of celeriac, or celery root. Try to select a celery root that is relatively smooth, so that it isn't too difficult to peel, and free of bruises. Once you peel this gnarled-looking knob (also called "knob celery"), it can be grated easily. Once grated, celeriac can be complemented by your favorite vinaigrette or a simple dressing of yogurt and fresh herbs. Try celeriac boiled and mashed, like mashed potatoes, or sliced thin and steamed with other vegetables. This is one vegetable you must always peel.

Breast-Protective Power Foods: Sunflower seed oil, Braggs Liquid Aminos or natural shoyu, lemon juice, garlic, shallots.

Basil Vinaigrette

(Approximately ¾ cup)

1 scallion
1½ tbsp extra virgin olive oil
2 tbsp flaxseed oil
1 tbsp mirin
5 tbsp fresh lemon juice (2–3 large lemons)
1 tbsp natural grainy mustard
1 tsp minced garlic
1 tsp fresh minced basil or oregano
2 pinches of sea salt

Clean and mince scallion. Combine ingredients in a food processor or blender until mixed. Serve over salad or cooked vegetables. For a thicker consistency, you can add 1 tbsp of any light miso such as sweet, mellow, or chickpea.

Combine Extra Virgin Olive Oil with Citrus Juice for Light and Flavorful Dressings

Honeybell Vinaigrette

(SERVES 4)

½ cup of honeybell orange juice, freshly squeezed
  (or substitute another sweet orange)
⅕ cup extra virgin olive oil
1 tsp lemon juice
1 minced shallot
⅓ cup cleaned and chopped mint
1 clove minced garlic
¾ tsp sea salt
ground pepper to taste

Combine ingredients in a food processor, or suribachi. Drizzle over julienne celery root and daikon radish strips, or any favorite salad ingredients. Toss, adjust seasonings, and enjoy.

> TIP: Look for Ajipon in Asian markets. The Japanese soy sauce is seasoned with citrus, and is less salty than most soy sauces. Ajipon complements seafood or vegetable salads beautifully.

Breast-Protective Power Foods: Extra virgin olive oil, flaxseed oil, lemon juice, garlic, scallion, basil.

Tri-Colore Vegetables with Marjoram Vinaigrette

(SERVES 4)

❦ *Steaming vegetables is preferable to boiling because the phytochemicals are often more protected by this cooking method. What could be simpler than filling a steamer basket with three of your favorite vegetables? The use of three different vegetables is an opportunity to introduce more variety into your diet—important in creating breast health. I especially love a fresh herbal vinaigrette drizzled over vegetables while they are still hot. I learned to "finish" vegetables this way while in France. Try it—you'll love it!*

⅓ lb each of fresh:
  cauliflower
  sugar snap beans
  yellow patty pan squash
sea salt

Vinaigrette

2 cloves minced garlic
½ tsp sea salt
1 generous tbsp minced fresh marjoram
¼ cup extra virgin olive oil
½ large, juicy lemon

Rinse vegetables in filtered water. In a steamer basket, add cauliflower florets, sugar snap beans, and sliced patty pan squash. Steam until tender, approximately 12 minutes.

While vegetables are steaming, grind garlic together with sea salt in a suribachi until pureed. Add minced marjoram leaves and continue to blend. Slowly add the olive oil, then the lemon juice. Blend together.

Add vinaigrette to steamed vegetables and toss, finishing with a little freshly ground pepper.

Tri-Colore Vegetables with Dijon Vinaigrette

(SERVES 2–4)

⅓ lb each of:
  beets
  carrots
  asparagus
sea salt

Scrub beets and carrots with a natural bristle vegetable brush. Slice beets very thin. Cut carrots into julienne strips. Rinse all vegetables. Place vegetables in a large stainless steel steamer basket. Add ⅛ tsp of sea salt. Cover, bring to boil, and steam for approximately 5–7 minutes. Carefully remove asparagus when they turn vivid emerald green (use a pair of tongs). You probably will want to leave the beets and carrots in to continue steaming for another couple of minutes. Test them using a knife. They should be just tender. Place the three vegetables, separately, on a pretty dish, and drizzle with vinaigrette.

Dijon Vinaigrette

3 tbsp red wine or herbed thyme vinegar
1½ tbsp extra virgin olive oil
1½ tbsp flaxseed oil
2 tbsp water
2 cloves of finely minced garlic
2 tbsp finely minced fresh parsley
1 tbsp Dijon mustard
sea salt and freshly ground pepper

Mix together all ingredients in a small bowl or suribachi. Salt and pepper to taste.

Breast-Protective Power Foods: Asparagus, beets, carrots, onions, extra virgin olive oil, flaxseed oil, garlic, parsley.

VEGETABLES

Your most significant anticancer ally is a variety of fresh vegetables and fruit. Eat at least five different vegetables daily.

Steamed Mixed Vegetables

❦ *Eating a variety of vegetables offers a wide spectrum of protective phytonutrients. Combine several vegetables and steam together.*

Ingredients	*Some other combinations*	
carrots	Brussels sprouts	corn
collard greens	cauliflower	carrots
summer squash	leeks	green peas
onions	onions	onions

Wash and cut vegetables. Cut dense vegetables like carrots and parsnips into julienne strips. Brussels sprouts and cauliflower need to be cut as thin as possible when steaming with more delicate vegetables such as leeks or onions. If you're combining corn and peas with carrots, you can mince or grate the carrots. After vegetables are cut, salt lightly with sea salt, and steam for 8–10 minutes.

Breast-Protective Power Foods: Collard greens, summer squash, carrots, onions, Brussels sprouts, cauliflower, leeks, corn, peas.

Broccoli and Shallots

(SERVES 4–6)

florets of 1 bunch of broccoli, rinsed
8 shallots, peeled and halved
2 pinches sea salt
2 tbsp flaxseed oil
umeboshi vinegar or lemon juice

Place broccoli in steamer basket. Toss in shallots. Sprinkle with sea salt. Steam for about 6–8 minutes or until broccoli is just tender. Drizzle with oil, add a little lemon juice and umeboshi vinegar after steaming.

Breast-Protective Power Foods: Broccoli, shallots, flaxseed oil, lemon.

Roasted Candied Carrots and Minced Leeks

(SERVES 8)

❧   *The sweetness of the roasted carrots is complemented by the unexpected, subtle, grassy spiciness of the tender leeks. This is a lovely, colorful dish to serve buffet style. The strong flavors are delicious and stay fresh for quite some time.*

> 2 tbsp filtered water
> 2 tsp sesame oil
> 6 large organic carrots cut into chunks, on the diagonal
> 1¼ tsp sea salt
> 2 tbsp honey
> 2 tbsp maple syrup
> 1 tsp cinnamon
> 2 cleaned and minced leeks
> 1 tsp umeboshi vinegar
> 1 tsp brown rice vinegar

Coat large pyrex baking dish (14 × 9 inches) well with water and 1 tsp of sesame oil. Place the carrot chunks in the baking dish and rub 1 tsp of oil on the carrots. Add 1 tbsp each of honey and maple syrup. Coat well.

In a preheated oven of 350°, roast the carrots for 45 minutes. Stir carrots and add 1 tsp of sea salt.

Continue cooking for 20 minutes. Remove from oven, add another tbsp each of honey and maple syrup. Coat well and stir. At this point you may want to add another tbsp of water to pan to prevent sticking. Add cinnamon, and another ¼ tsp of sea salt. Finish roasting for 20 minutes more.

Meanwhile, steam minced leeks for 5 minutes until just tender. Remove from steamer basket and put into small bowl. Season lightly with each vinegar.

When carrots are finished roasting, place in a large bowl to cool down. When carrots have cooled, mix together with leeks and serve.

Comment: Sesame oil (and olive oil) are the oils to use for gentle roasting or sautéing. Water used first in a baking dish (or sauté pan) creates a buffer between the heart source and oil, and helps to protect the oil.

Breast-Protective Power Foods: Carrots, leeks, sesame oil, cinnamon.

Turnips, Rutabagas, and Parsnips Medley

❦ *This recipe is very similar to a mashed vegetable dish served in Northern France, and goes well with roasted chicken, lamb, or Choucroute Garni Light with Tempeh. Season this hearty vegetable dish with a little organic butter or umeboshi paste.*

> spring or filtered water
> 1 turnip
> 1 rutabaga
> 1 or 2 parsnips
> 4–6 tsp umeboshi
>   paste
> ⅛ tsp salt

Clean vegetables using natural bristle brush. Don't peel. Cut into chunks, *barely* cover with water, and place lid on pot. Bring to a gentle boil. Cook for about 25–30 minutes. Vegetables are done cooking when you can pierce them with a knife or fork. Pour out water that is left in the pot.

You can mash the vegetables together right in the cooking pot. Season to taste with umeboshi paste and a little salt (for each cup of mashed vegetable, use about 1 tsp of umeboshi paste).

Breast-Protective Power Foods: Turnip, rutabagas, parsnips, umeboshi paste.

Chlorophyll-rich leafy greens are an abundant source of nutrients. Chlorophyll is known to be a blood builder and detoxifier of the colon and intestines. Second, very important for women is the often overlooked fact that the calcium content of leafy greens is actually higher and more absorbable than calcium from milk. Asian women consume greens at least twice daily, never drink milk, and do not get osteoporosis. One or more of the following delicious greens should be eaten daily. Simply prepare as suggested and with shoyu and lemon; umeboshi vinegar and lemon; brown rice vinegar and shoyu or umeboshi vinegar. Drizzle with a touch of fresh organic flaxseed oil before serving for added flavor and health benefits.

Crispy Blanched Cheese Cabbage

Slice Chinese cabbage thinly into ¼-inch pieces. Bring water to a boil and add the cabbage. After water returns to a boil, cook for 1 minute more, uncovered. Drain and serve with a touch of umeboshi vinegar and lemon.

> TIP: Blanch one of the following: collards, kale, bok choy, chopped broccoli, broccoli rabe, watercress, turnip greens, or mustard greens. Dress with your favorite condiments and fresh flaxseed oil. Enjoy!

Breast-Protective Power Food: Chinese cabbage.

Water Sautéed Vegetables

❦   *Water sautéing is a way to sauté vegetables avoiding the use of heated oils. I prefer this method over "non-stick sprays," which most likely contain oils that are not fresh and/or are processed in some way. You can also use vegetable or miso stock to sauté vegetables*

> 1–2 carrots
> 1 head of cauliflower
> 1 bunch of bok choy
> 1 medium onion
> 1 tsp natural shoyu or tamari
>   sauce
> Ginger root
> couple pinches of sea salt
> Walnut, sunflower, or flaxseed oil

Scrub carrots and cut into diagonals. Cut the diagonals into matchsticks. Rinse the cauliflower, separate, and cut into thin slices. Also rinse bok choy and cut the stems into ½-inch pieces. Break the leaves up into pieces with your hands. Peel and thinly slice the onion. Using a deep stainless steel skillet, heat a half inch of water along with tamari and 1 tsp of grated ginger juice (grate the ginger root, and squeeze juice by hand from the grated root), Add the cauliflower and stir over medium/high for 2 minutes. Add the carrots; stir for a couple of minutes, then add the bok choy stems. Cook for another couple of minutes. Next, add the onion slices. Sauté for 2–3 more minutes, add the bok choy leaves, and cover. Cook for 3 more minutes, add sea salt, ginger juice, and a drizzle of your favorite unheated oil.

Comment: Nonstick vegetable sprays are not a fresh, life-giving food. Utilize water sautéing instead, and drizzle fresh oils over food after cooking.

Breast-Protective Power Foods: Cauliflower, bok choy, carrots, onion, ginger, shoyu.

Broccoli and Leek Coulis

(SERVES 4)

❦ *A typical French approach for preparing vegetables, the "Coulis" is delicious and appealing. Create your own favorite vegetable combinations. Broccoli contains indole-3-carbinol, offering special protection against breast cancer.*

> 1 large leek (3 cups firmly packed)
> filtered water
> 3 cups broccoli cut into chunks
> 4 pieces of lightly steamed broccoli for garnish
> ¼ tsp sea salt
> 1 tbsp unroasted sesame tahini
> juice from 1 lemon
> 2 cloves of garlic

Cut roots off leeks. Dirt is usually deeply embedded in the layers of the leek, so to clean well, cut in half lengthwise for efficient rinsing. (Some cooks like to soak halved leeks in a large pot of water to remove dirt.) Next, simply cut into bite-sized chunks and rinse again. Rinse broccoli. In a medium-sized pot, bring enough water to a boil for cooking the vegetables. Add the leeks and broccoli chunks, *but wait to add the broccoli.* After 4 minutes or so, add the reserved broccoli. Four minutes later, until *just* soft (the broccoli should be bright emerald green), remove from heat and drain. Allow to cool for 15 minutes.

Reserve garnishing broccoli. Put the rest of the vegetables in a blender with remaining ingredients and puree. Adjust seasoning. Serve by placing coulis on each plate, with a bright green piece of broccoli on top.

For an appetizer serve surrounded by your favorite raw vegetables.

Comment: Leeks contain powerful immune-enhancing and antitumor allyl sulfides that increase the activity of protective enzymes. Include leeks often in soups, steamed vegetables, or elegant vegetable coulis.

Breast-Protective Power Foods: Leeks, broccoli, tahini, lemon juice, garlic.

Green Beans with Sesame Vinaigrette

(SERVES 4)

1 lb green beans

Vinaigrette

2 shallots
2 lemons
3 tbsp sesame oil
4 tbsp rice
   vinegar
2 tsp honey
1 tbsp mustard
sea salt

Wash and trim beans and blanch in lightly salted boiling water until bright green, approximately for 5 minutes. Peel and mince shallots. Combine the shallots with the rest of the vinaigrette ingredients in a food processor or suribachi. Adjust seasonings and toss through green beans. Serve and enjoy.

Breast-Protective Power Foods: Green beans, lemon juice, shallots, sesame oil.

Brussels Sprouts Piquant

(SERVES 3–4)

❦ *Brussels sprouts and savoy cabbage are the two cruciferous vegetables that contain the most indole-3-carbinol, the phytonutrient that is so protective for prevention of breast cancer. I love the taste of Brussels sprouts, and prepare them frequently.*

2 cups Brussels
sprouts
1 tsp rice vinegar
1 tsp umeboshi
vinegar

Wash and trim Brussels sprouts. Next, simply steam them in a steamer basket for 8 minutes. They should be a nice, vivid green, but cooked until just soft. As with all green vegetables, it is especially important not to overcook. Place them in a bowl and sprinkle lightly with the vinegars.

Sesame Brussels Sprouts

(SERVES 3–4)

2 cups Brussels sprouts
2 tsp sesame seeds
2–3 tsp shoyu or tamari sauce
1 tsp organic sesame oil

Wash Brussels sprouts and steam in a steamer basket for 8 minutes until just done—tender, but bright green. In a little skillet, on a gentle heat, very lightly stir sesame seeds until pale golden. Do not overroast.

Place Brussels sprouts in a bowl and add the oil and shoyu. Mix through and sprinkle sesame seeds on before serving.

TIP: Sesame seeds are a rich source of calcium and contain protective lignanphenols with antioxidant abilities.

Breast-Protective Power Foods: Brussels sprouts, sesame seeds and oil, shoyu.

Roasted Beets

(Serves 3–4)

❦   *Using water in the pan or dish with oil offers protection against the source of heat. (The water acts as a buffer between the oil and heat.) I like to dress roasted beets with a handful of lightly blanched minced leeks, and a tablespoon of finely minced organic orange peel to increase flavor and phytochemical protection.*

> 2 tsp each sesame oil and filtered water
> 1 lb small beets, thinly sliced
> 2 pinches sea salt

Add water and oil to Pyrex baking dish. Add beets and mix through with water-oil mixture. Bake in a 350° oven for about 30 minutes, stirring a couple of times. Serve as is, or let cool and serve on salad greens with dressing.

Comment: The sweetness of the roasted beets balance with the sodium in the meat to help reduce sugar cravings that may occur from eating meat. A roasted garnet yam is another option.

> TIP: I use a stainless steel "Mac" knife, available at better health food stores, or through catalogs. (See Resource Guide.)

Breast-Protective Power Foods: Beets.

Glazed Carrots

❦   *Cooking carotene-rich vegetables offers benefits for breast cancer prevention. Carrots are rich in carotenes.*

> 2–3-inch strip of kombu
> 4 carrots
> 1/8 tsp sea salt
> 1/2 cup filtered water
> 1 heaping tbsp barley malt

Soak the kombu until soft in a little water, just to cover. (Use the soaking water for plants.) Place the kombu in the bottom of a heavy pot.

Scrub the carrots and cut into thick julienne strips. Place the carrots on top of the kombu, add the salt and water, and bring to a boil. Lower the flame and cover. Cook over a medium-low flame for 15 minutes, until just soft.

Dilute the barley malt in a little carrot broth. Mix until the carrots are well coated.

Breast-Protective Power Foods: carrots, kombu.

Burdock Cooked in Apple Juice and Tamari

❦ *Burdock root tincture is sometimes utilized by herbalists and naturopaths for support in healing breast cancer. Include burdock root often, minced in soups, or as described in this recipe, along with whole grain salads as a condiment.*

> 2 burdock roots scrubbed and cut into 2-inch logs
> ½ cup filtered water
> ½ cup organic apple juice
> ⅓ cup shoyu or tamari sauce

Place burdock, water, apple juice, and tamari in a pressure cooker. Cover and bring to pressure on a medium flame. Cook on a medium flame for 7 minutes. Remove from heat and let pressure come down naturally. Remove burdock and cool. Serve with your favorite salad ingredients and vinaigrette or other salad dressing. Season with a touch of salt or 1 tbsp tamari.

Breast-Protective Power Foods: Burdock root, shoyu, or tamari sauce.

Sweet Winter Squash

❦ *Hokaido and delicata squash are two of my favorite fall/winter vegetables. Select only organic to ensure optimum taste and carotene content.*

> **Take any combination and amount of the following vegetables:**
> hokaido pumpkin
> kabocha squash

buttercup squash
delicata squash

Retain and scrub the skins of the vegetables with a natural bristle brush. An added feature of organic produce is the fact that the skin of the vegetable is richest in minerals, and need not be discarded because of pesticide sprays. Cut the vegetables into chunks, about 3 inches long and 1½ inches wide. The kabocha, buttercup, and hokaido can be cut narrower than the other vegetables for optimum cooking. Put the vegetables in a large steamer basket.

Cover the bottom of a large pot with ½ inch of water and place the basket into the pot. Cover and bring to a boil. Lower to medium and cook for 5 minutes. Reduce heat to medium-low setting and gently cook for another 15 minutes. Vegetables should be soft, but still firm. *Do not overcook*. Enjoy!

TIP: Squash can be sliced and spread out on a lightly oiled Pyrex baking dish (use sesame oil). Add 1–2 tbsp of water, the oil, and then the squash. Cover with foil and roast in a preheated oven for 45 minutes.

Breast-Protective Power Foods: Hokaido pumpkin, kabocha squash, buttercup squash, delicata squash.

> Choose the darkest green vegetables. The darker green they are the more cancer-inhibiting carotenoids they have.
> —*Frederick Kachik, Ph.D. Researcher,*
> *U.S. Department of Agriculture*

Greens Medley

⅓ kale, rinsed and cut
⅓ bok choy, rinsed and
   cut
⅓ dandelion greens,
   rinsed
1 tsp shoyu or tamari
   sauce
lemon juice
flaxseed oil

Rinse greens. In a steamer basket in a pot, put the kale and bok choy in the basket, and bring several cups of spring water in the pot to a boil. Cook until emerald green, approximately 2 or 3 minutes on a *gentle* boil. Add the dandelion greens during the last 30–60 seconds of cooking. Serve with a sprinkling of shoyu or umeboshi vinegar and a light squeeze of fresh lemon juice. Cleansing, nourishing, and protective! Also, dress greens with flaxseed oil to help assimilate carotenes.

Comment: Besides being rich in selenium, zinc, minerals, and antioxidants, dandelions contain a wide range of phytochemicals and phytosterols that are breast protective. Dandelions are known to actually increase interferon production and stop cancer promotion. Dark, leafy greens are also a rich source of calcium.

> TIP: Don't forget about delicious turnip greens. Try them as a substitute for dandelion greens in the "Greens Medley" dish. For specifics on cutting greens, *see* Chapter 8, "Nutrient-Dense Green Vegetables: Protective and Cleansing."

Breast-Protective Power Foods: Dandelion greens, kale, bok choy, shoyu, lemon juice, flaxseed oil.

SEAFOOD

Dilled Salmon in Miso-Lemon Sauce

❧ *Steaming salmon, my favorite cold water fish, preserves powerful fish oils (EPA and DHA) and also contributes to a tender, moist dish. Broiling, grilling, or sautéing cold water fish not only destroys protective oils, but creates potent carcinogens found in burned fats.*

3 tbsp sweet, mellow white, or chickpea miso
juice of 2 lemons
4 cloves garlic, peeled and minced
2 leeks, cleaned thoroughly, halved both horizontally and vertically
2 salmon fillets
4–5 sprigs of fresh cleaned dill

Mix miso, lemon juice, and garlic in a suribachi using a grinding motion. The sauce should be the consistency of a creamy salad dressing.

Line a stainless steel steamer basket with the leeks. Gently rinse salmon fillets in filtered water and place on bed of leeks. Pour sauce over salmon and leeks.

Place steamer containing fish and leeks in a large pot with a half inch of filtered water. Cover, bring water to a low boil, and steam for 15–20 minutes depending on thickness of steaks. Add dill during the last 3 minutes. Serve.

> TIP: The delicious sauce with this flavorful dish goes well with long grain boiled rice. Enjoy with a salad or lightly steamed vegetables for a gourmet meal.

Breast-Protective Power Foods: Salmon, leeks, lemon juice, dill, miso, garlic.

Fish in Papillotte with Fresh Thyme

(Serves 6)

❦ *This aromatic roasted fish in parchment is rich with niçoise flavors: olives, bay leaves, orange peel, shallots, and fresh thyme. The parchment ensures a juicy, gently cooked fish with lots of flavor.*

> 5 lb cod (1 cleaned whole fish or cod fillets)
> 1½ cups sliced shallots
> 2½ tbsp brown rice vinegar
> sea salt and freshly ground black pepper
> 2 tsp minced fresh thyme
> 8 pitted Niçoise black olives
> ½ organic orange peel, thinly minced
> 1 tbsp extra virgin olive oil
> 2 bay leaves
> 5 escarole leaves
> natural parchment paper
> ¼ cup chopped Italian parsley

Wash fish well and gently pat dry. Sauté shallots in vinegar on low medium for a few minutes until soft.

Sprinkle salt, pepper, and herbs inside and outside fish. Stuff inside of fish with shallots, olives, and orange peel. Rub outside with oil. Place bay leaves on top and cover with escarole leaves. Wrap in a large piece of parchment paper, large enough so that there is extra paper to roll the edges tightly closed. Put in a Pyrex dish and bake in a preheated 350° oven for 35 minutes. Remove the parchment and lettuce. Garnish with fresh parsley and thinly sliced wedges of orange and serve.

Delicious with arugula or fennel salad and herbed rice.

Comment: If you use fillets, simply spoon shallots and the rest of the ingredients over fish and wrap in parchment. The escarole leaves keep the fish moist.

Breast-Protective Power Foods: Cod, shallots, thyme, bay leaves, orange peel, parsley, escarole.

Spicy Shrimp Salad with Basil

(SERVES 2)

> 1 lb medium-sized cooked
>   shrimp
> 4–5 tbsp organic plain yogurt
> juice from 1 lemon
> 2 tbsp fresh minced basil
> couple pinches of cayenne pepper
> ½ tsp sea salt
> 2 tbsp minced scallions
> ½ cup finely chopped celery
> 1 ripe tomato
> lettuce

Cup shrimp in half, lengthwise. Remove tails from shrimp if they have not already been removed. Combine with the rest of the ingredients, except for the tomato and lettuce. Adjust the seasoning with salt, lemon, and cayenne pepper.

Rinse and dry lettuce, and put on a plate. Add the shrimp salad, add a little more minced fresh herbs for garnish, and surround with tomato wedges.

Comment: You can substitute cilantro or dill for the basil.

Breast-Protective Power Foods: Yogurt, lemon juice, basil, cayenne pepper, scallions, celery, yogurt.

Tuna with Coriander and Onions

(SERVES 4)

Inspired by Fish, The Basics, *by Shirley King.*

4 tuna steaks (6–10 ounces each)
3 medium-sized red onions, sliced thickly
4 cups fresh mixed greens (arugula, spinach, radiccio, etc.)

Marinade

1 tbsp coriander
juice from 1–2 limes
¾ tsp peppercorns
8 cloves garlic
1 tsp extra virgin olive oil
½ cup filtered water
2 tsp mellow or sweet white miso

Rinse fish and pat dry. Put onions and cleaned fish on a platter.

In a suribachi or food processor, grind gradually together marinade ingredients. The consistency should be thick.

Pour over fish and onions. Marinate for 2 hours. Turn fish after 1 hour.

Preheat oven to 450 for 10 minutes. Roast tuna and onions 4 minutes. Turn both onions and fish, and continue to roast another 4 minutes. Serve with wedges of lime over mixed greens.

Breast-Protective Power Foods: Tuna, red onions, garlic, extra virgin olive oil, miso.

Lightly Curried Scrod in Sweet Miso-Lime Sauce

(SERVES 4)

❦ *Cumin contains strong anticancer phytochemicals. The tomatoes and onions in this simple yet flavorful dish also offer protection against cancer.*

1–⅓ lbs scrod
6 cloves minced garlic
juice from 1 lime
⅓ cup Braggs Liquid Aminos
1½ tbsp sweet white miso
3–4 pinches of cumin
12 organic cherry tomatoes
⅓ cup very thinly sliced mild onion
½ tsp curry powder

Clean fish. Place in shallow sauce pan with garlic. Be sure to tuck half the sliced garlic under the fish to flavor liquid for sauce. Cover with lime juice and Braggs. Add cumin. Massage a thin layer of miso over fish. Cut tomatoes in half and place around fish with sliced onion. Add curry powder, cover, and bring to a gentle boil. Turn down and cook over medium-low gently for 15 minutes. Remove from pan right away to avoid an overcooked texture.

Serve with a light grain such as brown basmati rice or whole wheat couscous and plenty of vegetables, both in a salad and lightly steamed. The sauce is delicious. Spoon plenty over fish and grain.

Breast-Protective Power Foods: Garlic, miso, Braggs Liquid Aminos, cumin, onion, tomatoes.

Spicy Sardine Pita Pocket

(SERVES 3 or 4)

1 tin of sardines
3–4 thin slices of vidalia or other mild onion
1 cup mixed thinly sliced radishes and cucumber

sea salt
fresh dill, minced (optional)
1 cup arugula leaves
3 cloves pressed garlic
2 tbsp extra virgin olive oil
3 tbsp lemon juice
3 tsp Dijon natural mustard
ground pepper

Sprinkle onion, radishes, and cucumber with a little sea salt. Set aside for 20–30 minutes. (Optional: Add minced fresh dill.) Clean arugula well. Pat dry and set aside.

Prepare Dijon vinaigrette by combining garlic, olive oil, lemon juice, and mustard in a suribachi or small bowl.

Drain liquid from onion, radishes, and cucumbers. Combine all vegetables in a bowl with the vinaigrette, season with ground pepper, and adjust salt.

Fill pita bread with salad vegetables and sardines by dividing equally. Garnish with lemon wedges and serve.

TIP: Look for Crown Prince sardines. *See* the Resource Guide.

Breast-Protective Power Foods: Sardines, garlic, lemon juice, extra-virgin olive oil, arugula, onions, radishes, cucumbers.

Stove-Top Swordfish Steaks

(Serves 2)

❦ *If you want a healthy dinner that is simple and easy to prepare, pick up some fresh swordfish on your way home and try this wonderful dish. I garnish each serving with garlic slices.*

½ cup Braggs Liquid
   Aminos
juice from 1 lemon
12 large cloves of garlic
½ tsp chili powder
2 swordfish steaks, ½ lb
   each

Combine Braggs, lemon juice, and thinly sliced garlic cloves in skillet. Sprinkle chili powder on each side of swordfish. Cook uncovered on medium heat 5 minutes per side.

Comment: Braggs Liquid Aminos is available in most all health food stores and should be a staple of any kitchen. *Braggs is a substitute for soy sauce that is nonfermented, so it's a safe choice for women who are sensitive to fermented products such as soy sauce.* What is Braggs? It is concentrated vegetable protein in a liquid form, 100% natural.

Breast-Protective Power Foods: Lemon juice, Braggs Liquid Aminos, garlic, chili powder.

Yosenabe

(SERVES 4)

🍃 *Burdock root, known as "Gobo" in Oriental markets, excels in blocking cancers initiated by radiation or chemicals, and prevents breast tumors from developing. Burdock is an ideal anticancer food, and can be used in any dish you would use cooked carrot. I like Burdock slow-cooked to bring out its rich, earthy taste.*

1 burdock root, cut into thin matchsticks
8 shiitake mushrooms
3 tbsp shoyu or tamari sauce
1 3-inch strip kombu
1 lb mackerel (or equal amount of tempeh or tofu)
florets from medium bunch of broccoli or equivalent amount
   of sliced cabbage
1 small sliced onion
1 medium carrot, cut into strips (about 1 cup)
¾ cup of very thinly sliced daikon
1 medium leek, cleaned and sliced lengthwise

Sauce

juice of 2–3 lemons
4 tbsp chickpea or mellow white miso
¾ cup freshly grated ginger
2 finely minced scallions
4 cloves minced garlic

Scrub burdock root well with a natural bristle vegetable brush available in your health food store. Reconstitute mushrooms in mixture of shoyu and ½ cup water. Soak for ½ hour until very soft. Drain mushrooms and retain soaking liquid. Lightly wipe kombu with clean, damp cloth, barely cover with water, and soak for 15 minutes or until soft. Drain kombu and place it in a very large stainless steel skillet. Artfully arrange fish, vegetables, and mushrooms in separate sections. Add ½ cup of shiitake soaking liquid to contents of skillet.

Sauce

Blend lemon juice, garlic, and miso in suribachi until it has a syrupy consistency. You may need to add a tbsp of water if your lemons are small. Pour sauce over everything. Cover pan and bring to a simmer. Simmer over medium heat for 4 minutes. Turn down and cook over medium-low for 40 minutes. Finish dish with lots of ginger juice by squeezing (by hand) freshly grated ginger over food. Garnish with minced scallions before serving.

Watercress salad goes well with this hearty winter stew.

Breast-Protective Power Foods: Mackerel, broccoli, cabbage, tempeh, tofu, onion, carrot, daikon, burdock root, shiitake mushrooms, shoyu, kombu, leeks, lemon, miso, ginger, scallions, garlic.

Thai Lemon Grass Shrimp and Noodles in Broth

(SERVES 4)

1 cup cilantro leaves
1–2 green jalapeño peppers cut in half, seeds removed
6 slices fresh ginger
juice from 1 lime
1½ stalks lemon grass cut into 1-inch pieces
1 tbsp shoyu or tamari sauce
sea salt and pepper
2 lbs jumbo fresh shrimp
2 cups snow peas
½ cup minced garlic, crushed in a suribachi
juice of 2 limes
1½ packages (8.8 ounces per package) of udon noodles,
    cooked according to instructions

Broth Ingredients

shrimp shells from cleaned shrimp
1 stalk of celery
1 carrot
1 small onion
1 bay leaf
2 tbsp shoyu
3 tbsp mirin
5 cups filtered water

Bring broth ingredients to a boil. Cook on medium for 30 minutes. Drain out vegetables and shrimp shells. Set aside.

Clean the cilantro and mince half. Simmer together the broth, jalapeño, ginger, half the lime juice, and ½ cup cilantro with the lemon grass for 15 minutes. Add the shoyu, salt, and pepper. Taste and adjust seasonings. Add the shrimp and cook over medium heat for 3 minutes. Add the snow peas and garlic. Cook for another 3 minutes. Add the remaining minced cilantro and lime juice. Put noodles in four bowls. Ladle a portion of broth in each bowl. Top with shrimp and garnish with a little minced cilantro. Serve with a fresh salad and peanut dressing.

Breast-Protective Power Foods: Peppers, cilantro, ginger, lemon grass, shoyu, garlic, onion.

Shrimp and Avocado Salad with Cilantro

(SERVES 2)

🍴 *This is a typical French "starter" course, which I livened up with fusion vinaigrette—Asian miso with Latin cilantro and cayenne.*

1 tomato
1 ripe avocado
juice of 1 lemon
juice of ½ lime
½ cup extra virgin olive oil
½ handful of cleaned and minced cilantro
sea salt
½ lb medium shrimp, shelled and deveined

ground pepper
1 tsp mellow white miso
pinch of cayenne pepper

Briefly dip tomato in boiling water. Set aside to cool. Peel and mash avocado and mix together, in a bowl with the lemon and lime juice, cayenne pepper, extra virgin olive oil, cilantro, and a few pinches of sea salt. Peel, seed, and chop tomato. Steam or boil the shrimp for 3 minutes until opaque. Let cook for 10 minutes. Combine chopped tomato, shrimp, and avocado dressing. Adjust seasonings, add ground pepper, and serve over butter lettuce with lemon wedges. Very delicious and simple! Serve immediately.

Breast-Protective Power Foods: Tomato, extra virgin olive oil, avocado, lemon juice, cilantro, miso, cayenne.

Pesto Sauce

(SERVES 4)

🐛   *Although pesto sauce is usually served over pasta, this delicious sauce also works well over fish (or tofu).*
Simply add sauce to fish right at the end of the cooking process. It's most flavorful when not overcooked.

¾ cup loosely packed basil
½ cup pine nuts
4 tbsp extra virgin olive oil
4 cloves minced garlic
2 tbsp mellow miso

Wash basil and pine nuts. Remove stems from basil. Combine all ingredients on low speed in blender until creamy.

Breast-Protective Power Foods: Basil, extra virgin olive oil, garlic, miso, pine nuts.

GRAINS

Gingered Wild Rice Pilaf with Mixed Vegetables

(SERVES 4)

❦ *This dish is a wonderful combination of vivid and original flavors. Be sure to prepare right before serving for the freshest flavors.*

Rice

  4 cups filtered water
  1 cup wild rice
  ⅛ tsp sea salt

Mixed Vegetables

  ¼ tsp untoasted sesame oil
  2 tbsp filtered water
  1 clove sliced garlic
  2 cups mixed julienned celery, 2 thinly sliced on the diagonal
      scallions, and thinly sliced onion
  ⅓ tsp curry powder
  Herbamare® natural vegetable salt to taste
  ½ cup of one of the following vegetables, blanched and set
      aside:
      lima beans or green shelled soybeans (flash-frozen *green*
      soybeans are available in many Asian markets)

To Finish Pilaf

  2 tbsp grated fresh ginger
  2 tbsp flaxseed oil
  additional Herbamare® to taste

Bring water for rice to a rolling boil. Add salt and rinsed rice, loosely cover and cook for 45–50 minutes. Remove from heat. Drain, fluff with fork. Cover with a bamboo mat and set aside. In a sauté pan, lightly coat with a thin layer of sesame oil. Add water, garlic, and 2 cups of mixed vegetables. Sauté gently for 10 minutes. Add seasonings and continue to sauté for 5 more minutes. Combine rice and blanched peas, limas, or soybeans with sautéed vegetables. Lightly heat through for a couple of minutes. Add Herbamare to taste. Take freshly grated ginger and squeeze juice over rice pilaf (using hands). Taste, and add more if needed. Take off heat. Fluff with fork. Right before serving, mix through flax seed oil to finish dish.

Breast-Protective Power Foods: Celery, scallion, garlic, sesame oil, lima beans, green soybeans, ginger, flaxseed oil.

Basmati Rice with Mushrooms and Onions

(SERVES 4)

🌿 *My mother inspired many of my rice recipes, especially those with mushrooms. One of my favorite dishes she cooked was rice with mushrooms and onions.*

> 10 dried shiitake mushrooms
> 2⅓ cup + 1 tbsp filtered
>   water
> 3 tbsp shoyu or tamari sauce
> 1 cup brown basmati rice
> sea salt
> 1 tsp organic sesame oil
> 1 large thinly sliced onion
> Herbamane® natural
>   seasoning
> 2 scallions, cleaned and diced
> 2 tbsp organic walnut oil

Rinse mushrooms and bring ⅓ cup water to a boil. Place mushrooms, water, and shoyu into a small bowl (when the rice is finished cooking, the mushrooms will be reconstituted).

Bring 2 cups of water, rinsed rice, and ⅛ tsp of salt to a boil in a covered pot. Turn down and cook gently on low for about 40 minutes. When the rice is done—the aroma and tender texture will be apparent—fluff with a fork and immediately remove from heat. Cover with a bamboo mat or towel and set aside.

When mushrooms are soft, slice very thin. Put sliced mushrooms back into shoyu/water marinade.

Brush a skillet lightly with sesame oil. Add 1 tbsp water and the onion. Sauté onions on a medium-low heat with a couple of pinches of salt and Herbamane®.

Squeeze the marinade out of the mushrooms and set aside.

When the onions are tender, add the mushrooms, rice, and scallions. Toss throughout several generous pinches of Herbamane® and walnut oil.

Comments: Don't overcook rice. Serve as soon as possible when done. Keeping rice hot for a long time affects flavor and texture, just like with pasta.

Breast-Protective Power Foods: Brown rice, shiitake mushrooms, shoyu, onion, sesame oil, walnut oil, scallions.

Quinoa Salad with Carrot Miso Dressing

(SERVES 4)

2 cups cooked organic carrots
⅓ cup cooking broth from carrots
2 tbsp sesame butter
2 tbsp organic sesame oil
1 tbsp shoyu or tamari sauce
2 tbsp mellow white or barley miso
⅛ tsp sea salt

Scrub carrots and cut into ½-inch slices and just cover with filtered water. Gently boil, covered until tender. Don't overcook. Set aside and let cool. Transfer carrots with the rest of ingredients (except for cooking broth) into a blender. Puree, adding a small amount of broth to get desired consistency. Serve over cooked quinoa or brown rice on a bed of lettuce surrounded by steamed cauliflower and broccoli, garnished with crisp celery sticks and alfalfa sprouts.

Comment: Large carrots are the sweetest. The flavor of organic carrots really is sweeter than the nonorganic variety, and truly helps to make this simple recipe outstanding.

Breast-Protective Power Foods: Carrots, sesame butter, sesame oil, shoyu, miso.

Rice and Black Soybeans Garnished with Scallions

(SERVES 4)

❦   *Black soybeans and brown rice are a delicious, aromatic, homestyle dish enjoyed in Japan, often served in bento boxes. A technique used frequently by macrobiotic chefs is to dry-roast the beans in a skillet for a few minutes, stirring to prevent burning. Dry-roasting beans helps to cut down on cooking time because it helps to soften the beans. Boiling black soybeans is very time-consuming, because the beans are very hard and require almost 3 hours of cooking time. This is one of those dishes, wholesome and fragrant, that makes you glad you have a pressure cooker!*

> 2 cups short-grain brown rice
> ½ cup black soybeans
> 2¾ cup of filtered water
> ⅛ tsp sea salt
> 2–3 cleaned and finely minced scallions

Wash the rice, drain, and put into a pressure cooker. Clean the beans by putting them on a clean, damp dish towel. Pat gently with towel to remove dust. It is not recommended that soybeans be washed, because the skins peel off. After the beans have been cleaned, dry-roast in a hot skillet. The inside of the bean will be light brown in color when they are ready to pressure-cook.

Combine roasted beans, rice, water, and sea salt in a pressure cooker. Slowly bring up pressure. After you've brought it up to full pressure, lower the flame and cook for about 50 minutes. Bring the pressure down, and allow rice and beans to sit for several minutes. Remove from pot and garnish with scallions. Enjoy!

Breast-Protective Power Foods: Brown rice, black soybeans, scallions.

Barley and Shiitake Salad with Dill Vinaigrette

❦ *In macrobiotics, barley is thought of as the lightest grain, suitable for even the warmest days of summer.*

1 cup hulled and washed barley
3 cups + 2 tbsp filtered water
sea salt
½ chopped onion
ground pepper
9–12 fresh shiitake mushrooms, washed, diced, and patted dry
shoyu or tamari sauce to taste
½ cup thinly chopped scallions
½ cup carrot, scrubbed and diced small

Dill Vinaigrette

¼–⅓ cup lemon juice
2 tbsp extra virgin olive oil
1 clove garlic, minced
1 tbsp fresh, chopped dill
⅛ tsp sea salt

Bring 1 cup barley, 3 cups water, and ⅛ tsp of salt to a boil. Reduce heat and simmer for about 1 hour. Transfer to a bowl and let cool. Add 2 tbsp water to a pan. Water sauté carrot and onion until just soft. Season lightly with sea salt and ground pepper. Put shiitake mushrooms in a small pot. Mix equally half shoyu, and half water. Bring to a boil and turn down. Cover. Cook over medium-low heat for 15 minutes. Uncover and drain.

Make dressing ingredients and mix well. Combine dressing, barley, mushrooms, and scallions.

Breast-Protective Power Foods: Barley, shiitake mushrooms, onion, carrots, scallions, cilantro, lemon juice, extra virgin olive oil, dill.

Spanish Rice Salad with Roasted Onions

(Serves 4)

🍂 *Joyous summer corn and tomatoes, favorite foods of everyone, combine well with tomatillos, spices and roasted onions for a light and flavorful rice salad. Green tomatoes (or tomatillos) contain potent anti-cancer chemicals.*

2 large white onions
natural parchment paper
filtered water
2 tsp sesame oil
sea salt
2 tbsp balsamic vinegar
1½ cups brown rice
10 tomatillos
1 serrano chili, deseeded and minced (handle only with gloves—
   can burn skin and eyes)
4 cloves of minced garlic
2 cobs of fresh corn
2 minced scallions
1½ tsp umeboshi vinegar
½ tsp white pepper
2 ripe tomatoes
3 pinches of chili powder
3 pinches of cumin
3 pinches of cayenne pepper (don't touch with fingers—can burn
   eyes)

Preheat oven to 375°. Peel onions and cut into bite-sized pieces. In a large Pyrex baking dish cover with parchment paper and add 2 tbsp of water and sesame oil. Rub oil and water mixture over paper and on onion pieces. Add a couple pinches of sea salt, and roast uncovered for 30 minutes. Mix onions, add balsamic vinegar and a pinch more of salt, and roast for an additional 30–40 minutes or until lightly golden.

Cook rice in 2 cups of water with a pinch of salt. Bring to a boil, turn down, and continue to cook for 45 minutes. When finished cooking, remove from pot, and put into large bowl. Fluff with a fork and cover with a dish towel or bamboo mat and set aside.

Peel and rinse tomatillos. Cut into bite-sized pieces. You should wear rubber gloves to prepare chili, because it is extremely hot and *can burn fingers and eyes*. Deseed and finely mince chili. Add chili, tomatillos, and garlic to a sauté pan with a tablespoon of water. Add a couple pinches of salt. Sauté over medium-high for approximately 8 minutes. Don't sauté too long or the tomatillos will become mushy. Put tomatillos in bowl and set aside.

Take corn off cob and water sauté in a pan with 2 tsp of water, 2 minced scallions, umeboshi vinegar, and white pepper for about 4 minutes. Remove from pan and set aside in a small bowl.

Quickly submerge tomatoes in boiling water. Let cool, and the peel will easily remove. Discard the seeds and cut into chunks. Put into a small bowl with a few pinches of sea salt. Set aside.

When rice has cooled, combine all ingredients with remaining seasonings and serve.

Comment: Natural parchment paper, available in most health food stores, isn't treated with harmful chemicals. Be sure to avoid parchment paper that is not chemical-free.

Breast-Protective Power Foods: Brown rice, onions, tomatoes, corn, tomatillos, chili pepper, scallion, garlic, cumin, cayenne, sesame oil.

Millet and Leek Miso Soup

4–5 dried shiitake mushrooms
2:1 water-shoyu soaking mixture
¼ cup reconstituted wakame (seaweed)
5–6 cups filtered water
⅓ cup millet
1 cup minced leeks
⅓ cup light barley miso
3 tbsp shoyu or tamari sauce (or to taste)

Rinse mushrooms. Soak in water-shoyu mixture for 30 minutes. Slice thinly and discard stems.

Wipe wakame sea vegetable lightly with a clean damp cloth. Soak wakame in water to reconstitute, approximately 10–15 minutes. Cut out rib and discard. Chop wakame.

Combine water, millet, and wakame in a pot. Bring to a gentle boil and simmer for 25–30 minutes.

Carefully clean leeks by discarding top third and roots. Cut in half length-wise. Mince each half. Place minced leeks in a bowl of clean water and whoosh around. Discard water and rinse again. Repeat process about 4 times to make sure there is no sand residue. Mince leeks and add, with mushrooms, to soup mixture.

Puree miso with some soup broth and add mixture back to soup.

Heat gently for 3 minutes. Generally avoid boiling, as it can destroy enzymes.

Breast-Protective Power Foods: Millet, shiitake mushrooms, wakame, miso, shoyu, leeks.

SOY FOODS

Tempeh Sandwich Spread

(SERVES 3 or 4)

꽃 *Genistein, an isoflavone found in soybeans, has been noted by researchers as being ten times more powerful than previously thought. For more information on phytochemicals in soybeans, see Chapter 7, "Soybeans Protect Against Breast Cancer."*

Fermented soy foods, such as tempeh and miso, have been found to offer the most breast-protective benefits.

> 1 8-oz package tempeh (cut into 2-inch cubes)
> 1 medium-small chopped mild onion
> 2 small cloves of finely minced garlic
> 1 small bay leaf
> 1–2 tbsp fresh lemon juice
> ½ cup filtered water
> 2 tbsp light barley or chickpea miso
> ¼ tsp grated ginger juice
> 2 tbsp unroasted organic tahini
> ⅓ cup finely minced celery
> ½ cup finely minced Jerusalem artichoke
>   (optional)
> few pinches of sea salt
> couple pinches of Herbamare® natural
>   seasoning

Place tempeh, onion, garlic and bay leaf in a small pot. Just cover with water, bring to a boil, lower heat, and simmer uncovered for 20 minutes. Tempeh should be soft (but not mushy) and there should be a little water left. Put Tempeh, along with all remaining cooking liquid (some will have evaporated), in a small bowl and the rest of the ingredients. Mash until mixed. Salad should resemble tuna fish salad. Adjust seasonings and serve in a pita with lettuce.

Breast-Protective Power Foods: Tempeh, onion, garlic, bay leaf, lemon juice, miso, ginger, tahini, celery.

Oven-Barbecued Tofu

(SERVES 4)

1 1-lb block extra firm tofu
¾ cup natural barbecue sauce sweetened with honey
1 tbsp filtered water

Preheat oven to 350°. Slice the tofu. You should end up with about 10–12 slices from a block of tofu. In a large Pyrex baking dish, arrange the tofu. Make sure the slices don't overlap. Cover carefully with the barbecue sauce so that each piece has a light "coating" of sauce. Coat well. Lightly spoon just a little water around the periphery of the tofu to prevent sticking after baking. Cover tightly in foil. Roast for 20 minutes, remove foil, and bake for an additional 5–10 minutes.

Comment: Oven barbecued tofu is excellent in sandwiches or salads the following day. Look for a barbecue sauce that does not contain oil to avoid rancid, processed oils. (*See* the Resource Guide for my favorite, natural, oil-free, honey-sweetened barbeque sauce.)

> TIP: If you have a local Asian market, look for frozen green soybeans. Simply cook a small handful until just tender, in lightly boiling water. Sprinkle the beans over the oven-barbecued tofu the last few minutes of cooking. Shake a few drops of Tabasco sauce over the tofu and beans for seasoning, and continue to bake for about 5 minutes. Enjoy a home-style Chinese dish, full of flavor, with powerful health benefits.

Breast-Protective Power Food: Tofu.

Soybean Casserole with Chicken

(Serves 6)

❦   A great "rainy Sunday" fall or winter one-pot meal, Soybean Casserole, a Chinese home-style dish, is deeply rich and flavorful. I love the delicious flavors of slowly cooked soybeans combined with mushrooms and a little organic chicken, flavored richly with tahini and light miso.

It's tempting to pressure-cook this tough little bean, but slow cooking without the use of a pressure cooker makes the health benefits of the soybean more potent. In fact, pressure cooking soybeans greatly decreases the benefits of isoflavones.

If you are a vegetarian, simply leave out the chicken. It tastes great with or without the meat.

> 2½ cups soaked soybeans
> 2-inch piece of kombu
> filtered water
> 1 lb organic skinless chicken thighs (bone in) (about 4 pieces)
> 2–3 peeled and sliced shallots
> 12 shiitake mushrooms
> 1 tbsp shoyu or tamari sauce
> ⅔ cup sliced carrots (diagonal cut)
> 1 tbsp organic unroasted sesame tahini
> 1 tbsp sweet white miso
> 1–2-inch piece ginger root

Rinse soybeans and soak overnight in water. Lightly wipe kombu with a clean damp cloth and reconstitute in a couple of tablespoons of water until soft. Rinse soybeans and put in a heavy, large pot with softened kombu and 6 cups of fresh water. Bring to a boil, skimming off foam that will develop. Turn down to medium-high 15 minutes later, partially cover, and simmer for an hour. Add the chicken and shallots, with 3 additional cups of water. Bring to a boil, turn down to medium, partially covered, and cook for an additional hour. Stir gently once or twice while cooking.

Rinse shiitake mushrooms. Reconstitute in ⅓ cup of hot water and add shoyu. When mushrooms soften, discard hard stems (or save them to use later in vegetable stock) and cut mushrooms in half. Add mushrooms, carrots, salt and 2 cups of water to the soybeans. Mix gently, partially covered, and cook for the final hour. Ten minutes before done, puree the tahini and miso in a little liquid from the beans, and add to casserole. Mix gently. Grate ginger root, and squeeze juice from grated ginger (using hands) into casserole for garnish. If you don't have ginger, try minced scallions for garnish.

> TIP: Leftover soybeans from this delicious recipe make a great sand-
> wich spread.

Breast-Protective Power Foods: Soybeans, shiitake mushrooms, shoyu,
tahini, shallots, kombu, carrots, ginger.

Tempeh Fra Diavlo Sauce with Roasted Garlic

(Serves 4)

❦ *The Scotch bonnet is a potent little pepper, powerfully hot and powerfully
protective. Hot peppers contain capsicin, an anti-oxidant. When hot peppers are
combined with garlic, the phytonutrients in the garlic become even more protective.
Handle hot peppers carefully, using gloves.*

> 1 8-oz package soy tempeh
> ⅔ cup red wine
> 4 chopped shallots
> 3 pinches dried marjoram
> sea salt
> 2 cups sliced fennel
> Ground black pepper
> Parchment paper
> Filtered water
> 1 32-oz jar spaghetti sauce
> 1 Scotch bonnet pepper
> 1 head roasted garlic (*see* recipe on page 000)
> 4 pitted and sliced black olives
> 1 sweet red pepper
> 4¼ tsp extra virgin olive oil

Preheat oven to 365°.

Marinate tempeh in wine, 2 chopped shallots, marjoram, and 3–4 pinches
of salt for 1 hour. Crumble tempeh up, and mix into the wine and herbs. Mix
again in 30 minutes to ensure coverage. In another small Pyrex dish put
fennel, 2 sliced shallots, ½ tsp salt, and ground pepper on a sheet of parchment
paper. Add 2 tbsp water and roast uncovered at 350° for 40 minutes. When
tempeh has finished marinating, drain wine, add ⅓ jar of spaghetti sauce, and

minced Scotch bonnet without the seeds. *Caution: This is a fiery hot pepper that can burn skin and eyes; wear rubber gloves while deseeding and mincing.* Add ½ cup water to tempeh, sauce, and red pepper. Mix well and roast at 350° for ½ hour. When tempeh is finished, remove from oven and set aside. Preheat oven to 500°. On a small piece of parchment paper in a baking dish, lay halved, deseeded red pepper skin side up. Roast for 20 minutes until skin is charred. Let cool. Peel pepper.

Combine tempeh, sauce, fennel, garlic, olives, and remaining sauce in jar. Dice red pepper and add. Heat on medium-low, add additional salt to taste. Prepare pasta, drain, dress with additional extra virgin olive oil and salt. Serve with tempeh fra diavlo sauce. Drizzle a little unheated extra virgin olive oil on each serving and enjoy.

Breast-Protective Power Foods: Tempeh, fennel, garlic, spaghetti sauce, Scotch bonnet pepper, shallots, marjoram, extra virgin olive oil.

Herbed Tofu Salad with Horseradish

(SERVES 3–4)

🌿   *Freshly grated horseradish gives a spicy dimension to this tofu salad with a variety of crisp vegetables. Horseradish is a member of the cabbage family, and contains many phytochemicals that help to protect against cancer.*

> 6 cups filtered water
> 1 lb tofu
> 10 radishes
> 3 tbsp fresh horseradish, grated
> 2 scallions
> 2 tbsp umeboshi vinegar
> 2 tbsp extra virgin olive oil
> 2 tbsp flaxseed oil blend
> 3 tbsp fresh dill, minced

Bring water to boil. Quickly submerge tofu in water for 10 seconds. Remove and let cool. Clean and chop radishes. Grate horseradish after first removing skin. Use small holes for grating (to avoid watery eyes, keep face away from grater). Combine all ingredients, except for dill, in a blender. Purée. Add dill, mix, and serve. Garnish with additional fresh dill.

Stuff a pita pocket with this crisp, spicy salad, or enjoy it as a side dish with rice or pasta.

Breast-Protective Power Foods: Tofu, scallions, radishes, extra virgin olive oil, flaxseed oil, horseradish, dill.

Baked Tofu in Miso Tahini Sauce

(Serves 3–4)

❦ *Simple and delicious, Baked Tofu in Miso Tahini Sauce is a great way to save time in the kitchen. Double the recipe and make enough for a couple of meals. Be sure to garnish with freshly chopped scallions.*

1 tbsp mellow white miso
2 tbsp organic unroasted tahini
1 tbsp filtered water
1-lb package of organic tofu
minced scallions for garnishing

In a suribachi or a small bowl, mix miso and tahini with water until blended. Cut tofu into 12 slices and arrange on a Pyrex dish. Spread the miso tahini over the tofu and roast in a preheated 350° oven for 10–15 minutes. Remove from oven, garnish, and serve. Excellent for sandwiches.

Breast-Protective Power Foods: Tofu, miso, tahini, scallions.

Slow-Roasted Tempeh with Sundried Tomatoes and Fennel

1 cup sundried tomatoes
filtered water
2½ tbsp white miso
1 block tempeh
¾ cup fennel, cleaned and sliced into 4-inch lengths
4–6 garlic cloves, cut into slices
6 natural pitted black olives
sea salt

ground pepper
pinches of thyme, rosemary, and oregano
extra virgin olive oil

Reconstitute tomatoes with 1 cup of water. Soak for at least 10 minutes. Mix liquid from tomatoes with miso. (Use ½ to ⅔ cup tomato liquid for mixing with miso.) Preheat oven to 375°.

Cut block of tempeh into thirds. Cut each section in half to create a thinner slice. Take tempeh slices and fennel, and place in a small casserole with garlic. Place reconstituted tomatoes and miso tomato broth on tempeh-fennel combination. Add olives, herbs, and seasonings. Cover casserole and roast for 45 minutes covered, and 20 minutes uncovered.

Adjust seasonings and drizzle with extra virgin olive oil. Serve with salad and quinoa.

Comment: You need a sharp, pointed knife to cut tempeh into thin slices, which is the best way to use it in casseroles.

Breast-Protective Power Foods: Tempeh, tomatoes, fennel, garlic, miso, olive oil, thyme, rosemary, oregano.

Miso-Scallion Spread for Sandwiches

❦ *This delicious miso scallion spread is an alternative to butter (high in saturated fat) or mayonnaise with hydrogenated fat or rancid canola oil. Try it with chicken, turkey, soy bologna, or tempeh sandwiches. The spicy scallions are immunoprotective, and full of breast-healthy phytonutrients. Sesame seeds provide a wonderful source of EFAs.*

When selecting bread, be sure you look for whole wheat bread, as opposed to cracked wheat. The less processed the grain, the healthier.

1 tbsp mellow white or sweet white miso
3 tbsp organic unroasted sesame tahini
1–2 tbsp filtered water
2 tbsp finely minced scallions

Gradually blend miso and tahini in a little bowl. Stir in a small amount of water for a thinner mixture—look for a texture similar to that of Dijon mustard. Add minced scallions and continue to blend. Delicious on bread with tempeh or tofu sandwiches.

Breast-Protective Power Foods: Tahini, miso, scallions.

Choucroute Garni Light

(SERVES 8)

❦ *Throughout France, a favorite "rustic" dish, Choucroute Garni, is often served. Parisians are very fond of this traditional dish, sauerkraut with various sausages and juniper berries cooked in wine, sharing it with friends, and plenty of white wine.*

I've created a healthier version of this hearty French dish.

The Cabbage

approximately 2½ tbsp balsamic vinegar
1 tbsp filtered water
1 small head sliced and rinsed cabbage (approximately 8 cups)
1 tsp sea salt
8–10 juniper berries (optional)
5 bay leaves
2 cups organic low-salt sauerkraut, rinsed quickly, with liquid squeezed out
ground pepper

In a large sauté pan, put 1 tbsp vinegar and 1 tbsp water, and cabbage. Cook 4 minutes over high heat. Add the salt and stir constantly. Add remaining vinegar, juniper berries, bay leaves, and sauerkraut. Stir, turn down to medium, and cook for 3 minutes more. Add freshly ground pepper and mix. Cover and remove from heat.

The Sausage

1 10-oz package vegetarian soy sausage links
2 tbsp filtered water
1 cup sliced onions
3 sliced shallots
½ tsp sea salt
½ tsp paprika

Cut sausage links into halves or thirds. In a separate sauté pan, put water, onions, and shallots. Sauté over high heat for 3 minutes. Salt lightly and stir. Turn down to medium heat, add sausage and paprika, stirring well. Sauté over medium heat for 4 minutes. Sausage will begin to lightly brown. Turn down to medium-low for another 4 minutes.

Combine cabbage, sauerkraut and sausage, and serve.

Comment: Traditionally this dish is served with mashed potatoes and perhaps baked apples or sauce. To create a lighter balance, I recommend serving it with a salad and a quickly cooked green vegetable.

> Juniper berries are valued as a blood cleanser and as being helpful in stimulating the liver. Valued since Ancient Egyptian and Roman times, juniper berries can be used in stuffings, cooked with meat, and crushed with salt to flavor green vegetables and cabbage.

Breast-Protective Power Foods: Cabbage, sauerkraut, juniper berries, soy sausage, shallots, paprika.

POULTRY AND MEAT

Moroccan Garbanzo Stew with Lamb

(Serves 6–8)

❧ *Vegetables, beans, and herbs, with a small quantity of meat for essential amino acids, combine to make a satisfying and nutritionally complete one-pot meal. Eating meat in condiment-size portions keeps saturated fats to a minimum. This is perhaps why traditional cultures have fewer instances of cancer, heart disease, and osteoporosis than we do in the West. A small amount of meat from time to time offers a complete source of amino acids and provides Vitamin B12.*

   6 loin lamb chops or equivalent in stewing lamb (with bones)
   1 15-oz can organic diced tomatoes
   3 cups cooked garbanzo beans
   2 bay leaves
   filtered water
   1½ tsp sea salt
   5 small white onions
   8 cloves peeled garlic
   5 sprigs parsley
   2 minced and seeded jalapeño peppers
   1½ tsp cinnamon
   ½ tsp turmeric
   ½ tsp coriander
   ½ tsp cumin seed
   ¾ lb cauliflower (2 cups florets)
   ¾ lb green beans (2 cups cut in half)
   ½ lb carrots (1 cup)
   1 tbsp kuzu

Prepare lamb by carefully trimming and discarding fat. Cut into bite-sized pieces. Add lamb, lamb bones, canned tomatoes, garbanzo beans, bay leaves, and 2 cups water. Bring to a slow boil in an uncovered pot. Turn down to medium. Cook for about 1½ hours, stirring occasionally. Add 1 tsp salt and stir.

Peel onions and cut in half. Mince garlic. In a large pot, add 2 tbsp water, garlic, 2 sprigs of chopped parsley, and onions. Water sauté on high for about 5–10 minutes. Turn down to medium-high and add the minced peppers, seasonings, and ½ tsp salt. Stir. Add the cauliflower and green beans and sauté, stirring gently. Cut carrots on the diagonal into bite-sized pieces. Add carrots and sauté for 20 minutes.

After lamb and garbanzo beans have been cooking for about an hour, add the vegetable mixture to the pot.

In a small bowl with 2 tbsp of water, add kuzu root carefully to dissolve. *Make sure the stew is bubbling before you add the dissolved kuzu.* Stir kuzu gently into stew to thicken. Serve with whole wheat couscous and salad.

Caution: Handle jalapeños only with gloved hands; these are very hot peppers that can burn skin and eyes.

Breast-Protective Power Foods: Garbanzo beans, lamb, green beans, cauliflower, onions, carrots, tomatoes, garlic, parsley, peppers, bay leaves, cinnamon, turmeric, cumin, coriander.

Parchment Roasted Chicken Rosemary

(Serves 6)

❦   *Roasting chicken or lamb in parchment ensures a juicy, flavorful dish. The herbs, garlic, shallots, etc., seem more flavorful as well. Phytochemicals in turmeric have been widely researched and found to be a stronger antioxidant than Vitamin C. In traditional medicine, turmeric has been used for many centuries to treat cancer and to relieve pain. Turmeric protects against DNA damage. The American Institute for Cancer Research, in a 1996 conference, summarized several studies showing turmeric to be beneficial in treating cancers of the breast, skin, and colon in laboratory animals.*

⅔ cups Braggs Liquid Aminos
2 lemons
½ tsp turmeric
½ tsp freshly ground pepper
6–8 cloves sliced and/or crushed garlic
½–⅓ cup chopped fresh rosemary
2½ lbs skinless free-range chicken breasts

Combine Braggs Liquid Aminos, juice from lemons, and seasonings with rinsed chicken. Marinate chicken for about 3 hours, turning several times in marinade. Discard marinade.

Take a separate piece of natural parchment paper (available from health food stores) for each chicken breast, and fold in half. Each *halved* sheet should be large enough to enclose the chicken. Be sure each package also contains plenty of the garlic and rosemary. Fold the parchment paper over each piece of chicken, and fold edges together to form a packet.

In a preheated oven of 385°, roast chicken for 20–25 minutes. (Test with knife to be sure inside of chicken is not pink.) Serve with salad, vegetables, and a little grain (½–1 cup of cooked grain per person).

Comment: Rosemary is a powerful antioxidant, especially breast- and liver-protective.

Breast-Protective Power Foods: Braggs Liquid Aminos, lemons, turmeric, garlic, rosemary.

Roasted Loin Lamb Chops and Sage in Parchment

(Serves 4)

¾ cup freshly squeezed lemon juice
3–4 tbsp Braggs Liquid Aminos
2 cloves elephant garlic, sliced thin
4 organic loin lamb chops
4 tbsp fresh sage, finely chopped

Combine lemon, Braggs Liquid Aminos, and garlic. Marinate lamb chops for 1 hour, turning occasionally. Discard marinade. Place one lamb chop on a 15-inch length of parchment paper. Put some garlic and rosemary on top. Bring short sides of parchment together, roll, and fold. Close remaining ends in a similar fashion. When done correctly, the chop should be completely enclosed with space between the chop and the parchment paper on all sides and on top. This enhances the cooking process. Repeat for the remaining chops. Place in a Pyrex baking dish and roast uncovered in a 350° oven for 20 minutes. Garnish with finely minced sage.

Comment: Look for Coleman's brand naturally raised lamb.

Breast-Protective Power Foods: Lamb, lemon juice, Braggs Liquid Aminos, garlic, sage.

Roasted Red Pepper Turkey Burgers

(SERVES 3–4)

❦ *Traveling to Budapest was intriguing. I have a strong memory of richly mosaiced, elaborate antique public baths, including radioactive waters and sulfur baths! Equally imprinted on my memory is a cuisine redolent with red pepper and lots of paprika.*
Creating this dish, I was inspired by the wonderful flavors of Budapest.

> 1¼ lbs low-fat ground turkey
> ½ small red pepper
> 1 heaping tbsp finely minced celery
> ⅔ cup diced onion
> sea salt
> ground black pepper
> 2–3 cloves minced garlic
> ¾ tsp paprika
> 2 tbsp honey- or maple syrup–sweetened barbecue sauce

Put ground turkey in a large bowl. Roast red pepper under the broiler in a preheated oven for about 7 minutes, or until the pepper skin is wrinkled and charred. After the pepper cools, peel off the skin, chop, and add to turkey. In a small pan, add 1 tsp filtered water. Sauté the celery and onion on medium-high. Add a couple pinches of salt and ground black pepper. Sauté, stirring constantly, for approximately 10 minutes. Combine garlic, paprika, sautéed vegetables, ¼ tsp sea salt, ground black pepper, and barbecue sauce gently to the ground turkey and red pepper. Form into burgers.
Cook burgers in a 475° oven on a Pyrex dish, uncovered, about 6 minutes per side. Serve over wilted dandelion greens.

Breast-Protective Power Foods: Red pepper, onion, garlic, celery, paprika.

When selecting lean cuts of beef, be aware that adjustments have to be made in cooking.

Tips for Cooking Lean Cuts of Beef

- Reduce cooking time. Avoid cooking to well-done stage.
- Preheat oven to ensure proper cooking.
- Try marinades with citrus; they help to tenderize.
- Use moist cooking methods. (Cover pan, cook in parchment.)

People who eat roasted meat, which cooks at a much lower temperature than grilling or frying, have no increased risk of stomach cancer. Studies from the American Health Foundation found that people who ate their meat rare and in low quantities had the lowest rate of cancer. Be aware, however, that the juice that bubbles on the bottom of the roasting pan is high in carcinogens.

Thai Flank Steak Salad

Steak and Marinade

1½ lbs rump or flank steak (select naturally raised, hormone-free beef)
⅓ cup minced lemon grass (approximately 3 stalks)
2 chopped and seeded serrano or jalapeño peppers
4–6 cloves minced garlic
⅓ cup organic ketchup
⅓ cup Braggs Liquid Aminos
1 tbsp dark brown honey
1 tbsp rice vinegar
1–2 tbsp Worcestershire sauce (optional)
ground pepper (optional)

Salad

Red lettuce, washed and drained
2 scallions, thinly sliced
1 stalk lemon grass, finely minced
1 mild Maui or vidalia onion
2 ripe tomatoes
2 serrano or jalapeño peppers, thinly sliced
2 tbsp minced cilantro
4 red radishes

Peanut Dressing

3 tbsp sesame oil
juice from 1 lime

1 tsp honey
3 tbsp water
⅓ cup ground peanuts
⅛ tsp sea salt

Combine marinade ingredients. Marinate steak, turning every hour, for 3 hours. Preheat oven to 400°. Cover meat with foil, in a roasting pan, and cook 25-30 minutes. Cut onions and tomatoes into wedges. Arrange lettuce on a platter with the rest of the salad ingredients. When steak is done, slice thinly and place over salad ingredients.

Combine peanut dressing ingredients in a small food processor or surbachi. Lightly salt, spoon dressing over steak and salad, and enjoy.

Caution: Handle serrano/jalapeno peppers only with gloved hands; these very hot peppers can burn skin and eyes.

TIP: I use my flaxseed grinder occasionally for grinding peanuts or other nuts.

Chicken Salad with Grapes and Turmeric

(Serves 4–6)

❦ *If you like chicken salad, you'll love this one! The turmeric and other spices provide a "Moroccan twist," and the grapes give this savory dish an unexpected dimension.*

Chicken

2 cups vegetable broth or filtered water
3 skinless chicken breasts, on the bone, split in the middle
4 cloves peeled garlic
1 chili pepper
1 bay leaf
1 coarsley chopped onion
½ celery stalk, cut into chunks
6 black peppercorns

Salad

½–¾ cup sliced almonds
¾ cup finely chopped bok choy stalks (the white part)
1 cup seedless organic red grapes cut in half
1 cup organic plain yogurt
½–¾ tsp turmeric
sea salt to taste
ground pepper
4 cups watercress

Place all chicken ingredients in a shallow pan and bring to a boil. Reduce heat to medium-low and cook for about 20–25 minutes. Remove from heat and cover. Allow chicken to cool until you can handle it without burning your fingers. Remove from bones and slice the chicken into bite-sized pieces.

Combine all the salad ingredients except for the watercress while the chicken is a little lukewarm, to blend flavors. Adjust seasonings by adding the turmeric and the salt and ground pepper to taste.

Clean and dry the watercress, and serve the chicken salad on watercress.

TIP: Try bok choy stalks diced into your favorite salads instead of celery, to increase your intake of breast-protective cruciferous vegetables.

Breast-Protective Power Foods: Almonds, bok choy, red grapes, yogurt, turmeric, watercress, garlic, chili pepper, onion, celery.

Marjoram Roasted Lamb Shanks

(SERVES 2)

❦ *Marjoram-scented roast lamb—the flavors were meant to go together. Enjoy this version of lamb shanks, slow roasted in a clay pot, which contains far less fat than most others.*

The vegetables in this dish serve as a rack on which to roast the lamb shanks, so the fat content is reduced; they are not eaten.

1 large carrot
1 large onion
1 rib of celery
2 shallots

sea salt
1 cup red wine
2 lamb shanks
sprigs of marjoram

Marinade

4 cloves minced garlic
1 tsp salt
2 tsp minced fresh
   rosemary
3 tbsp minced fresh
   marjoram
4 tbsp extra virgin olive oil
ground pepper
sprigs of marjoram

Submerge the clay pot in water in the sink for 2–3 hours. In a suribachi, combine the minced garlic with 1 tsp sea salt. Blend until pureed. Add minced herbs and olive oil and mix until well blended. Trim fat from lamb shanks and massage marinade into the lamb. Add ground pepper. Let meat marinate for approximately 5 hours, covered, in the refrigerator. Turn once, after 2½ hours, and rub marinade over meat.

Scrub carrot and cut in half. Cut onion into chunks. Clean and cut celery into half, length-wise. Peel shallots. Add all vegetables to the clay roaster with a few pinches of sea salt. Add red wine.

Place lamb shanks on top of cut vegetables so the vegetables make a kind of rack for the meat to sit on. This will allow fat to drip off the meat while cooking, preventing it from cooking in fat. Add sprigs of marjoram and place in 400° oven, covered. Roast for 1 hour.

Optional: Refresh lamb before serving with "gremolata," 2 tbsp each of minced fresh parsley and marjoram, grated zest from ½ lemon, 1 clove minced garlic, a few pinches of sea salt. Spoon gremolata over the lamb.

Breast-Protective Power Foods: Lamb, garlic, rosemary, extra virgin olive oil, marjoram, celery, carrots, onions, shallots.

VEGAN

Tex-Mex Chili Vegetarian Style

(SERVES 6–8)

❦ *If you want to include more soy into your diet, try "second-generation" soy foods such as the textured vegetable protein in this spicy chili dish. Second-generation soy foods offer a wide range of possibilities for the chef and still offer powerful health benefits.*

1 cup dried pinto beans, soaked 8 hours
3-inch piece kombu seaweed
4–5 cups filtered water
2 bay leaves
½ tsp extra virgin olive oil
1 medium onion, chopped
3–4 large cloves minced garlic
1 10-oz package vegetarian soy sausage
1¼ tsp cumin
3½ tsp chili powder
1-lb can organic whole peeled tomatoes
¼ tsp sea salt
¼ tsp paprika
freshly ground pepper to taste
1 tbsp red miso
1 tsp honey
chopped fresh cilantro and onion for garnish

Drain the beans. Wipe kombu lightly with damp cloth. Place beans and kombu in a 4-quart pot with 3 quarts of water. Beans should be covered with water. In 10 minutes, kombu will be reconstituted. Add bay leaves to beans and bring to boil. Reduce heat, stir occasionally, and simmer uncovered for an hour. Skim off the foam that gathers every 15 minutes or so on the surface of cooking beans. Option: Pressure-cook beans for 20 minutes.

Put 2 tbsp of water and olive oil in a 4-quart pot. Begin sautéing onions and garlic on low, adding salt. While onions and garlic are becoming soft, crumble the sausage into pot along with garlic and onions. As the sausage cooks, add the cumin and chili powder. Break apart the tomatoes and add with juice to sausage. Mix cooked beans into sausage, tomatoes, and additional spices along with an additional cup of filtered water. Stir well and cook uncovered over low for 30 minutes.

Puree miso in a small bowl or suribachi with some cooking liquid from tomatoes and spice mixture, and add to chili along with the honey. Adjust seasonings and serve garnished with cilantro and onion.

Breast-Protective Power Foods: Pinto beans, soy sausage, red miso, kombu, garlic, bay leaves, paprika, cilantro, onion, extra virgin olive oil, cumin.

Tomato Soy Sausage Stew Topped with Basil Purée

(SERVES 4)

Roasted Tomatoes

6 ripe tomatoes
6 cloves garlic, finely minced
1 tbsp extra virgin olive oil
1 tbsp water
3 tbsp fresh rosemary
¼–½ tsp dried oregano
sea salt and ground pepper to taste

Stew

½ cup basil leaves
¼ cup extra virgin olive oil
1 10-oz package soy Italian sausage links
2 cloves garlic, finely minced
2 Anaheim, or other chili peppers, cored, seeded, and chopped
Roasted Tomatoes, according to above recipe

Preheat oven to 250°. Slice tomatoes and arrange on Pyrex baking dish with garlic, oil, water, rosemary, oregano, salt, and pepper. Roast uncovered approximately 60 minutes until tender. Remove from oven and set aside to cool. When cool enough to handle, remove skins from tomatoes and transfer meat (insides) to large bowl. Chop the tomatoes and set aside with juices. Taste and adjust salt and pepper.

In a food processor, chop the basil leaves. Add 2 tbsp of olive oil and puree. Remove from food processor and transfer to bowl.

Cut sausage into bite-sized pieces. Add 2 tbsp water to a stainless steel skillet. On low heat, sauté sausages, turning every few minutes. Turn up to medium heat last couple of minutes. Cook sausages approximately 15 minutes. Remove sausages from pan and set aside.

In the same skillet that the sausage cooked in, put in about 2 tbsp water and garlic and peppers. Cook gently over low heat to release aroma. Sauté in this light way for about 4 minutes. Add tomatoes and broth. Heat together for 2 minutes; add sausages.

Delicious over brown rice, with the basil puree drizzled over the top. Serve with a large salad.

Caution: Don't handle without gloves—this hot pepper can burn skin and eyes.

Breast-Protective Power Foods: Soy sausage, basil, extra virgin olive oil, garlic, chili or anaheim pepper, tomatoes, rosemary, oregano.

Savory Seitan with Sage

(SERVES 4)

🌱 *Seitan, a high-protein food, is eaten regularly by people who practice macrobiotics. It is made from wheat gluten and can be purchased in the refrigerator section of your health food store. Sage, an underused herb, offers protective phytochemicals that have antioxidant and antitumor abilities.*

   1 tbsp spring or filtered water
   2 small chopped onions
   3 cloves fresh minced garlic
   couple pinches of sea salt
   1 package ready-made seitan, about 1–1½ lbs
   4 tbsp mirin (Japanese cooking wine, macrobiotic section
      of health food store)
   2 tbsp shoyu or tamari sauce
   garlic salt (to taste)
   white pepper (to taste)
   2 tbsp fresh minced sage leaves

In a large skillet heat water medium-high. Sauté onions and fresh garlic 3–4 minutes. Stir until light golden. Add sea salt, to taste. Put seitan in skillet;

add mirin. Continue to stir-fry over medium-high. Mix well. Add shoyu and garlic salt, pepper, and fresh sage. Continue to stir well. Serve with salad, steamed vegetables with vinaigrette, and brown rice.

Breast-Protective Power Foods: Garlic, onions, shoyu, sage.

DESSERTS

For Your Information
- *Agar*—A sea vegetable with protective qualities that is used for gelatins and aspics in natural foods cuisine.
- *Kuzu*—A root used for centuries as a powerful medicine that can calm an aching stomach, get rid of a headache, and more. Often used in place of flour or cornstarch as a thickener in natural foods cuisine.
- *Rice syrup*—A sweetener made from rice that is not as concentrated as maple syrup, or honey. Because it doesn't raise the blood sugar as high as other sweeteners, it is often used in macrobiotic cooking for desserts.

Mocha Soy Custard

(Serves 4)

❧ *This is a delicious, creamy pudding that children love.*

> 1 tbsp kuzu
> filtered water
> 2 tbsp Yannoh grain coffee
> 4 cups soy milk
> sea salt
> ½ cup rice syrup
> 2 tbsp agar powder
> ¼ tsp almond extract

Dissolve kuzu in 2 tbsp of water. In a bowl, dissolve grain coffee in 3 tbsp of water. Heat soy milk in medium pot with a pinch of sea salt and almond extract. Add the dissolved grain coffee. Slowly dissolve the rice syrup into mixture. Cook over low heat until the syrup is dissolved completely. Next dissolve the agar, and allow to cook over a low flame for approximately 20 minutes until flakes are completely dissolved. Be sure to stir constantly. Add the dissolved kuzu, stirring well. Stir for 5 minutes, over low heat, until mixture thickens. Pour into heat-resistant bowls and cool. Put into the refrigerator and chill until set, approximately 3 hours.

Breast-Protective Power Food: Soy milk.

Apple Crunch

(SERVES 8)

❦ *This is my favorite apple crisp recipe—not too sweet, with a delicious, crunchy oatmeal topping. The hazel nuts make it special.*

Topping

1½ cups rolled oats
½ tsp sea salt
2½ cups flour (white, whole wheat, or oat)
½ cup chopped hazelnuts
⅓ cup butter (softened at room temperature)
⅓ to ½ cup maple syrup or rice syrup

Filling

6 medium, organic, unpeeled Macoun apples, cored and sliced
½ cup maple syrup
1 tbsp kuzu (optional)

Topping: Combine oats, salt, flour, and nuts in mixing bowl. Add butter and mix by hand until uniformly and slightly crumbly. Add syrup and vanilla and mix by hand until consistency of a dry cookie dough (it breaks apart easily). Spread into a shallow baking dish and bake uncovered at 375° for about 15 minutes or until light brown, turning frequently.

Filling: In medium pot, cook apples with syrup and salt, uncovered on medium heat, until tender. (Add a little water if necessary to supplement the naturally occurring juices.) If juice is thin, dissolve kuzu in 2 tbsp water, add to cooking fruit, and stir until thick. Serve in pretty bowls with topping.

Comment: Butter can't be beat for baking. It is the most stable fat when heated, and also happens to taste just right in pastries and deserts. Bake with butter (instead of canola or safflower oils). Just make sure your butter is organic!

> TIP: Desserts containing oats, such as this apple crisp, are high in fiber, which helps to balance the sweetness of the maple syrup.

Breast-Protective Power Foods: Oats, hazelnuts, apples.

Stoney Hill Banana Bread

(YIELD: 1 LOAF)

❦ *This recipe was contributed by my friend, Rachel Nickerson Luna, an artist, writer, and baker par excellence! I recommend all of Rachel's creations, including her biscotti, pies, banana bread, books, and paintings—not necessarily in that order.*

⅓ cup softened butter
¾ cup dark honey
2 eggs
1 cup (2 or 3) ripe bananas
1½ cups unbleached flour
1 tsp baking soda
¼ cup wheat germ
½ cup walnuts

Preheat oven to 350°. Cream together butter and honey. Add eggs and bananas. Sift together flour and soda and add to banana mixture with wheat germ and walnuts, stirring until ingredients are blended. Pour batter into buttered loaf pan. Bake at 350° for approximately 45 minutes or until top splits and a knife inserted in the middle comes out clean. Remove from pan and cool on rack.

> TIP: Purchase walnuts in shells for EFA freshness. Crack open nuts right before baking to ensure complete protection against rancidity.

Breast-Protective Power Foods: Bananas, walnuts.

Almond Amazake Pudding

(Serves 1–2)

1 tsp kuzu
1 tsp filtered water
1 cup almond
   amazake

In a small cup or bowl, dissolve kuzu in water. Stir well to dissolve. Put amazake in a small stainless steel or enamel pot. Bring to a bubbly, low boil. Stir kuzu in, mixing gently. In about 30–60 seconds the kuzu will act as a thickening agent, creating a creamy pudding consistency. Put pudding into a dessert bowl and cook. You can refrigerate to moderately chill before serving.

Cherry Apple Kanten

(Serves 4)

❦   *This is a natural foods version of aspic, made with agar flakes, which are a type of sea vegetable. This pudding is popular in Japan.*

16 oz organic cherry apple juice
2 tbsp agar flakes
pinch of sea salt

Combine the juice, agar, and salt in a pot. Bring contents to a boil, stirring constantly to dissolve the agar flakes. Reduce heat and simmer for 10–15 minutes, stirring continuously. Remember, patience is required for dissolving agar. Remove from heat when agar is dissolved. Place in a shallow container and refrigerate until mixture gels, about 1 to 1½ hours.

Breast-Protective Power Food: Agar flakes.

Brown Rice Pudding

(SERVES 4)

¾ cup chopped almonds
1 cup filtered water
3 tbsp organic unroasted sesame tahini
4 cups cooked long-grain brown rice
4 cups organic soy milk
5 tbsp rice or maple syrup
2 tsp vanilla flavoring

Preheat oven to 350°. Cook almonds in 1 cup water over medium-high heat for a couple of minutes and blend together with tahini. Stir rice, soy milk, maple syrup, and tahini almond mixture together, with vanilla, in a pot with a lid. Bring to boil over medium heat. Simmer uncovered for 10 minutes. Place mixture in a baking dish with lid and bake in the oven for 45 minutes. Remove lid abut 5 minutes before the end (after 40 minutes of baking) to brown the top. Serve warm or chilled.

Breast-Protective Power Foods: Brown rice, almonds, tahini, soy milk.

Baked Apples

2 organic Macoun apples
½ cup maple syrup
2 tsp cinnamon
2 pinches sea salt

Preheat oven to 375°. Core apples, but do not peel.
Place in a small baking dish with a little bit of water, approximately ⅛ of an inch. Drizzle maple syrup over apples and into the core. Sprinkle cinnamon on apples. Bake uncovered for 50 minutes, basting with the juice once or twice.

TIP: Too rushed to bake an apple? Try one of the delicious, organic apple sauces in jars from the health food store. My favorites: apple-raspberry or apple-cherry.

Breast-Protective Power Foods: Apples, cinnamon.

Mock Coffee Flan with Raspberry Sauce

(SERVES 6)

4 cups soy milk
¾ cup rice syrup
2 heaping tbsp agar flakes
3 tbsp Yannoh organic grain coffee
pinch of salt
1 tsp almond extract
filtered water
organic raspberry jam

Bring soy milk and rice syrup to a low boil in a small pot, add agar, and stir until dissolved, approximately 20 minutes. Separately dilute Yannoh in 3 tbsp heated soy milk, and add salt and almond extract and stir. Add Yannoh and soy milk, salt, and almond extract to pot with soy milk, rice syrup, and agar. Dilute kuzu in 2 tbsp water and add to flan mixture, while *maintaining low boil*.

Stir until blended, approximately 3 more minutes. Remove flan from heat, and pour through a small mesh strainer into 6 individual dessert bowls and refrigerate until jelled, approximately 2 hours.

In a separate pot, dilute 6 tbsp of raspberry jam in 6–8 tbsp of water and stir until blended. *After dessert has jelled*, spoon raspberry sauce on top of flan.

Breast-Protective Power Foods: Soy milk, agar.

BEVERAGES

Teeccino caffeine-free, herbal coffee is a wonderful option for your coffee pot or espresso maker. Yannoh is a delicious, instant natural grain coffee.

Grain Coffee

(Serves 1)

1 tbsp instant Yannoh organic grain coffee
2 tbsp soy milk
4 oz boiling, filtered water

In a large mug, mix Yannoh with soy milk. Add boiling water and mix well. Enjoy. Add additional Yannoh if you like a stronger taste.

Breast-Protective Power Food: Soy milk.

Hot Co-Co Mocha

(Serves 2)

2 cups soy milk
2 tbsp Yannoh organic grain coffee
2 tbsp cocoa powder (Chatfields unsweetened)
2–3 tsp rice syrup

Mix ingredients together in a little pot, heat and serve.

Comment: This drink is subtly sweetened with a natural sweetener, rice syrup. The light sweetness of rice syrup is not as over-powering as sugar.

Breast-Protective Power Food: Soy milk.

Summer Almond Amazake Shake

(SERVES 1)

❦ *You can combine another type of summer fruit in this shake. Try raspberries or a ripe, pitted peach in place of the strawberries, if you prefer.*

> 4 oz almond amazake
> ½ cup ice cubes
> ½ cup strawberries

Combine ingredients in a blender. Puree for several seconds and serve.

Breast-Protective Power Food: Strawberries.

PASTA

Pasta con Broccoli

(SERVES 2)

❦ *When you have a craving for pasta, try a recipe like this in which lightly cooked broccoli cuts down the amount of simple carbohydrate provided by the pasta. Reducing simple carbohydrates, and replacing them with complex carbohydrates is breast and heart protective, and also helps to prevent diabetes.*

> 1 8-oz package pasta
> 2 cups broccoli florets or chopped broccoli rabe
> ¼ cup extra virgin olive oil
> ¼ cup flaxseed oil
> 1–2 tsp umeboshi vinegar
> 4 cloves chopped garlic
> sea salt and ground pepper to taste
> fresh lemon juice

Cook pasta 8–12 minutes in boiling water. Set aside to drain.
Meanwhile, bring water to a boil and add broccoli (or broccoli rabe). Boil

for 3–4 minutes until bright green. Test with a fork to ensure tenderness. Do not overcook. Remove and drain in a strainer or colander.

Mix broccoli and pasta in a bowl with oils, umeboshi vinegar, garlic, salt, and pepper. Taste. Adjust seasonings, and add a little freshly squeezed lemon juice. Serve on a bed of mixed mesclun greens.

Comment: Umeboshi vinegar, made from umeboshi plums, is known to be alkalizing for the blood. The umeboshi plum is able to absorb excess acid that can arise from alcohol, overeating, or sugar. Try a teaspoon of umeboshi vinegar in a cup of kukicha tea next time you have a headache or indigestion.

TIP: Serve mesclun greens on the side.

Breast-Protective Power Foods: Broccoli, garlic, extra virgin olive oil, flaxseed oil, umeboshi vinegar, lemon juice.

Pasta Primavera with Oven-Roasted Tomatoes

(Serves 4)

1 lb pasta
3 cups of your favorite mixed vegetables, cut into bite-sized pieces. Use broccoli rabe, zucchini, peas, cauliflower, etc.
½ cup niçoise olives, pitted and sliced

Oven-Dried Tomatoes

24 plum tomatoes
18 shallots
2 tbsp filtered water
8 cloves garlic (with the peel still on)
4 tbsp extra virgin olive oil
2–3 tbsp finely minced fresh rosemary

To Finish Dish

¾ cup chopped fresh basil
3 tsp fennel seeds

freshly ground pepper
3 tbsp sea salt
4 tbsp flaxseed oil
2 tbsp brown-rice vinegar

Preheat oven to 250°. Halve tomatoes and shallots; leave skin on shallots. Put 2 tbsp of filtered water in a baking dish. Rub olive oil on tomatoes, shallots, and garlic. Drizzle remaining oil in baking dish. Place tomatoes and shallots skin side down in dish, with garlic. Bake until tomatoes are about ½ of their original size, for about 5 hours. They should still be a little juicy. Remove from oven and toss in chopped rosemary. Set aside to cool.

Cook pasta. Drain and place in a large bowl with vegetables, roasted tomatoes, and rosemary. Peel garlic and shallots (from the roasting pan); toss through.

Mix basil, fennel, pepper, salt, flaxseed oil, and vinegar through pasta. Toss and serve.

Breast-Protective Power Foods: Tomatoes, broccoli rabe, zucchini, peas, cauliflower, shallots, garlic, extra virgin olive oil, rosemary, flaxseed oil, fennel seeds, fresh basil.

Wild Yam Soba with Herbs and Lemon

(Serves 4)

1 lb wild yam soba noodles
2 tsp filtered water
6 cloves garlic, peeled and minced
6 shallots, peeled and minced
2 tsp extra virgin olive oil
2 tsp grated organic lemon zest
4 tsp fresh lemon juice
½ cup chopped Italian parsley
2 tsp sea salt
freshly ground pepper

Cook pasta until tender in a large pot of boiling water, for 7 minutes. Drain.

During the time the pasta is cooking, put water in a skillet. Add the garlic, shallots, and half of the olive oil (1 tsp). Stir constantly over medium high heat, for about a minute and a half.

Place the pasta in a large bowl. Add the rest of the ingredients, including the second tsp of olive oil and toss. Add freshly ground pepper and sea salt to taste, and toss well.

Breast-Protective Power Foods: Wild yam soba, extra virgin olive oil, shallots, garlic, lemon zest, lemon juice, Italian parsley.

Uncooked Tomato Sauce with Olives

(SERVES 2)

❦ *Serve this delicious, light, fresh tomato sauce when summer tomatoes are at their peak. I like to spoon this sauce over monk fish or lemon sole. The sauce is wonderful over pasta, but remember to eat smaller portions of pasta along with a large salad or serving of vegetables to reduce the amount of starch you consume.*

> 1 lb fresh ripe tomatoes
> 3 cloves of peeled and sliced garlic
> sea salt and ground pepper to taste
> 1½ tbsp fresh organic flaxseed oil
> 1½ tbsp extra virgin olive oil
> 4 tbsp chopped basil
> ½ tsp dried oregano
> 6 natural pitted black olives

Blanch tomatoes in boiling water for 4–5 seconds. Set aside to cool. Peel and cut in half. Put a strainer over a bowl; squeeze juice and seeds into the strainer.

Mince the garlic in a food processor. Add the tomatoes and a couple of pinches of salt with the strained juice and puree for a minute. Add one tbsp each of the flax and olive oil. Puree with fresh chopped basil. Add the dried oregano and puree for about 5 more seconds. Set aside in a glass bowl with the olives. Stir throughout and cover to marinade. Before serving, adjust seasoning, add ground pepper and sea salt to taste.

Comment: Be careful not to oversalt because olives provide a salty taste.

TIP: Be aware that most olives available in bins (such as in delis and ethnic markets) that are so-called gourmet in quality do contain preservatives. Select olives available from the natural food store.

Breast-Protective Power Foods: Tomatoes, olives, garlic, flaxseed oil, extra virgin olive oil, basil, oregano.

CHAPTER 20

Personal Care Guide

"The way to health is to have an aromatic bath and scented massage every day."

—*Hippocrates*

Reducing or eliminating over-the-counter medication for everyday problems like headache strengthens the immune system. Natural medicine is effective, and has the distinct advantage of protecting health without side effects. Conventional medicine can often be combined with the suggestions in this chapter, such as aromatherapy, reflexology, and exercise. When taking new herbs and supplements, be sure to let your physician know.

I have noticed that more physicians are becoming knowledgeable about, and recommending, natural medicines. For example, a woman who had plastic surgery scheduled told me that her surgeon recommended "arnica," a homeopathic remedy to promote healing and prevent bruising and swelling.

The following recommendations utilize essential oils, homeopathy, herbs, and lifestyle suggestions for some general conditions. Noted herbalist and nutritionist Donald Yance created a general, breast-healthy supplement program for *Total Breast Health*. Ann Katz, a dynamic woman who worked closely with Yance to help heal her breast cancer, used such a program and shares her inspiring story here. If you are actively healing breast cancer, you will need a program designed specifically for you.

☞ Sleep

Did you know that important immune-enhancing compounds are released during sleep? Sleep is an aid in both preventing and healing illness. Whether you are dealing with the common cold or breast cancer, immunity is greatly enhanced during deep levels of sleep. Many people become stressed out during the day. At bedtime, they find the events of the day racing through their minds. These recommendations are designed to help you "unwind" before bed, and to promote deep and restful sleep. Don't underestimate the value of daily exercise and fresh air to promote restful sleep.

Never eat before bed; instead, encourage your digestive organs to cleanse and rest at night. If you are going through a period of insomnia, having an early, light dinner can also help to promote sleep. Try using 10-12 drops of chamomile or lavender essential oil in 2 tablespoons of a base of almond oil and massage your entire body, after body brushing to promote a relaxing, deep sleep.

Many people report disturbing side effects, such as grogginess, headaches, poor memory, or even nausea, from over-the-counter (as well as prescription) sleeping pills. Homeopathic sleeping tables have no side effects. Try Quietude by Boiron, which is available in health food stores.

Natural Melatonin: Sleep in a Darkened Room

Melatonin, a sleep-inducing hormone produced by the pineal gland, is also (rather surprisingly) a breast-protective antioxidant. Melatonin has been found to prevent the promotional phase of mammary tumors in animals, and to protect against cellular replication of human breast cancer. Researchers believe that melatonin may help to keep estrogen levels from rising. Women who have estrogen-receptor-positive breast cancer have been found to exhibit low levels of melatonin. Increase melatonin levels naturally by being outside as much as possible in natural light. Sleep in a darkened room with no artificial light (night light or clock radio) to trigger melatonin release at night.

A Relaxing Bath

Epsom salts baths with Dr. Hauschka's lavender bath oil is my favorite way to relax, especially before bed. A way to guarantee instant sleep is to follow up with Haushka's lavender body oil and a cup of lemon balm or chamomile tea. Don't forget to sprinkle essential oil of lavender on your pillow!

Cold water bathing or showering has been found to support the immune system by stimulating T-cell production. Naturopathic physicians W. Boyle and A. Saine discussed hydrotherapy in their 1988 book, *Lectures in Naturopathic Hydrotherapy.*

Daytime Hydrotherapy to Revitalize

You can practice your own form of hydrotherapy by finishing a shower or bath with cold water, eliminating (or lowering) the hot water. It may sound strange, but it is certainly revitalizing to experience the refreshing rush of cool water. Another way to use this constitution strengthener is to step into a cool shower after working up a sweat— after aerobic exercise, for instance.

☞ Outlook: Relax and Lift Your Spirits!

Feeling Blue?

Did you know that, during the winter when days are short and the sky is dark, many women (and men) suffer from a winter depression called seasonal affective disorder (SAD)? This type of depression generally subsides in the spring, when the days once again become sun-filled. What can you do to avoid depression in the winter? Look for the Inner Balance catalog in the Resource Guide, and investigate its winter therapy light boxes, which use full-spectrum lightbulbs. Full-spectrum fluorescent tubes are also available for office use.

◆ Neroli (orange blossom) essential oil, used in a diffuser (10-12 drops in water) and/or as a massage oil (10 drops in 2 tbsp of base oil, such as almond oil) can help to lift spirits. Essential oil of orange (neroli is in this family) has been used for this purpose for centuries. Clary sage essential oil is especially beneficial for hormonal ups and downs. The use of clary sage is recommended for depression associated with PMS or menopause, and other symptoms of these conditions. Acupuncture is often beneficial for depression, promoting better relaxation, energy, sleep, and moods.

TIP: In a base of almond oil, add a few drops of clary sage for a wonderful, soothing, hormone-calming body oil. Just 5 drops of clary sage per 1 tsp of almond oil can help to alleviate PMS or peri-menopause, or menopause anxiety.

◆ Omega-3 deficiency can result in a greater tendency toward depression. In a study of fatty acids and the central nervous system, scientists at the National Institutes of Health found that seriously depressed patients had lower levels of omega-3 than mildly depressed or healthy patients. Be sure to include flaxseed oil in your diet to help prevent depression.

◆ Investigate St. John's Wort (scientific name, "hypericum") for depression. St. John's Wort, as described by Harold Bloomfield in his book *Hypericum and Depression,* has been effective for many people with depression. Look for Nature's Way St. John's Wort, standardized extract and whole herb in capsule form, and use Dr. Hauschka's St. John's Wort body oil as your daily massage oil.

◆ For anxiety, Nature's Way's Kava is an herb that promotes relaxation and is available in health food stores. Take one Kava softgel supplement two to three times a day.

In a Panic?

◆ The combination homeopathic remedy simply called "Nervousness" by Boiron, available in your health food store (non-habit-forming), helps control nervousness.

◆ A dose of nature is helpful for women healing breast cancer, as researchers at the University of Michigan School of Nursing at Ann Arbor found. Relaxing, outdoor activities like gardening, sitting in the park, and taking walks help women with breast cancer to set goals, concentrate on projects, and see them through.

☞ Body Brushing

Using a natural bristle brush, rub dry skin briskly starting at the feet, brushing upward, toward the heart. Be sure to massage lightly under the arms, inside thighs, behind the knees, and the groin. Best times for brushing: before bedtime, to ensure a deep and restful sleep, or just before showering. Combine 6 drops of chamomile (to sooth) and lavender (to relax and rejuvenate) in a base of 2 tablespoons of almond oil, and massage into skin. *See* the Resource Guide for a natural bristle body brush and essential oils.

☞ Breast Self-Exams

"Bless your breasts," as recommended by Dr. Christiane Northrup, during monthly self-exams. Become familiar with what your breasts feel like, so you can pick up any changes when you do your monthly self-exam. A week after your period, to avoid tenderness, is a good time to examine your breasts, but any time of the month is fine. Breast self-exam is especially important in women, under 50 because breast tissue is denser, which makes it difficult to image. Nearly one-third of all breast cancers are detected by women's self-examinations; most of those would not show up on a mammogram because of breast density or other reasons. Many experts believe that the death rate from breast cancer has been decreasing due, in part, to early detection.

TIP: For a nourishing, protective breast self-massage salve, try Hygiea's St. John's Wort and dandelion blossom salve while you are doing your breast self-exam. *(See* the Resource Guide.)

Check carefully under your arms and all over the breast area, in every direction. See if your breasts feel the same as they did the month before. Look for dimples, bulges, indentations, or a change in nipple direction. Check for spots that may be tender or feel tight. If you do detect a lump, check to see if the other breast is the same; it might be normal breast tissue. A hard, small lump—like a grain of rice—needs to be checked by your physician.

To facilitate breast self examination, you may want to investigate the FDA-approved Sensor Pad, a silicone-filled, soft pad that looks like a deflated balloon. Thirteen studies have shown that the Sensor Pad enables women to feel changes of shape in their breasts that they might otherwise miss. For more information on the Sensor Pad and how to order it, *see* the Resource Guide.

For a breast self-exam shower card, call the American Cancer Society at 1-800-ACS-2345. They also offer a free booklet on breast self-examination.

For a six-minute instructional video, *see* the Resource Guide.

☞ Breast Implants

The first comprehensive review of the scientific literature and confidential government and industry documents concludes that women with breast implants are at a high risk for breast cancer.

The study, published in the November issue of the peer-reviewed *International Journal of Occupational Medicine and Toxicology* (1995), presents a detailed analysis of the carcinogenic hazards of silicone gel and polyurethane breast implants.

"Risks of breast cancer have been ignored in the current controversy over implants," says Dr. Samuel Epstein, author of the study. "Evidence on the carcinogenicity of implants, particularly those wrapped in polyurethane foam, is strong. Recent epidemiological studies claimed as proof of safety are grossly flawed. Such studies would have even given a clean bill of health to asbestos." For information on health and legal issues with respect to breast implants, refer to the Resource Guide for the *Toxic Discovery Network Newsletter*.

☛ Colds and Flu

Recent scientific studies encourage the use of natural remedies that bolster immunity to treat colds and flu. Researchers are beginning to be concerned that after a lifetime of penicillin use, elderly people may become resistant to its effects. Thirty percent of all elderly people who get bacterial pneumonia die from it because it cannot be controlled bv antibiotics. Natural medicine not only is effective at relieving the symptoms of cold and flu, but also helps to fight the viruses, speeding up recovery time.

Natural Remedies

◆ Astragalus root: During the flu season, drink a cup of astragalus tea daily for an excellent preventative tonic. (Also *see* page 263, Mushrooms for Immunity, a soup recipe, for use of astragalus in soup.) Astragalus increases the production of interferon and generally encourages all phases of your immune system. *Power Tea*: Astragalus root is available from an herbalist or in the health food store (if it has a comprehensive herb section). Select a 12-25-gram slice of astragalus root. Boil in 1 cup of water for about 15 minutes, discard the root, and drink the tea. Fresh root tea is much more effective than astragalus tonic.

◆ Vitamin C: Avoid megadosing on vitamin C, which may cause excess levels of iron to build up. Megadoses of vitamin C can also interfere with some cancer treatments. Consuming vitamin C-rich foods, however, provides us with a safe level of vitamin C that is easily absorbed, as well as with other vitamins, phytochemicals, and nutrients that give us added protection.

Vitamin C-rich foods:

• Encourage the production of interferon, a protein in cells that helps to keep the virus from spreading.
• Stimulate infection-bashing T-cells.

Vitamin C-rich foods to include in your diet, especially when fighting a cold or flu, are kiwi fruit, strawberries, cantaloupe, grapefruit, and lemon juice in hot water. Don't forget that vegetables are another wonderful source of vitamin C, especially sweet red pepper, lightly steamed broccoli, kale, alfalfa sprouts (in salads), and cabbage. Raw garlic activates the immune system and is effective against microbial infections that cause colds and flu. Mince a couple of cloves of garlic into vinaigrette and soups, or sprinkle on salads. Be sure to consume some yogurt, because garlic is so strong it may actually eliminate some flora in your digestive system. Yogurt, rich in lactobacilli (and other protective organisms), will replenish friendly flora.

◆ Echinacea: As demonstrated by researchers at the Institute of Pharmaceutical Biology in Munich, echinacea strengthens the body's natural immune defenses. Studies have confirmed that 180 drops of a tincture of this popular cold and flu remedy, used daily, offer optimum recovery benefits. Compounds in the extract of echinacea strengthen the body's natural immune system in two ways:

• Echinacea's compounds enhance a protein called properdin, which neutralizes bacteria and viruses.
• It increases the number of phagocytes, the cells that find infectious agents and destroy them. Phagocytes also inhibit the proliferation of viruses.

◆ Elderberry: For complete information on this cold and flu fighter, look for Brigette Mar's booklet *Elder* (published by Keats). Israelis have been using elderberry for years, as shown in the work done by virologist Madeline Mumcuoglu, Ph.D. Dr. Mumcuoglu found that 90 percent of a group of patients suffering from the flu who drank elderberry extract recovered in just two to three days. The group of patients given a placebo took six days to recover. Elderberry works in two ways:

• Anthocyanins (fruit pigments) stop a threatening enzyme that the invading virus uses to infect cell membranes.
• Proteins in elderberry block dangerous hemagglutinin, which helps viruses get to healthy cells.

Look for Sambu Guard, a blend of elderberry fruit and flower extract with echinacea and vitamin C from Flora (*see* the Resource Guide).

◆ Tea Tree Oil: Oil from the leaves of the Australian *Melaleuca alternifolia* tree, commonly called Tea Tree Oil, has antibacterial and antiseptic properties. There are several ways to use this exotic, wonderful-smelling oil for treating colds and flu and stopping the spread of infection:

• In a small diffuser, add 8-10 drops of oil to several tablespoons of water. Light the candle and keep it beside you. (*See* the Resource Guide for essential oil supplies.)

- If you don't have a diffuser, add 10 drops of oil to a bowl of very hot water. Inhale the healing fumes, covering your head with a towel for added benefit.
- Put 10 drops of oil in a steam vaporizer.
- For a hot compress, fill the sink with hot water. Add several drops of oil. Take a clean washcloth and submerge in the water. Squeeze out excess liquid, and press on face and neck.

> TIP: Include shiitake mushrooms in your chicken soup for immune strength, and be sure to eat lots of onions and shallots—all of which possess antiviral and antiinflammatory benefits—for prevention of bronchitis and other infections.

◆ Boiron's Homeopathic Oscillococcium cold remedy, especially if taken early on, when initial symptoms of scratchy throat and sniffles appear, can dramatically shorten the duration of colds and flus. (*See* the Resource guide for ordering information.)

☞ Essential Oils For Lymphatic Rejuvenation

The esssential oils myrrh and ginger can be used to encourage the removal of stagnant conditions in the lymph: Add 6 drops each of myrrh and ginger into a base of 2 tbsp of almond oil. Rub into the breast and armpit area, and the sides of the neck.

More on Tea Tree Oil

◆ Lymphatic Recharge: Deanna Cross, an expert in the use of essential oils and aromatherapy, suggests keeping a bottle of tea tree oil in your bath or shower and to use it in the following manner: Dilute 10 drops of tea tree oil in a small amount of almond oil. Massage under armpit, where fatty tissue is, between armpit and breast. If you find that area is sore when you rub it, your lymph system is sluggish. Another great place to use tea tree oil is on the soles of your feet because all nerve endings (or meridians) are accessible on the soles. You can use the oil on your soles without diluting because the skin is tougher there. In fact, Christopher Hobbs suggested in his *Handbook for Herbal Healing*, tea tree oil is an excellent natural medicine for athlete's foot.

Bay Laurel

◆ According to Mindy Green, co-author of *Aromatherapy: A Complete Guide to the Healing Art*, bay laurel is also an excellent detoxifier. Use bay laurel with tea tree oil (as described), or by itself. The best variety is True Bay, or *Laurus nobilis*.

Lovemaking

◆ Ylang Ylang essential oil can raise your ester levels, reflected in your libido. Use this sweet smelling essential oil in a diffuser, or add 8-10 drops to a couple of tablespoons of almond oil to use as a body oil. (*See* the Resource Guide.)

◆ Creme de la Femme, developed by a woman doctor, is a natural vaginal lubricant, very effective, and completely hormone-free. This is an ideal product for women who are going through menopause and aren't taking hormone replacement therapy. (*See* Phillips Publishing Merchandising in the Resource Guide to order.)

☛ Deodorant: Think Twice About It

Evidence now available questions the safety of the chemicals present in deodorants, even the "natural" clear stones, available in health food stores. The use of commercial deodorants is of particular concern right after shaving when the pores are open around the root ducts of hairs, which are concentrated over the lymph system area. Try Dr. Haushka's gentle deodorant (*see* the Resource Guide).

TIP: On the day you are getting a mammogram, don't wear commercial antiperspirant with aluminum, since it interferes with mammography imaging. Even the clear deodorant stones contain aluminum.

☛ Environment

Avoid Bleached Paper Products

Breast Cancer Action News, a publication of the Canadian Breast Cancer Network (*see* the Resource Guide), has published information describing the problems associated with bleached paper products such as toilet paper, sanitary napkins, and tampons. Greenpeace researcher Joe Thornton says, "Stopping organochlorine pollution of our bodies and the environment should be a priority of breast cancer prevention strategies."

Did you know that most tampons and sanitary napkins are made from paper that has been treated with chlorine bleach? Look for Natracare, all-cotton feminine protection products that are made without harmful chlorine. Natracare tampons contain no fragrance, binders, or synthetics. (*See* the Resource Guide.)

> TIP: Many personal hygiene products containing talcum powder—soaps, deodorants, condoms, and contraceptive diaphragms, to name a few—may be risk factors in the development of ovarian cancer, according to the May 1997 *Bottom Line.* Talc particles travel through the cervix, line the uterus and fallopian tubes, and can slowly create serious problems in the ovaries.

☛ Exercise

Why is exercise thought to be so beneficial in offering protection against breast cancer? For one thing, it decreases the amount of estrogen a woman produces during her lifetime. I believe that exercise plays an important role in reducing stress and, in some cases, even alleviating depression. Many experts believe that anxiety and depression can weaken immunity, contributing to the onset of breast and other cancers. A study of Radcliffe graduates by Dr. Rose Frisch from Harvard University actually found that young women who exercised most—the teenage girls who were most active were most protected against breast cancer as adults. Exercise offers the following breast-protective benefits:

- Reduces insulin levels.
- May delay menarche in young girls (early menarch is linked to increased risk of breast cancer).
- Reduces the frequency of ovulation.
- Helps to prevent obesity.
- Helps to prevent abdominal fat (which increases estrogen).
- Relieves stress and depression.
- Encourages restful sleep and helps prevent insomnia.

Just four hours of moderate exercise a week reduced breast cancer risk 37 percent, researchers reported in May 1997 in the *New England Journal of Medicine*, after following 25,624 women for thirteen years. That finding was supported in a smaller study by Dr. Leslie Bernstein, a researcher at the

University of Southern California School of Medicine in Los Angeles. Dr. Bernstein evaluated 1,000 women and found that those who engaged in 3.8 hours of exercise per week were less than half as likely to develop breast cancer as sedentary women.

A study from Norway noted that women who are inactive have higher triglycerides than more active women. Higher triglyerides may encourage greater exposure to estrogen, which may promote breast cancer.

Researchers at Loma Linda University in California found that exercise can boost defense against disease. Protection against malignancies was increased by simply a 45-minute brisk walk five times a week. If you do aerobic exercise in the morning, your metabolism increases, helping to burn calories.

An invaluable result of exercise, sweating, helps to increase detoxification. Try using a sauna or steam bath or other opportunities to release pesticides and other toxins.

The healing powers of castor oil have been known for thousands of years. Castor oil has been used in folk medicine to detoxify the lymphatic and digestive systems and to "attract" immune-enhancing cells. Mindy Green suggests combining a few drops of lavender oil with castor oil to offer additional benefits. The Women to Women Clinic in Maine is a great resource for products to make the process easy. (*See* the Resource Guide.)

TIP: Carefully warm a cotton flannel cloth soaked in castor oil in the oven to just above body temperature. Place the cloth over the area for cleansing (breast, liver, intestines), and cover with a towel or hot water bottle. For more information on castor oil, read Edgar Cayce's *Encyclopedia of Healing* (Warner Books, 1986.)

☞ Breathing

Proper breathing—deep breathing, with emphasis on breathing through your nose, fully filling up your lungs with air—can enhance relaxation and help to promote aerobic capacity while exercising. Studying meditation and yoga will encourage better breathing habits. Deep, full breathing also supports the lymphatic system, which is breast protective. Body brushing also aids breath work by increasing circulation. Dr. Hauschka's Dwarf Pine Body Oil is a wonderful, warming body massage oil that is great to use before or after exercise, and helps promote deeper breathing.

Smoking causes breathing problems, lung cancer, and breast cancer. Lung cancer takes more women's lives each year than any other cancer, including breast cancer. Lung problems can begin as early as the teenage years. Smoking during those years poses a significantly increased risk of breast cancer. Studies show that the greater the incidence of smoking, the greater the incidence of breast cancer. If you smoke, it is time to realize that smoking does indeed contribute to breast cancer. Smoking also contributes to heart disease—the Number 1 cause of death among women. If you are interested in qutting smoking, investigate acupuncture. A skilled accupuncturist can easily help you to quit in just one or two sessions.

Many people are sensitive to dust, mites, and other household pollutants. Plants are very helpful in filtering toxins from the air. Even chemicals from new carpets or drapes can be filtered by common household plants such as English ivy. Retired NASA scientists Bill Wolverton, Ph.D., of Wolverton Environmental Services Inc. in Picayune, Mississippi, recommends the following plants as best for cleaning the air: palms, the peace lily, and Boston ferns. Boston ferns can detoxify 1,800 micrograms of formaldehyde from the air in just one hour.

For nontoxic paint, mildew cleaners, and household products, refer to NEEDS in the Resource Guide. Special vacuums for hypoallergenic people and a variety of air filters are also available.

Avoid trailing pesticides into your home. Remove shoes when you enter to ensure that you are not bringing harmful chemicals into your home.

☛ Hair Manageability

Make sure you are getting enough flaxseed oil and protein. After adding flaxseed oil to my diet, I was amazed at how much better my hair looked and felt. Phyto hair products from France—my favorite shampoos, conditioners, and styling products—are all natural. (*See* the Resource Guide.)

To reduce dry hair and skin, get a filter to remove chlorine from your shower (*see* the Resource Guide).

Temporary hair loss can occur as a result of chemotherapy. A diet rich in fresh vegetables (especially onions, leeks, chives, and garlic), fruit, whole grains, and protective oils, along with adequate protein at each meal, helps hair growth.

> TIP: Chemotherapy also causes nausea, which can make eating difficult. To reduce nausea, try umeboshi vinegar on vegetables, Eden's ume extract *(see* the Resource Guide) in teas, and fresh ginger root juice added to soups, salads, grains, and fish.

☞ For Skin Beauty

For soft, beautiful skin, supplement regularly with flaxseed oil, and eat plenty of fresh, green vegetables. The chlorophyll in the vegetables helps to cleanse the blood, which encourages clear skin. Avoiding fried foods is basic to blemish-free skin. Drinking plenty of water is another helpful way to nourish skin and prevent dry skin in the winter.

Collagen, which helps create firm skin and softens wrinkles, is formed by vitamin C. Make kiwi your favorite fruit—one kiwi contains 74.5 mg. of vitamin C.

I love Dr. Hauschka's facial pack, which is used after cleansing and gently steaming the face. I also use the skin creme liquid (in the summer) and rose or creme pack (in colder months). *See* the Resource Guide.

For healing scars and burns: Break an aloe leaf and apply the clear, soothing juice inside to a cooking burn or to a healing wound or scar. Aloe can both soothe pain and speed the healing process. Women undergoing radiation treatment report that aloe is extremely soothing to radiation burns.

☞ Headache

◆ A natural diet, free from chemicals, food additives, and food colorings, is fundamental to preventing migraines and headaches. Also, omega-3 fatty acids offer significant relief in the frequency and intensity of migraines, so don't forget to supplement with flaxseed oil. Eliminating chocolate can be helpful to headache sufferers.

◆ The isoflavones in soy appeared to help people who suffer from one type of migraine headache called HHT (hereditary hemorrhagic telanyicctasia), researchers at Yale University School of Medicine discovered in 1997. A study is under way to determine whether isoflavones can relieve headaches in non-HHT patients.

◆ Power tea: Soothing tea for relief of headache: 1 teaspoon of kuzu (medicinal root starch available in macrobiotic section of health food store), dissolved in 2 tbsp of filtered water. Add a cup of very hot water, and 1 teaspoon of organic soy sauce. Stir and sip slowly.

◆ Try using Dr. Hauschka's sage foot bath. Combining a hot foot bath with a cold compress on the head helps to reduce the volume of blood flow in the head by constricting blood vessels. This in turn helps to reduce the pain.

◆ An epsom salts bath is another option to reduce headache pain. Usually headaches are triggered by overindulgence in food or wine, or even exposure to allergens in food (like chocolate). Environmental allergens, like paint fumes, can also trigger headaches. You might want to investigate the NEEDS mail order catalog to order hypoallergenic paint and cleaning supplies (see the Resource Guide). Soaking in a hot epsom salt bath assists in the elimination of toxins through the skin. The magnesium in the epsom salts is absorbed through the skin, assisting in relaxation and even in promoting sleep.

◆ Another power tea: Yarrow tea, drunk hot while in the bath, promotes sweating, which aids in the release of toxins.

◆ Feverfew, an herb that has a long history of use, is often effective against headaches, even migraines. Use 125 milligrams per day. As always, quality is of the utmost importance.

> TIP: When I begin to get a headache, I do a careful body brushing, then mix 6 drops each of rosemary and lavender essential oils in about 2 tbsp of almond oil base. I use this body oil to massage thoroughly all over my body. I dab Extra Strength Tiger Balm lightly on my temples.

☛ Alleviating Breast Pain

Poor diet, stress, and high alcohol and coffee consumption all contribute to mastalgia, or breast pain. Improving diet and reducing stress help the body to utilize essential fatty acids that can be healing for this condition. Eliminate harmful fats and oils like excessive saturated fat, fried foods, trans-fats, and processed supermarket oils, and consume flaxseed sesame, and sunflower oils and protective fats from cold water fish like salmon and tuna. It can take as long as three or four months to see results from cutting back on coffee, alcohol, and saturated fat, but it is worth it. As a supplement, investigate evening primrose oil, under the guidance of your nutritionist or physician. Look for Nature's Way EFAMOL Evening Primrose Oil capsules in your health food store. EFAMOL PMS Control contains specially selected vitamins, including a high level of vitamin B6, which helps to alleviate the bloating and breast tenderness associated with PMS. On each of the ten days before menstruation, take 5 capsules of EFAMOL PMS Control. You can continue taking EFAMOL Evening Primrose Oil as directed on the label. (See the Resource Guide for ordering information.)

> TIP: To decrease benign breast lumps, eliminate coffee.

☞ Low Energy

◆ Flaxseed oil is an energy-producing supplement. Sun Wellness Chlorella (in tablets or granules) is also a wonderful, natural source of energy; simply stir into fresh vegetable juices, shakes, or water. Eat more good-quality protein for greater energy. (*See* the Resource Guide.)

◆ Essential oil of grapefruit extract in a diffuser can give you a lift, as can Dr. Hauschka's lemon bath and lemon body oil. Enough exercise and enough sleep are imperative. Try chlorella in juice or water for an energy boost.

☞ Memory Aid

◆ Try essential oil of rosemary in your diffuser, as a body oil, or both. Another helpful tip is to drink green tea with several drops of ginko biloba tincture. The phytonutrient-rich caffeine in the tea complements the ginko.

☞ Prayer, Meditation, And Support Groups

◆ Both prayer and meditation have been documented in research to be powerfully enhancing for the immune system.

Inner Work: Attitude Is Key

Prayer, meditation, therapy, and support groups have all been shown to aid women with breast cancer. Research has shown that praying for oneself as well as praying for other people is an aid in healing. Women with breast cancer who attend support groups have been shown to live up to eighteen months longer, according to David Spiegal, M.D., from Stanford University. One-quarter of the forty-two grants awarded to scientists in 1997 by the National Institute of Health's Office of Alternative Medicine were for studies of the mind-body connection.

☞ For Efficient Digestion

Morning Sickness or Nausea

Use New Chapter's Ginger Capsules to alleviate morning sickness. In her *Health Wisdom for Women* newsletter, Christiane Northrup, M.D., recommends keeping ginger capsules right next to the bed, along with a glass of water. In the morning, take 5-15 capsules upon awakening. Ginger capsules can be taken with meals throughout the day. Dr. Northrup recommends taking up to 5 capsules every three hours, as needed.

> TIP: New Chapter's Ginger Capsules can also be used to alleviate nausea from chemotherapy.

Constipation

Select grains over pasta. Drink plenty of water, and take acidophilus. My favorite is PB8 (*see* the Resource Guide). A great remedy for constipation is simply to grind a couple of tablespoons of flaxseeds and cover in water. Soak flaxseeds for approximately 2-8 hours, and mix into juice or water. The mucilage in the water and flaxseed mixture acts as a lubricant in the intestines, and the fiber from the flaxseeds helps as well.

☞ For Relief From Symptoms of PMS or Menopause

You may want to investigate natural progesterone cream for relief from symptoms of PMS or menopause. The progesterone level used in "Fem-Gest" (*see* the Resource Guide) is recommended by John Lee, M.D. (author of *Progesterone: The Many Roles of a Remarkable Hormone*), and used in his clinical studies. Fem-Gest can also be used for osteoporosis. Natural progesterone cream may help to rebuild bone loss, as Dr. Lee's work has indicated.

Although there have been no reports of any health problems associated with progesterone cream, I encourage you to find a knowledgeable health care professional to work with you in using natural progesterone.

☞ Reflexology

Did you know that all the points for organ detoxification and healing are in your big toe? Reflexology expert Kim Godon recommends pressing the big toe for healing pressure points, which actually affect all the organs in your body.

☞ The Value of Sunshine

While it's obviously imperative not to sunbathe in the noonday sun, studies show sunlight can be beneficial for everyone, especially for women, for the vitamin D our bodies manufacture when sunlight reacts with the cholesterol found in the skin.

Studies in the United States and Soviet Union have documented that women living in areas with the most hours of sunlight have markedly lower rates of breast cancer. A study of 133 women done in 1997 at the Northern California Cancer Center found vitamin D from sun exposure linked to a reduced rate of breast cancer.

Vitamin D also helps to balance blood sugar, and researchers have found that low levels of vitamin D may contribute significantly to glucose intolerance. Chromium, zinc, magnesium, taurine, vitamin C, and vitamin D are nutrients that the body needs to use sugar effectively.

Skin cancer, of course, is a concern, so moderation is key. However, the increase in breast and other cancers dramatically exceeds that of skin cancer. A 1993 article in *Preventative Medicine* documented the fact that, the closer people live to the Equator, the lower cancer rates are. While more research is needed on vitamin D and breast cancer, scientists suspect that this drop in cancer rates is linked to the increase in the amount of sunlight absorbed by people who live closer to the Equator. A study performed at Boston University Medical Center (led by Dr. Michael Holick) determined that in the winter, especially in the Northern latitudes, it is not possible to obtain vitamin D from sunlight. Graduate students sat in the sun for five hours a day during the winter in Boston, and it was found that no vitamin Dw as made from November to February. Consume extra fish in the winter to assure adequate levels of natural vitamin D.

Exposure to sunlight each day also helps in preventing breast cancer by increasing levels of the body's natural, breast-protective melatonin production.

Dr. Michael Jansen, author of *The Vitamin Revolution,* points out that people who do not wear sunscreen only need about 5-10 minutes of sun for just a few days a week to obtain adequate exposure to UV rays for the body to be able to make vitamin D. Those who wear sunscreen of SPF 15, however, will have to get an hour and a half of sun daily, according to Dr. Jansen.

TIP: Fish such as sardines (with bones), herring, and tuna, as well as organic eggs and liver, are good sources of vitamin D.

Sunlight is also important for preventing osteoporosis. Dr. Alan Gaby, author of *Preventing and Reversing Osteoporosis,* recommends regular exposure to sunlight for reasonable periods of time to avoid vitamin D deficiency. Supplementing with vitamin D in large doses is not advised, since it can cause toxic effects. For people unable to go outdoor much, or in the winter, Dr. Gaby and Dr. Northrup recommend supplementing with low doses of vitamin

D, about 200-400 units daily as part of a multivitamin mineral program. Animal studies show that vitamin D supplementation is not advisable during pregnancy, because it may cause birth defects. Be sure to include more vitamin D-rich foods in the winter. Make tea with organic egg shells in the water, and if you are not a vegetarian, cook soup with organic beef, lamb, or chicken bones.

Exercise caution when using sun blocks. Studies indicate a correlation between higher rates of skin and breast cancer and increased use of sun block, including a 1993 article called "Rising Trends in Melanoma" in the *Annals of Epidemiology*.

Use skin blocks (as natural as possible) in moderation, making frequent use of hats and umbrellas, and above all, avoid direct exposure to the sun during the hottest time of the day.

Look for Aloe Gator Sun Block Lotion, available in some health food stores (*see* the Resource Guide).

☞ Weight Loss

Research has shown that a weight gain of 10 pounds after the age of thirty was linked to a 23% increase in breast cancer, and a gain of 20 pounds was associated with a 52% increase. A nutrient-dense, whole foods diet, healing sleep, rejuvenating exercise, and fresh air and sunlight comprise an important foundation for breast health.

◆ Flaxseed oil can provide energy for exercise, and for a metabolism boost, which aids in burning calories. Try 2 tablespoons of organic flaxseed oil daily. Be sure to exercise on a regular basis to increase metabolism. Oshadi (*see* the Resource Guide) makes a combination essential oil for massage that is a weight loss/cellulite aid. Add more protein and vegetables to your diet and reduce portions of whole grains and pasta.

◆ Green tea helps to burn calories.

◆ Robert Crayhon, author of *Nutrition Made Simple*, suggests that CoQ10 can help overweight people to lose weight. "Some studies show half of the overweight population may be in need of CoQ10 to lose weight efficiently," according to Crayhon.

A study published in the Journal of the American Medical Association (November 5,1997) examining 95,000 women found an increased risk of breast cancer with every pound gained after age eighteen. The use of estrogen, combined with weight gain, seemed to lead to an even greater risk.

☞ Supplements and Herbs

It is really important when healing breast cancer to have an individualized program, designed specifically for you. A knowledgeable herbalist, nutritionist, or naturopath will be able to take all of your needs into account. Do you have any allergies? What kind of breast cancer do you have? Are you undergoing chemotherapy or radiation treatment? What is your age?

These questions and others are best discussed with an informed expert so that you will be taking the right vitamins and herbs for your specific needs.

Donald Yance is an expert in both nutrition and use of herbs. I have asked him to design a good, general program for most women to follow for prevention.

Master Herbalist and Nutritionist Donald Yance on Supplements for the Prevention of Breast Cancer

Donald Yance, a member of the American Herbalist Guide, certified nutritionist, and master herbalist, works closely with many physicians aware of nutritional concerns, as well as maintaining his own active practice in Norwalk, Connecticut. One of Yance's areas of expertise is working with medical doctors to develop individualized nutritional programs for people with cancer. Yance is also involved in two research programs at the Columbia-Presbyterian Medical Center Hospital with women who have breast cancer and cannot take hormone replacement therapy. One is examining how to reduce symptoms of menopause; the second is a study of herbal treatments for fibroid tumors. Many women with whom Yance has worked have healed breast cancer by employing dietary, lifestyle (exercise), and supplemental programs he individualized for them. Yance acknowledges how strongly linked a fresh, whole foods, organic diet is with the healing of cancer—no matter what kind of cancer. He firmly believes nutrients such as vitamins, minerals, and essential fatty acids are best consumed directly from the foods we eat, not from pills or capsules. This ensures consumption of the most effective nutrients, fresh and completely balanced. For instance, it's preferable to obtain beta-carotene from food sources, as opposed to isolating it and larking it as a supplement, because it's available within the complete spectrum of all carotenoids. In other words, a healthy balance of vitamins and minerals can be obtained from a whole foods diet. As a practical matter for many women, however, supplementation is indicated.

Although Yance strongly recommends that women who are actively healing breast cancer seek the help of a certified nutritionist or naturopath for an individualized program including fresh flaxseed and extra virgin olive oil, he recommends the following supplement program for women who want to prevent breast cancer.

- Multivitamin: 2-4 per day, preferably New Chapter Every Woman. New Chapter is a completely natural vitamin. New Chapter also does not provide megadoses of vitamins, which means its multi is very easily absorbed by the body and does not create imbalances.
- 100-300 micrograms daily of OPC grape seed extract.
- Alpha-lipoic acid: 100-300 milligrams daily. Raises intercellular glutathione, and is rich in sulfur. Protects genes and expression of genes. Increases utilization of vitamin C.
- Selenium: Between 100 and 400 micrograms daily. If the diet is rich in whole foods and a wide variety of foods, less can be taken.
- New Chapter Life Shield Antioxidant: One each day.
- Beta-Carotene Plus: Contains 160 milligrams per gram of beta-carotene, including other carotenoids of plant origin. Each drop represents 15,000 IU of non-toxic vitamin A activity. Suggested dose: 2-6 drops daily with meals (*see* the Resource Guide for Madison Botanicals).
- Doctor's Choice for Women: Two or three capsules a day. Contains a wide range of nutrients from foods. Manufactured by Enzymatic Therapies (*see* the Resource Guide).
- Harmonizer soy product (see the Resource Guide).
- CoQ10 supplementation, 50-200 milligrams daily.
- Rebalance hormones by use of dietary changes and aggressive exercise.

Yance also makes two general recommendations to all women interested in preventing breast cancer: Get enough sleep, and reduce exposure to enviromental toxins. Yance recommends sleeping in a darkened room at night and getting adequate sunlight during the day to increase melatonin production. Decreased levels of melatonin have been correlated with increased rates of breast cancer. From Yance's experience of treating many people with various types of cancers, he suspects that most cancers are environmentally induced. He recommends reducing toxins by consuming organic food and replacing chemical products with more natural ones.

Ann Katz's Rebirth

Ann Katz, a client of Yance's, shares with us her experience of utilizing diet, herbs, supplements, and lifestyle changes in her successful treatment of breast cancer.

In 1993, Ann Katz had been going through extensive fertility treatments for four long years and suffering disappointing miscarriages, was hoping the current *in vitro* treatment would be successful and result in a full-term pregnancy. The past year had been particularly poignant, owing to the terrible loss of Ann's mother. On October 24, while they were making love, Ann's husband discovered a lump in her breast.

Ann, who had been going to New York City daily for blood tests and sonograms connected to her fertility treatments at Cornell, rose at her usual time the following morning—4 A.M.—so she could keep her doctor's appointment in Manhattan and be back in Connecticut at her office by 9 A.M. When Ann's doctor looked at the lump, he recommended that she see a specialist right away. Ann was seen by a doctor at Yale (in New Haven) that same day. The mammogram indicated that there was a problem, and a biopsy was performed.

On Friday morning, Ann returned to New York City for egg retrieval. Afterward, she and Edward drove to Yale to learn the results of the biopsy: malignant. Because Ann was still feeling the effects of calming medication from the egg retrieval procedure that same morning at Cornell, she seemed to hear the shocking news through a haze that absorbed much of the initial fear. To make life seem even more painful, Cornell called on Monday to say none of the eggs was viable. But on Friday, after long days filled with disappointment, an unexpected call from Ann's fertility doctor restored hope: The initial report about her eggs had been wrong. One had survived. Her doctor informed her that the embryo was going to be frozen, which gave Ann a lot of hope.

Life is not a series of coincidences, Ann told me. It was no accident, for example, that just one month before the breast cancer diagnosis in October 1993, Ann had attended a conference at the Kripalu Meditation and Yoga Center for the first time. Ann believes that God gave her the tool—meditation—to deal, spiritually and physically, with what was happening to her. "God gives us all the tools to make good and healthy choices for ourselves, free from political and even familial restrictions—objective choices," Ann told me.

Ann began practicing yoga and meditation as soon as she returned from Kripalu, and they soon became daily practices. After the diagnosis of breast cancer, she began a workshop with Bernie Seigal, M.D., and also found herbalist and nutritionist Donald Yance. Her new program began.

A New Life

"The year before the lump appeared, I was really experiencing a very dark side of my soul," Ann said. "I felt I had no control over anything. I couldn't conceive, my mother died, and I was working at a job I didn't like while my husband was starting his own business. The fertility treatments involved a lot of hormones, and also were invasive. All those aspects of my life, especially the loss of my mother and the miscarriages, were just too much.

"When I was diagnosed with breast cancer, I knew I had to change my life," Ann continued. "What I had been doing before wasn't working. I also realized I had to make peace in my life if I were going to die. I was confronted with my own mortality. I realized, too, if I was going to survive, I would have to be making some changes. The changes Donnie recommended to me, initially to prepare for surgery, I was eager to implement." Ann's surgery was initially scheduled for November 1993.

Before her diagnosis, Ann drank 6-8 cups of decaffeinated coffee each day. She still drank coffee with caffeine at regular intervals (between fertility treatments), but had mostly switched to decaf for fertility reasons.

Ann drank alcohol moderately, perhaps a couple of drinks each week. She ate margarine on a regular basis, didn't buy organic eggs, dairy, meat, or pesticide-free produce. She was receiving a huge onslaught of estrogen, between the hormones for fertility treatment and those in the animal products she was consuming, besides being exposed to the pesticides in nonorganic fruits and vegetables. Ann also was drinking unfiltered water. She ate processed foods like individually wrapped slices of cheese. "I really wasn't label conscious at that time," Ann says. "Now, of course, I am." She also had a fairly high intake of ice cream, milk, and cheese. "All this changed after diagnosis," Ann told me.

One of the interesting consequences of Ann's dietary improvements occurred in the early weeks of her diagnosis. Ann twice had to donate blood for the surgery, and her doctor gave her iron pills. It was Ann's understanding that supplemenhng with iron could prevent antioxidants and other nutrients from being absorbed. Deciding not to take the iron, Ann relied instead on an enormous amount of fresh, leafy green vegetables—all organic—to build up her iron (and other nutrients) naturally. "Three times a day, I ate broccoli, broccoli rabe, kale, bok choy, collard greens, or dandelions," Ann said. "My green vegetable intake, along with other healthy foods, gave me a great blood profile, showing no iron deficiency."

Ann added, "In fact, when I had chemotherapy, I was frustrated because they kept increasing the dosage. The white blood cell count has to go below a certain point for them to know the chemo is working. My white blood count was strong because of my nutritious diet and the supplement program I was on." Ann's solution, at Bernie Seigal's recommendation, was to meditate on the number of white blood cells that the doctor wanted so that the chemo would not be increased. It worked.

Ann's diet now includes the following: organic yogurt with acidophilus, horrnone-free eggs, use of diluted miso or vegetable broth for sautéing, olive oil, Udo's Choice Oil, green vegetables, cruciferous vegetables, yams, tofu, tempeh, soy products, Bragg's Liquid Aminos, sea vegetables (kelp, wakame); shiitake mushroom broth with astragalus, and the use of soy powder in a special shake I find delicious.

"Use soy powder, yogurt—be sure it's organic—and strawberries, honey-dew, or cantaloupe, along with a couple of ice cubes," Ann explains. "I love it."

"Once or twice a week, I have a little organic chicken, red meat, or turkey," Ann says. Ann also eats salmon, trout, and snapper. Her multi-vitamin is Every Women II by New Chapter, and she takes an antioxidant formula called Clinical Nutrients by Phyto Pharmica, calcium D-glucarate, and Reishi 5, along with the other herbs and supplements personally designed for her bio-chemistry by Donald Yance.

A couple of Ann's favorite cleansing tips, also suggested by Yance, are:

Cleanse A: Watermelon Morning Cleanse.

Eat watermelon in the morning before 11 A.M. "The rind of the melon can be boiled for tea, but I didn't bother. I found this to be a great bowel cleanse," Ann said.

Cleanse B: Spring or Fall Cleanse (great for immune strength).

Include the following foods, which have a healing and cleansing effect, daily: asparagus, beets, fresh horseradish, pears, apples, and milk thistle seeds (small dried seeds, similar to flaxseeds, which can be lightly browned in the oven and sprinkled on foods like cereal).

Milk thistle strengthens the liver. Place milk thistle in a heavy-duty pepper grinder and grind into soups, vegetables, and grain dishes. Milk thistle seeds are available from Mountain Rose Herbs (see the Resource Guide).

The embryo that had been frozen when Ann was diagnosed with breast cancer did not survive the thaw. "Accepting that the fertility treatments were not working happened when I found out the embryo didn't thaw," Ann told me. "It was at that point I had closure on that segment of my life. I was able to accept that the in vitro just wasn't working." Ann and her husband went on to adopt a beautiful baby boy.

Today, Ann still lives in Connecticut. She has left corporate life behind, and has a yoga and meditation practice that specializes in cancer support. (*See* the Resource Guide.) Ann searched deeply for answers, both within herself and from the spiritual writings of Buddhism and Judaism. Ann's diagnosis of breast cancer was a watershed experience, giving her the tools to make healthier decisions for herself. Ann's cancer remains in remission.

Resource Guide

Products

Aeron Life-Cycles—Hormone testing; results are returned directly to consumer within 5–7 working days (1-800-631-7900).

Aloe Gator Suncare—natural sunscreen (1-800-531-5731).

Bio-Nutritional Formulas (1-800-950-8484)

Fem-Gest Progesterone Cream—A transdermal cream of natural progesterone.

Iso-Gen Soy Extract Tablets

Coenzyme Q10—50 mg and 150 mg

Osteo-Gest Calcium Formula (containing calcium hydroxyapatite, phosphorus [calcium to phosphorus 2:1], and vitamin D)

Bountiful Gardens—organic seeds. (1-707-459-6410)

Castor Oil Kits—Complete, including "fomentek" bag. Women to Women Clinic (1-207-846-6163).

Crown Prince—Full line of natural, canned fish products; no additives or fillers. Available in health food stores (1-800-255-5063).

Low-Sodium Pink Salmon

Norwegian Brisling Sardines in Pure Olive Oil

Solid White Natural Albacore Tuna in Water—No Salt Added (No hydrolyzed vegetable protein, which is an additive found in almost all traditional canned tuna, containing naturally high levels of MSG).

Delk Pharmacy—Natural hormones. Information you can discuss with your OB-GYN (1-615-388-3952).

Eden Products—Superior organic, natural soybean products (from soybeans not genetically engineered) and other natural foods. Available in health food stores. For more information, call 517-456-7424. In Canada, 1-800-248-0320.

Full line of miso	Shiitake mushrooms
Shoyu	Green tea
Tamari	Kukicha tea
Tomato products	Pickled daikon radish
Sauerkraut	Soba noodles
Sea vegetables	Udon noodles
Umeboshi vinegar, paste, and concentrate	Parsley garlic finbows
	Tekka (burdock root and miso condiment)
Yannoh	
Edensoy Original	Dandelion root concentrate

Flora—In United States, call 1-800-498-3610. In Canada, call **Flora Distributors**, 1-604-436-6000. In Europe, Salus Haus GmbH & Co., 011-49-8062-9010.

Full line of organic oils, bottled in opaque glass, complete with pressing date. Flax, sunflower, walnut, extra virgin olive oil, sesame, pumpkin, safflower, and almond oil. Udo's Choice Perfected Oil Blend—A blend of certified organic flax, sunflower, and sesame oils.

Flor-Essence Tea

Sambu: Guard for colds or flu. Elderberry fruit concentrate with elder flower, echinacea and vitamin C.

Udo's Choice Digestive Enzyme Blend.

Udo's Choice Beyond Greens

Fats That Heal, Fats That Kill by Udo Erasmus (Alive Books, Vancouver), 1993.

Fungi Perfecti—Mushroom tea, made from powered fruit bodies of relshi, shiitake, maitake and zhuling (close relative to maitake, with antitumor activity) (1-206-426-9292).

Goldmine Natural Food—Maitake mushrooms and other natural foods (1-800-475-3663).

Dr. Hauschka—Full line of pure, natural cosmetics, body and bath oils, skin care products, and a newsletter (1-800-243-1117). In Canada: Oasis Distributors (514-286-9146).

Health Circulator—Excellent lymphatic rejuvenator developed by NASA (1-972-596-0299).

Hygieia—Organic herbal breast massage salves. Fresh picked herbs, blossoms and plants; infused olive oil salves (1-413-528-6085).

Dandelion with evergreen oil

Evergreen, hemlock, and poke massage salve

St. John's Wort (hypericum) and dandelion blossom massage salve.

"Kidzherbs"—thirteen packets of organically grown seeds, and forty-page book of cartoon and botanical illustrations for children (1-541-846-6704); $14.95 for book and herbs.

Meyerberg Goat's Milk Products—Available in grocer and health food stores. For more information, call 1-800-343-1185.

Miracle Exclusives—Nut and seed grinders for flax seed; grain and flour mills (1-800-645-6360).

Mountain Rose Herbs—Milk thistle seeds, mail-order herbal supplies, cello bags (vegetable cellulose, biodegradable) for food storage (1-800 879-3337).

Natural Lifestyle Supplies (1-800-752-2775)
> 4-cup glass stovetop teapot
> Diffuser for electric burners

Nature's Way Products—available in health food stores. Call 1-800-962-8873 for product information.
> EFAMOL Evening Primrose Oil
> EFAMOL PMS Control with vitamins, including B6
> Femaprin Vitex Extract (Chaste Tree)
> Kava Extract softgel capsules
> TRU-OPCs, Dr. Jack Masquelier's Patented OPC Formula

NEEDS (National Ecological and Environmental Delivery System) Home Shopping Service—Natural mail-order pharmacy specializing in nutritional, herbal, and homeopathic supplements and hypoallergenic products. (1-800-634-1380)
> Harmonizer soy product
> Air purifiers
> Filtration vacuums
> Toxin-free products: mildew control, paint, primers, stains, adhesives and specialty coatings
> Candida formulas
> Boiron's Quitede, Nervousness, and Oscillococcium cold remedy
> Carlson's Dry Vitamin E
> Carlson's Easy Soy
> Champion Juicer

Herb Pharm Tonics: Liver, Burdock Blend, and Eleuthero Licorice Compound

Johnny's Selected Seeds—Organic seeds. (1-207-437-9294)

New Chapter—Provides fully-grown, 100% whole food nutrients, with safe potencies. Available in health food stores (1-800-543-7279).
> Every Woman multivitamin
> Ocean Herbs: purest and most valuable sea vegetables (brown algae, alaria, red algae, and dulse) in a vegicap
> Ginger Capsules and Extract Syrup

Lifeshield Antioxidant with protective herbal extracts, such as turmeric Reishi 5 Extract Combination

Nichols Garden Nursery—Organic seeds. (1-514-928-9280)

NO RAD Corporation—Computer radiation shields. 1549 11th Street, Santa Monica, CA 90401 (1-800-262-3260).

Nutrition Now (1-800-929-0418)

Acidophilus PB8

Phillips Publishing Merchandising (1-800-705-5559)

Creme de la Femme—Nonhormonal vaginal lubricant

Phyto Hair Products—An all natural, herbal based, extremely effective French natural product line for hair (1-800-648-0349).

Primavera Life—Aromatherapy supplies. Highest quality essential oils (1-707-996-1888; fax, 1-707-996-7888). Consumer catalog and educational materials.

Provisions—Middle Eastern cous cous. Mail order from Seattle, Washington (1-800-943-6262).

Horizon Herbs—A source for organic purslane and other seeds. (1-541-846-6704).

Rainbow Light Organic Herbal Tinctures—Catalog available. (1-800-635-1233). Liv-A-Gen Tonic with milk thistle

Real Salt—Chemical-free natural mineral salt with wholesome trace minerals (1-435-529-7922)

Sensor Pad—To facilitate a thorough breast self exam. (1-800-356-6911) www.APC.NET/IPI

Special-Teas—Herbal tea blends, custom mixed (1-203-921-1428).

Sara's Natural Barbeque Sauce—Sugar and oil free. Mail order (1-914-434-2404).

The Sprout House—Newsletter, books, seeds, and sprouting supplies. (1-413-528-5200)

Sun Wellness, Inc.—Sun chlorella granules or tablets (1-800-829-2828)

Sur La Table—Oleificio Chianti extra virgin olive oil bottled in green glass (1-800-243-0852).

Teeccino—Caffeine-free herbal coffee for brewing, Teeccino can be made in a filter drip (with unbleached filters), an expresso maker or percolator, and is available in a variety of delicious flavors (chocolate mint, hazelnut, or original) (1-805-966-0999).

UniTea Herbs—Excellent herbal teas, including "Immuni Tea" with Astragalus (1-303-443-1248).

Walnut Acres—Source for organic flax seeds (1-800-433-3998).

Water Filtration—Multi-Pure water filters (1-573-581-2446).

Whole Foods Cooking and Consultation

Myrna Baye (1-203-325-1142)

Yoga Instruction and Meditation

Ann Katz (1-203-226-2701)

Practitioners

Complementary Medicine

Alan Cohen, M.D.—Milford, CT (1-203-877-1936)
Dixie Mills, M.D.—Women to Women Clinic (1-207-846-6163)
Michael Schacter, M.D.—Suffern, NY (1-914-368-4700)
Marvin Schweitzer, N.D.—Naturopathic Physician, Norwalk, CT (1-203-847-2788)

Acupuncture

Dr. George Wu—New York, NY (1-212-213-8139) Buffalo, NY (1-718-833-0296)

Master Herbalist and Nutritionist

Donald Yance—Norwalk, CT (1-203-849-8522)

Bach Flower Remedies and Nutrition

Carolyn Heller-West, M.A., M.N.S.—Phone consultations. Riverdale, NY (1-718-601-1774)

Life-Choice Consulting

Sue Kipperman—Personal and professional coaching together with hands-on healing therapy helping to facilitate lifestyle changes. Westport, CT (203-227-1308)

Nutrition

Robert Crayhon—New Rochelle, NY (1-914-632-4565)
Joan Friedrich—Bronxville, NY (1-914-423-3531)
Dina Khader—Mount Kisco, NY (1-914-242-0124)

Chiropractic

Dr. Michael McGlynn—Norwalk, CT (1-203-846-4466)
Dr. James D. Murphy—Mexico, MO (1-573-581-2446)

Bibliography

Suggested Reading

Austin, N. D., and Cathy Hitchcock; *Breast Cancer: What You Should Know (But May Not Be Told) About Prevention, Diagnosis, and Treatment*, Prima Publishing (Rocklin, CA), 1994.

Bertolli, Paul, and Alice Waters; *Chez Panisse Cooking*, Random House (New York), 1988.

Cayce, Edgar, and B. Ernest Frejer; *The Edgar Cayce Companion*, A.R.E. Press (Virginia Beach, VA), 1995.

Cichoke, Anthony J.; *Enzymes and Enzyme Therapy: How to Jump Start Your Way to Lifelong Good Health*, Keats Publishing (New Canaan, CT), 1994.

Erasmus, Udo; *Fats That Heal, Fats That Kill*, Alive Books (Vancouver), 1993.

Gittleman, Ann Louise; *Before the Challenge*, Harper (San Francisco), 1998.

Gladstar, Rosemary; *Herbal Healing for Women*, Fireside (New York), 1993.

Haas, Elson M.; *The Detox Diet*, Celestial Arts (Berkley, CA), 1996.

Hobbs, Christopher; *Foundations of Health: Healing With Herbs and Foods*, Botanica Press (Santa Cruz, CA), 1992.

Joseph, Barbara; *My Healing from Breast Cancer*, Keats Publishing (New Canaan, CT), 1996.

Keville, Kathi, and Mindy Green; *Aromatherapy, A Complete Guide to the Healing Art*, The Crossing Press (Freedom, CA), 1995.

King, Shirley; *Fish the Basics*, Chapters Publishing (Shelburne, VT), 1996.

Laux, Marcus, N.D., and Christine Collins; *Natural Woman, Natural Menopause*, Harper Collins (New York), 1997.

Lee, J. R.; *Progesterone: The Multiple Rules of a Remarkable Hormone*, BLL Publishing (Sebastapol, CA), 1993.

Lee, John, M.D. *What Your Doctor May Not Tell You About Menopause*, Warner Books (New York) 1996

Love, Susan M.; *Dr. Susan Love's Breast Book*, Addison-Wesley (Reading, MA), 1990.

McCully, Kilmer, M.D.; *The Homocysteine Revolution*, Keats Publishing (New Canaan, CT), 1997.

Madison, Deborah, with Edward Espe Brown, *The Green Cook Book*, Bantam (New York), 1987.

Michnovicz, Jon J., with Diane S. Klein; *How to Reduce Your Risk of Breast Cancer*, Warner Books (New York), 1994.

Mindell, Earl; *Soy Miracle*, Simon and Schuster (New York), 1995.

Northrup, Christiane; *Women's Bodies, Women's Wisdom*, Bantam Books (New York), 1994.

Pelton, Ross, Taffy Clarke Pelton, and Vinton C. Vint; *How to Prevent Breast Cancer*, Fireside Publishing (New York), 1995.

Pressman, Alan H., and Sheila Buff; *The GSH Phenomenon: Nature's Most Powerful Antioxidant and Healing Agent*, St. Martin's Press (New York), 1997.

Romano, Rita; *Dining in the Raw, Cooking with "The Buff,"* Kensington Publishing (New York), 1997.

Schulick, Paul; *Ginger: Common Spice and Wonder Drug*, Herbal Free Press Ltd. (Brattleboro, VT), 1993 (1-800-903-9104).

Schwitters, Bert (in collaboration with Jack Masquellier); *OPCs in Practice: The Hidden Story of Proanthocyanidins, Nature's Most Powerful and Patented Antioxidant*, Alpha Omega Editrice, Via San Damaso 23, 00165 Roma, Italy, 1996. Phone—39-6630398; Fax—39-6632196.

Smith, Lendon; *How to Raise a Healthy Child*, M. Evans (New York), 1996.

Ullman, Dana; *The Consumer's Guide to Homepathy*, J. P. Tarcher (New York), 1996.

Wargo, John; *Our Children's Toxic Legacy*, Yale University Press (New Haven, CT), 1996.

Waters, Alice; *Chez Panisse Vegetables*, HarperCollins (New York), 1996.

Weed, Susun; *Breast Cancer? Breast Health! The Wise Woman Way*, Ashtree Publishing (Woodstock, NY), 1996.

Winter, Ruth; *A Consumer's Guide to Medicines in Food*, Crown Trade Paperbacks, (New York), 1995.

Worwood, Valerie Ann; *The Complete Book of Essential Oils and Aromatherapy*, New World Library (San Rafael, CA), 1991.

Magazines

Alive Magazine (7436 Fraser Park Drive, Burnaby, BC V6J5B9 Canada).
Healthy and Natural (1-800-883-8894).
Mamm (1-212-242-2143; mamm@poz.com).
Natural Health Magazine. (Boston Common Press, 17 Station St., Brookline, MA 02146).
Total Health Magazine (1-800-788-7806).
Townsend Letter for Doctors and Patients (1-360-385-6021).
Yoga Journal (1-510-841-9200).

Newsletters

The American Herb Association Quarterly Newsletter (P.O. Box 1673, Nevada City, CA 95959.)

Berkeley Wellness Letter (University of California, P.O. Box 420148, Palm Coast, FL 32142.)

Breast Cancer Action (1-415-243-3996).

Center for Science in the Public Interest (CSPI) For Nutrition Action Health Letter, write to: CSPI, 1875 Connecticut Avenue, N.W., Suite, 300, Washinton, DC 20009-5728 (1-202-332-9110).

Health Action Network Society Newsletter and information service (1-604-435-0512.)

Health and Healing Newsletter Edited by Julian Whitaker, M.D., Phillips Publishing (1-800-539-8219).

HerbGram (P.O. Box 201660, Austin, TX 78720).

The National Council Against Health Fraud Newsletter (P.O. Box 1276, Loma Linda, CA 92354).

Prescription for Healthy Living Edited by James Balch, M.D., and Jolle Martin Root, N.C. (1-800-289-9222.)

Toxic Discovery Network Breast implant newsletter. (1-573-445-0861).

Tufts University Diet & Nutrition Letter (P.O. BOX 57834, Boulder, CO 80321-7834).

Menopause

A Friend Indeed (Box 515, Place du Parc Station, Montreal, Canada H2W2P1).

Menopause News (1-415-567-2368).

Midlife Zest (1-805-964-2252).

Women's Health

Harvard's Women Health Watch (1-800-829-5921).

Health Wisdom for Women Newsletter by Christiane Northrup, Phillips Publishing. (1-800-211-8561).

Women In Health (1-818-594-1572).

Women's Health Advocate Newsletter (1-800-829-5876).

Women's Health Letter (1-818-798-0638).

Astrology and Healing

Lightworks by Luana Collins Rubin (1-303-516-1615).

Catalogs

As We Change Menopause Catalog (1-800-203-5585).

Becoming Inc. Breast Cancer catalog (1-800-980-9085).

Harmony Catalog Products in harmony with the earth. (1-800-869-3446)

Convection oven made in Italy

Full-spectrum nature light bulbs; 60, 75, 100, 150 watts

3-way bulbs; 50, 100, and 150 watts

Seventh-generation chlorine-free paper products and cleaners

Bleach and treatment-free sheets, blankets, quilts, mattress covers, robes, and bras

Pure laundry soap (100% natural, organic ingredients)

Food storage bags made without plastic

Fresh citrus juicer, stainless steel construction

Natural slipcovers and throw pillows free of formaldehyde, dyes, and bleach

All natural bed systems (mattress and bed springs)

Cell phone shield to dramatically reduce radiation

Cedar rolls (natural moth repellent) for drawers and closets

Natracare bleach-free sanitary napkins and tampons

Inner Balance Catalog Natural healing and wellness (1-800-482-3608).

Creating a Healthy Home video—information on how to make your kitchen and home healthier places.

Soft heat sauna

Turbo shower filter

Winter therapy lightbox

Full-spectrum fluorescent tubes

Pressure cooker

Body brush with handle

Sounds True Over 300 audio and video tapes for the inner life (1-800-333-9185).

Booklets

Herbs for the Liver and Hayfever (Gladstar, Rosemary; Sage, P.O. Box 420, East Barre, Vermont 05649).

"Phytochemicals in Teas and Rosemary and Their Cancer Preventive Properties," Ito, Chi-Gang, et al., in *Food Phytochemicals in Cancer Prevention II: Teas, Spices and Herbs*, American Chemical Society, Washington, D.C., 1994.

The Cultivation of Organic Medicinal Herbs and Plants and other booklets by Richard A. Cech AGH, available on assorted topics such as milk thistle, burdock, herbs of the Mediterranean and more. Catalog and growing guide available from Horizon Herbs, (1-541-846-6704), e-mail—herbseed@chatlink.com.

Additional Information

Alternative Cancer Therapies—For information, contact Susan Silberstein, Ph.D., Center for Alternative Cancer Education, Box 48, Wynnewood, PA 19096 (1-610-642-4810).

American Association of Naturopathic Physicians—Naturopaths receive four years of medical training, complemented by in-depth information on herbs, supplements, and nutrition. Referral service for naturopaths (1-206-323-7610).

Breast Cancer Action News—A Publication by the Canadian Breast Cancer Network (1-613-788-3311).

Breast Self-Exam videotape—Available for $25.00 in English, Spanish, or Haitian from CRW Enterprises, P.O. Box 2228, Woodbridge, VA 221930. If you cannot afford to purchase a copy, you can request one from the American Cancer Society by calling 1-800-ACS-2345.

Cancer Prevention Coalition—For a report on the carcinogenicity of polyurethane foam, send $10 to CPC, 520 N. Michigan Ave., #410, Chicago, IL 60611 (1-312-467-0600).

Demeter Association Inc.—Certifiers of organically grown and produced yogurt from humanely treated animals (1-818-843-5521).

Free Report on Nutrients in Organic Food From Doctors' Data—P.O. Box 111, West Chicago, IL 60185-9986.

Mothers Supporting Daughters with Breast Cancer (MSDBC)—(1-401-778-1982).

National Alliance of Breast Cancer Organizations (1-800-719-9154).

Naturopathic Medical Schools—Bastyr College, 144 N.E. 54th Street, Seattle, WA 98105.

Ontario College of Naturopathic Medicine—60 Berl Avenue, Toronto, Ontario M84 3C7, Canada.*

Pesticide Hotline—U.S. Environmental Protection Agency, NPTN, Texas Tech. University, Thompson Hall, Room S129, Lubbock, TX 79430. (1-800-858-7378) Mon-Fri 8 a.m-6 p.m. (EST).

"Pesticides Breast Cancer Link"—Articles and bibliography for $5 from New York Campaign Against Pesticides, P.O. Box 6005, Albany, NY 12206-0005.

Lymphatics

For lymphatic drainage massage: The Upledger Institute, Inc. (1-800-233-5880).

*Especially recommended.

For lymphatic health and rejuevenation:
Dr. Marika von Viczay
Isis Health and Rejuevenation Center
Asherville, NC 28880
(1-704-253-8371)

Organochlorines

For information on organochlorines and breast cancer:

Greenpeace	OR Greenpeace (Canada)
1017 West Jackson	185 Spadina Avenue
Chicago, IL 60607	Toronto, Ontario, MST 2C6
(1-312-666-3305)	(1-416-345-8408)

Mammography

For an accredited mammography facility:
American College of Radiology (1-800-ACR-LINE).
National Cancer Institute (1-800-4-CANCER).
Mammography Screening: A Decision-Making Guide; $6.00 from the Center for Medical Consumers, 237 Thompson Street, New York, NY 10012.

Donald Yance, Nutritionist and Master Herbalist

Product Recommendations:
• Alpha-lipoic acid
• Selenium
Specific Companies:
• Beta-Carotene Plus, distributed by Puget Consumer's Co-Op (1-206-547-1222).
　• Doctor's Choice for Women, Enzymatic Therapies (1-800-553-2370).
　• Harmonizer Soy Product (1-800-643-1380).
　• Life Shield Antioxidant, New Chapter (1-800-543-7279).
　• Multi-vitamin, New Chapter (1-800-543-7279).
　• OPC grape seed extract, Nature's Way (1-800-962-8873).

AMAS Test

Early cancer screening test (non-invasive). (1-800-9-CATEST)

Foundations

American Menopause Foundation (1-212-714-2398).

The Broda-Barnes Foundation Directory of medical doctors for hypothyroidism and proper testing (1-203-261-2101).

The Foundation for Preventive Oncology, Inc. Institute for Hormone Research An independent foundation dedicated to the prevention of cancer through scientific research, preventive medicine, and public education (1-212-683-7070).

Herb Research Foundation Non-profit library providing accurate botanical information with an advisory board of eighteen leading medicinal plant experts. Offers over 185 information packets including breast cancer, menopause, and phytosterols. (1-303-449-02265).

National Wildlife Foundation, Washington, DC. *Danger on Tap*, The Government's Failure to Enforce the Federal Safe Drinking Water Act.

Organization Dedicated to the Preservation of Healing Medicinal Plants Request brochure: United Plant Savers (1-802-479-9825).

Organizations

African American Breast Cancer Alliance—Support groups and information, Minneapolis, MN (1-612-644-7119).

American College of Radiology—Mammography Accreditation Dept. (1-800-227-6440)

American Holistic Medical Association—Help with complementary approaches, national referral directory (1-919-787-5181).

American Institute for Cancer Research Nutrition Hotline—(1-800-843-8114)

Cancer Care Inc.—Free professional counseling, information, referrals, and practical help. New York (1-800-813-4673).

Citizens for Health—Information about genetically engineered foods. Website: www.citizens.org (1-800-357-2211).

Consumer's Health and Medical information Center—Current information on the latest treatments for both standard and alternative treatment. P.O. Box 390, Clearwater, FL 33517.

ECaP (Exceptional Cancer Patients)—Founded by Bernie Siegel, M.D. Network for emotional support groups, Middletown, CT (1-203-343-5950).

Food and Water Inc.—Information on protecting the food and water supply (1-800-EAT-SAFE).

Herbal Educational Services—P.O. Box 57, Swans Island, ME 04685 (1-800-252-0688).

Memorial Sloan-Kettering Cancer Center—(1-800-525-2225)

National Alliance of Breast Cancer Organizations—(1-888-80-NABCO).

National Institute for Cancer Research—(1-800-843-8114)

Oldways Preservation and Exchange Trust—Preserving traditions and fostering cultural exchange in the fields of nutrition, cooking and agriculture. Cambridge, MA (1-617-621-3000).

The Organic Foods Production Association of North America (or PANA)—Publication and membership available. P.O. Box 1078, Greenfield, MA 01301 (1-413-774-7511).

Physician Referral Services—American Association of Naturopathic Physicians, P.O. Box 20386, Seattle, WA 98112.

Rosenthal Center for Alternative/Complementary Medicine—College of Physicians and Surgeons, Columbia University, New York City (1-212-305-4755; Fax, 1-212-305-1495).

Santa Barbara Breast Cancer Institute—Breast health resources. (1-805-565-2244)

Susan Komen Breast Cancer Foundation—(1-800-I'M AWARE).

USDA'S Meat and Poutlry hotline—Information regarding safe food handling (1-800-535-4555)

Y-ME National Breast Cancer Organization—(1-800-221-2141).

References

Introduction: Creating Breast Health

"Assays for Potentially Anti-Carcinogenic Phytochemical in Flax Seed"; report issued by the Midwest Research Institute, Kansas City, MO, 1993.

Bland, Jeffrey S., Ph.D.; "Natural Healing"; *Delicious!*, September 1997.

Brody, Jane; "What Is a Woman to Do to Avoid Breast Cancer? Plenty, New Studies Suggest"; *New York Times*, May 28, 1997.

Brody, Jane; "Transfatty Acids Tied to Risk of Breast Cancer"; *New York Times*, October 14, 1997.

Cancer and Steroid Hormone Study of the Centers for Disease Control and the National Institute of Child Health and Human Development, 1986: "Oral Contraceptive Use and the Risk of Breast Cancer"; *New England Journal of Medicine* 315:405-411.

"Editorial: Postmenopausal Hormone Replacement Therapy—Time for a Reappraisal?"; *New England Journal of Medicine* 336, June 19, 1997.

Erasmus, Udo; *Fats That Heal, Fats That Kill*; Alive Books (Vancouver), 1993.

"Food, Nutrition, and the Prevention of Cancer: A Global Perspective"; American Institute for Cancer Research and the World Cancer Research Fund, December 1997.

Grodstein, Francine, Meier J. Stampfer, Graham A. Colditz, et al.; "Postmenopausal Hormone Therapy and Mortality"; *New England Journal of Medicine* 336:1769-1775, June 19, 1997.

La Vecchia, Carlo, Silvia Franceschi, Adriano DeCarlo, Attilio Giacosa, and Upworth; "Olive Oil and Breast Cancer Risk in Italy"; *Nutrition Research Newsletter*, Vol. 15, No. 2, p.12(1), February 1996.

Lubin, J. H., B. E. Burns, W. J. Blot, R. G. Ziegler, A. W. Lees, and J. F. Fraumeni; "Dietary Factors and Breast Cancer Risk"; *International Journal of Cancer* 28:685-689, 1981.

Normura, A. M., B. E. Henderson, and J. Lee; "Breast Cancer and Diet Among the Japanese in Hawaii"; *American Journal Clinical Nutrition* 31:2020-2025, 1978.

Phillips, R. L.; "Role of Lifestyle and Dietary Habits in Risk of Cancer Among Seventh Day Adventists"; *Cancer Research* 35:3513, 1975.

Report of President Clinton's Presidential Special Commission on Breast Cancer, 1997.

Trichopoulos, Dimitrios, M.D., and Loren Lipworth (Department of Epidemiology and Center for Cancer Prevention, Harvard School of Public Health, Boston, MA); "The Role of Diet in the Etiology of Breast Cancer."; In: *Seventh European Nutrition Conference*, Vienna, May 1995, Editors Austrian Nutrition Society K. Wildham, J. Leibetseder, and M. Bavernfried.

Weatherall, Sir David, and David Weatherhill; *Science and the Quiet Art: The Role of Medical Research in Health Care*; W.W. Norton (New York), 1995.

Chapter 1: The Effects of Fats and Oils on Breast Cancer

American Health, March 1997. Nutrition Update, "The Fat You Don't Know About."

American Heart Association Report, Summer 1997. Leading scientific authorities call into question population-wide limits on egg consumption.

Austin, N.D., and Cathy Hitchcock; *Breast Cancer: What You Should Know (But May Not Be Told) About Prevention, Diagnosis, and Treatment*; Prima Publishing, (Rocklin, CA) 1994.

Aviram, M., and K. Eigs; "Dietary Olive Oil Reduces Low-Density Lipoprotein Uptake by Macrophages and Decreases the Susceptibility of the Lipoprotein to Undergo Lipid Peroxidation"; *Annals of Nutrition and Metabolism* 37:75-89, 1995.

Awad, A. B.; "Transfatty Acids in Tumor Development and the Host Survival"; *Journal of the National Cancer Institute* 67:189-92, 1981.

Bang, Ho, J. Dyerberg, and N. Hjorne; "The Composition of Food Consumed by Greenland Eskimos"; *Acta Med. Scand.* 200:69-73, 1976.

Baxevanis, C. N. et al.; "Elevated PGE2 Production by Monocytes Is Responsible for the Depressed Levels of Natural Killer and Lymphokine-Activated Killer Cell Function in Patients with Breast Cancer"; *Cancer* 72:441-501, 1993.

Bougnoux, P.; "Alpha-Linolenic Acid Content of Adipose Breast Tissue: A Host Determinant Risk of Early Metastases in Breast Tissue"; *British Journal of Cancer* 70:330-334, 1994.

Brisson, G. J.; *Lipids in Human Nutrition*; Burgess (New Jersey), 1981.

Brody, Jane E., "Women's Heart Risk Linked to Kinds of Fats, Not Total"; *New York Times*, Nov. 20, 1997.

Cave, W., et al.; "Dietary Omega-3 Polyunsaturated Fats and Breast Cancer"; *Supplement to Nutrition*, 12:1, 1996.

Cohen, Leonard A., Diane D. Thompson, Yoshichi Maeura, Keewhan Choi, Michael E. Blank, and David P. Rose; "Dietary Fat and Mammary Cancer. I: Promoting

Effects of Different Dietary Fats on N-Nitrosomethylurea-Induced Rat Mammary Tumorigenesis"; *Journal of the National Cancer Institute* 77:33-42, 1986.

"Consumption of Olive Oil and Specific Food Groups in Relation to Breast Cancer Risk in Greece"; *Journal of the National Cancer Institute* 87, No. 2; January 1, 1995.

Durbec, J. P., G. Chevillotte, J. M. Bidart, P. Berthezene, and H. Sarles; "Diet, Alcohol, Tobacco, and Risk of Cancer of the Pancreas: A Case-Control Study"; *British Journal of Cancer* 47:463-70, 1983.

Erasmus, Udo; *Fats That Heal, Fats That Kill*; Alive Publishers (Vancouver), 1993.

Erasmus, Udo; "The Value of Fresh Flax Oil"; and "Additional Studies Show Omega-3 Inhibits Tumor Formation Without Harming Normal Cells"; *Lipid Letter*, Issue no. 3.

Falk, R. T., L .W. Pickle, E. T. Fontham, P. Correa, J. F. Fraumeni; "Life-Style Risk Factors for Pancreatic Cancer in Louisiana: A Case-Control Study"; *American Journal of Epidemiology*. 128:324-36, 1988.

Fortes, Cristina, Francesco Forastiere, Fabrizio Anatra, and Giovanni Schmid; "Re: Consumption of Olive Oil and Specific Food Groups in Relation to Breast Cancer Risk in Greece" (correspondence); *Journal of the National Cancer Institute;* Vol. 87, No. 13, 1995.

Horrobin, David F.; *New Approaches to Cancer Treatment: Unsaturated Lipids and Photodynamic Therapy;* Churchill Communications Europe (London), 1991.

Johnson, Mireille; *The Cuisine of the Sun*, Vintage Books (New York), 1976.

Karmali, R. A.; "Omega-3 Fatty Acids and Cancer"; *Journal of Internal Medicine* 225 (Suppl. 1, 1989):197-200.

Kelley, D. S.; "Alpha-Linolenic Acid and Immune Response"; *Nutrition* 8:215-17, 1992.

Kohlmeier, Lenore, et al.; "Adipose Transfatty Acids and Breast Cancer in the European Community Multicenter Study on Antioxidants, Myocardial Infarction, and Breast Cancer"; *Cancer Epidemiology, Biomarkers, and Prevention*, September 1997.

Knekt, P., D. Albanes, R. Seppanen, et al.; "Dietary Fat and Risk of Breast Cancer"; *American Journal of Clinical Nutrition* 52:903-908, 1990.

Kort, W. J., Ineke M. Weijjma, Amelie M. Bijma, William P. Van Schalkwyk, Antoine J. Vergroesen, and Dick L. Westbroek; "Omega 3 Fatty Acids Inhibiting the Growth of a Transplantable Rat Mammary Adneocarcinoma"; *Journal of the National Cancer Institute*, Vol. 79, September 1987.

Kurmat, J., R. A .Marsh, and J. Fuchs; "Effect of Omega 3 Fatty Acids on Growth of Rat Mammary Tumor"; *Journal of the National Cancer Institute* 33:477, 1984.

Landa, M. C., N. Frago, and A. Tres; "Diet and Risk of Breast Cancer in Spain"; *European Journal of Cancer Prevention* 3:313-20, 1994.

La Vecchia, C., E . Negri, S. Franceschi, A. DeCarli, A. Glacosa, and L. Lipworth; "Olive Oil, Dietary Fats, and the Risk of Breast Cancer"; *Cancer, Causes, Control* 6:545-50, 1995.

La Vecchia, C., E.. Negri, S. Franceschi, A. DeCarli, A. Glacosa, and L. Lipworth; "Olive Oil and Breast Cancer Risk in Italy"; *Nutrition Research Newsletter*, Vol. 15, No. 2, p.12(1), February 1996.

Leak, A.; "Cardiovascular Effects of Omega-3 Fatty Acids"; *New England Journal of Medicine* 318:549-557; 1988.

Linder, M. C.; *Nutrition and Metabolism of Fats in Nutritional Biochemistry and Metabolism with Clinical Application*, M. C. Linder, ed. Elsevier (London), pp. 476-505, 1991.

Mack, T. M., M. C. Yu, R. Hanisch, and B. E. Henderson; "Pancreas Cancer and Smoking, Beverage Consumption, and Past Medical History"; *Journal National Cancer Institute* 76:49-60, 1986.

Martin-Moreno, J. M., W. C. Willett, L. Gorgojo, et al.; "Dietary Fat, Olive Oil Intake, and Breast Cancer Risk"; *International Journal of Cancer* 58:774-80, 1994.

Nielson, N. H. and J. P. Hansen; "Breast Cancer in Greenland: Selected Epidemiological, Clinical, and Histological Features"; *Journal of Cancer Research and Clinical Oncology* 98:287-299, 1980.

Northrup, Christiane; "Creating Breast Health: A Holistic Approach to Breast Wellness Based on Diet, Nutrition, and Self Knowing"; 1994; audio tape available from Sounds True Audio, 1-800-333-9185.

Papadopoulos, G., and D. Boskou; "Antioxidant Effect of Natural Phenols in Olive Oil"; *Journal of the American Oil and Chemical Society* 9:669-671, 1991.

Pelton, Ross, Taffy Clarke Pelton, and Vinton C. Vint; *How to Prevent Breast Cancer: A Lifestyle Guide for the Prevention of Breast Cancer and Its Recurrence with an Investigation of the Critical Risk Factors"*; Fireside Publishing (New York), 1995.

Qu, Y. H. et al.; "Genotoxicity of Heated Cooking Oil Vapors"; *Mutation Research* 298:105-111, 1992.

Raloff, J.; "This Fat May Aid the Spread of Breast Cancer"; *Science News*, November 1994.

Reddy, B. S., and Y. Maeura; "Tumor Promotion by Dietary Fat in Azoxymethan-Induced Colon Carcinogenesis in Female F344 Rats: Influence of Amount and Source of Dietary Fat"; *Journal of the National Cancer Institute* 72:745-50, 1984.

Richardson, S., and M. Gerber; "Nutritional Factors and Breast Cancer: A Case-Control Study in a French Mediterranean Region." In: *Epidemiology of Diet and Cancer* (M.J. Hill, A. Giacosa, P. J. Caygill, eds.), Ellis Horwood, (Chichester, UK) pp. 353-377, 1994.

Richardson, S., M. Gerber, and S. Cenee; "The Role of Fat, Animal Protein, and Vitamin Consumption in Breast Cancer: A Case-Control Study in Southern France." *International Journal of Cancer* 48:1-9, 1991.

Rockwell, Sally, ed.; "Canola (Rape Seed) Oil"; *Allergy Alert*, September-October 1996 (P.O. Box 3165, Seattle, WA, 98103, 206-547-1814).

Rose, D. P., and M. A. Hatala; "Dietary Fatty Acids and Breast Cancer Invasion and Metastasis"; *Nutr. Cancer* 21:103-11, 1994.

Sake, C.; "Promises, Promises"; *Muscle and Fitness*, August 1997.

Setchell, K. D. R., and H. Aldercreutz; "Mammalian Lignans and Phytoestrogens: Recent Studies on Their Formation, Metabolism, and Biological Role in Health and Disease." In: *Role of Gut Flora in Toxicology and Cancer*, I. R. Rowland (ed.), (London), Academic Press, pp. 315-343.

Shields, P. G. et al.; "Mutagens from Heated Chinese and U.S. Cooking Oils"; *Journal of the National Cancer Institute* 87:836-841, 1995.

Supplement to Nutrition 12:1, 1996.

Synderwine, E. G.; "The Food-Derived Heterocyclic Amines and Breast Cancer: A 1995 Perspective"; *Recent Results in Cancer Research* 140:17-25, 1995.

Tinsley, I. J., J. A. Schmitz, and D. A. Pierce; "Influence of Dietary Fatty Acids on the Incidence of Mammary Tumors in the C3H Mouse; *Cancer Research* 41:1460-65, 1981.

Trichopoulou, A., K. Katsouyanni, et al.; "Consumption of Olive Oil and Specific Food Groups in Relation to Breast Cancer Risk in Greece"; *Journal of the National Cancer Institute* 87:110-16, 1995.

Trichopoulou, Antonia, Klea Katsouyanni, Sherri Stuver, Lia Tzala, Charalambox Gnardellis, Eric Rimm, and Dimitrios Trichopoulos; "Consumption of Olive Oil and Specific Food Groups in Relation to Breast Cancer Risk in Greece"; *Journal of the National Cancer Institute*; Vol. 87, No. 2, January 18, 1995.

Trichopoulou, Antonia; "Editorial: Olive Oil and Breast Cancer"; *Cancer Causes and Control*, Vol. 6, p. 475, 1995.

Weil, Andrew; *Spontaneous Healing*; Fawcett Columbine, (New York), 1996.

Whitaker, Julian; *Dr. Whitaker's Guide to Natural Healing*, Prima Publishing, (Rocklin, CA) 1996.

Yu, S. Z., R. F. Lu, D. D. Xu, et al.; "A Case-Control Study of Dietary and Nondietary Risk Factors for Breast Cancer in Shanghai"; *Cancer Research* 50:5017-5021, 1990.

Chapter 3: The New Millennium:
Challenging the Myth of the Low-Fat Diet

Bang, H. O., J. Dyerberg, and Neilsen A. Brondum; "Plasma Lipids and Lipoprotein Pattern in Greenlandic West Coast Eskimos"; *The Lancet* 1:1143, 1971.

"Benefits Found in Asian Fish Diet." *New York Times*; July 4, 1997.

Brody, Jane E.; "Personal Health: Fat and Health"; *New York Times*, February 1996.

Brody, Jane E.; "Personal Health: Preventing Breast Cancer"; *New York Times*, May 7, 1997.

Byrne, C., et al.; *Journal of Nutrition* 126:2757-64, 1996.

Cobias, L., et al.; "Lipid Lipoprotein and Hemostatic Effects of Fish vs. Fish Oil in W-3 Fatty Acids in Mildly Hyperlipidemic Males"; *American Journal of Clinical Nutrition* 53:1210-16, 1991.

Crayhon, Robert,; "Nutrition in Depth: The Age of Carbohydrates Is Over"; *Total Health*, Vol. 19, No. 3, 1997.

Franceschi, Silvia, Adriano Favero, Adriano DeCarlo, Eva Negri, Carlo La Vecchia, Monica Ferraroni, Antonio Russo, Simonetta Salvini, Dino Amadori, Ettore Conti, Maurizio Montella, and Attilio Giacosa; "Intake of Macronutrients and Risk of Breast Cancer"; *The Lancet*, Vol. 347(9012), p. 1351(6), May 18, 1996.

Karmali, R. A. "Omega-3 Fatty Acids and Cancer"; *Journal of Internal Medicine* 225(Suppl. 1):197-200, 1989.

Karmali, R. A. et al.; "Plant and Marine Omega-3 Fatty Acids Inhibit Experimental Metastasis of Rat Mammary Adnocarcinoma Cells" *Prostaglandins, Leukotrienes, and Essential Fatty Acids* 48:309, 1993.

Kurfield, D. M., C. B. Welch, L. M. Cloud, et al.; "Inhibition of DMBA-Induced Mammary Tumorigenesis by Caloric Restriction in Rats Fed High Fat Diet"; *International Journal of Cancer* 43:922-925, 1989.

Landa, M. C., N. Frago, and A. Tres; "Diet and Risk of Breast Cancer in Spain"; *Gur. J. Cancer Pres.* 3:313-20, 1994.

La Vecchia, Carlo, Eva Negri, Silvia Franceschi, Andriano DeCarlo, Attilio Giacosa, and Upworth; "Olive Oil and Breast Cancer Risk in Italy"; *Nutrition Research Newsletter*, Vol.15, No. 2, p.12(1), February 1996.

Lee, H. P.; "Dietary Effects on Breast Cancer Risk in Singapore"; *The Lancet* 337:1197-1200, 1991.

Martin-Moreno, J. M., W. C. Willett, L. Gorgoso, et al.; "Dietary Fat, Olive Oil Intake, and Breast Cancer Risk"; *International Journal of Cancer* 58:774-80, 1994.

National Research Council, *Diet, Nutrition, and Cancer*; National Academy Press (Washington, DC), 1982.

Rudin, Donald, and Clara Felix; *Omega 3 Oils to Improve Mental Health, Fight Degenerative Diseases, and Extend Your Life*; Avery Publishing Group (New York), 1996.

Trichopoulou, Antonia, Klea Katsouyanni, Sherri Stuver, Lia Tzala, Charalambox Gnardellis, Eric Rimm, Dimitrios Trichopoulos; "Consumption of Olive Oil and Specific Food Groups in Relation to Breast Cancer Risk in Greece"; *Journal of the National Cancer Institute*; Vol. 87, No. 2, January 18, 1995.

Trichopoulos, Dimitrios, and Loren Lipworth (Department of Epidemiology and Center for Cancer Prevention, Harvard School of Public Health, Boston, MA); "The Role of Diet in the Etiology of Breast Cancer"; In: *Seventh European Nutrition Conference*, Vienna, May 1995, Editors Austrian Nutrition Society K. Wildham, J. Leibetseder, and M. Bavernfried.

Chapter 4: The Importance of Organic Food

"Are Toxic Fertilizers Poisoning Our Food?"; *Delicious!*; October 1997.

"Benefits Found in Asian Fish Diet"; *New York Times*; July 4, 1997.

"Breast Cancer and Pesticides"; *Soil and Health*; January 1994.

"EcoCancers"; *Science News*; July 3, 1993.

Falck, et al.; "Pesticides and Polychlorinated Biphenyl Residues in Human Breast Lipids, and Their Relation to Breast Cancer"; *Archives of Environmental Health* 47:143-46, 1992.

Hill, Michael J.; In: *Role of Gut Flora in Toxicity and Cancer*, I. R. Rowland, ed. Academic Press (London), p. 461 1988.

"Pesticides in the Diets of Infants and Children?"; *National Academy of Sciences Report,* 1993.

Roloff, Janet; "EcoCancers"; *Science News;* October 1993.

Smith, Bob L.; "Organic Foods vs. Supermarket Foods: Element Levels"; *Journal of Applied Nutrition* 45(11):35-29, 1993.

"The Environmental Link to Breast Cancer"; *Ms. Magazine;* May-June 1993.

Weil, Andrew; "Pollutants Linked to Breast Cancer"; *Natural Health,* November-December 1993.

Whole Foods, March 1996. (rBGH milk and cancer)

Chapter 5: Raw Foods and Juices Provide Protective Enzymes

Cichoke, Anthony J.; *Enzymes and Enzyme Therapy: How to Jump Start Your Way to Lifelong Good Health,* Keats Publishing (New Canaan, CT), 1994.

Erasmus, Udo; *Fats That Heal, Fats That Kill;* Alive Books (Vancouver), 1993.

Gonzales, M. D.; "The Importance of Pancreatic Enzymes and Alternative Cancer Therapy"; lecture delivered at the Open Center, New York City, 1995.

Romano, Rita; *Dining in the Raw, Cooking with "The Buff";* Prato Publications (Prato, Italy), 1996.

Total Health, Vol. 19, No. 4, Fall 1997.

Chapter 6: Flaxseed and Flaxseed Oil: Nature's Superfoods for Breast Health

Aldercreutz, H., and T. Focais; "Determination of Urinary Lignans and Phytoestrogen Metabolites, Potential Anti-Estrogens and Anti-Carcinogens in Urine of Women on Various Habitual Diets"; *Journal of Steroid Biochemistry* 25:791-97, 1986.

Lampe, J. W., et al.; "Urinary Lignan and Isoflavonoid Excretion in Premenopausal Women Consuming Flax Seed Powder"; *American Journal of Clinical Nutrition* 60:122-128.

Obermeyer, W. R., S. M. Musser, J. M. Betz, R. E. Casey, A. E. Pohland, and S.W. Page; "Chemical Studies of Phytoestrogens and Related Compounds in Dietary Supplements: Flax and Chaparral"; *Journal of Experimental Biology and Medicine,* 998:6, 1995.

Rudin, Donald, and Clara Felix; *Omega 3 Oils to Improve Mental Health, Fight Degenerative Disease, and Extend Your Life;* Avery Publishing Group (Garden City, NY), 1996.

Serraino, M., and L. U. Thompson; "Flax Seed Supplementation on Early Markers of Colon Carcinogenesis"; *Cancer Letters* 63:159-165, 1992.

Serraino, M., and L. U. Thompson; "The Effect of Flax Seed Supplementation on Early Risk Markers for Mammary Carcinogenesis"; *Cancer Letters* 60:122-128, 1991.

Serraino, M., and L. U. Thompson; "The Effect of Flax Seed Supplementation on the Inhibition and Promotional Stages of Mammary Carcinogensis"; *Nutrition and Cancer* 17:153-59, 1992.

Setchell, K. D. R.; "Discovery and Potential Clinical Importance of Mammalian Lignans"; In *Flax Seed in Human Nutrition*, S. C. Cunnane and L. U. Thompson, ed. ADCS Press (Champaign, IL), 1995.

Stevens, L. J., S. Zentall, et al.; "Essential Fatty Acid Metabolism in Boys with Attention Deficit Disorder"; *The American Journal of Clinical Nutrition* 62:761, 1995.

Thompson, L. U.; "Effects of Flax Seed on Breast and Colon Cancers"; Department of Nutrition Sciences, University of Toronto, 1991.

Thompson, Lillian, and M. Serraino; "Lignans in Flax Seed and Breast Carcinogenesis"; Department of Nutritional Sciences, University of Toronto, 1989.

Thompson, L. U., D. Robb, M. Serraino, and F. Cheung; "Mammalian Lignan Production from Various Foods"; *Nutrition and Cancer* 16:43-52, 1991.

Am. J. Clin. Nutr. 59(6) :1304-09, 1994.

Carcinogens 17(6):1343-48, 1996.

J. Am. Soc. Nephrol. 5(3):487, 1994.

Kidney Int. 48(2):475-80, 1995.

Nutrition Science News, Vol. 2, No. 7, July 1997.

Prostaglandins Lekot Essent. Fatty Acids 54(6):451-55, 1996.

Chapter 7: Soybeans Protect Against Breast Cancer

Aldercreutz, H., R. Heikkinen, M. Woods, et al.; "Excretion of the Lignans Enterolactone and Enterodiol and of Equol in Omniverous and Vegetarian Postmenopausal Women and in Women with Breast Cancer"; *The Lancet*, December 1 1, 1982, p. 1295-1299.

Angier, Natalie; "New Respect for Estrogen's Influence"; *New York Times*, June 24, 1997.

Avila, Raphael; "The Super Isoflavones"; *Energy Times*, February 1997.

Baggott, J. E., T. Ha, W. H. Vaughn, et al.; "Effect of Miso (Japanese Soy Bean Paste) and NaCl on DMBA-Induced Rat Mammary Tumors"; *Nutrition and Cancer* 14:103-109, 1990.

Barnes, S., C. Grubbs, K. D. R. Setchell, and J. Carlson; "Soy Beans Inhibit Mammary Tumors in Models of Breast Cancer"; *Mutagens and Carcinogens in the Diet*, 1990, p. 239-253.

Barnes, S.; "Effect of Genistein on *In Vitro* and *In Vivo* Models of Cancer"; *Journal of Nutrition* 125:77S-83S, 1995.

Brylawaki, R.; "Tofu Chic: The Role of Soy Beans in Breast Cancer Prevention"; *Oncology Times* 14, July 1990.

Coward, L., N. C. Barnes, K. D. R. Setchell, and S. Barnes; "Genistein, Daidzein, and Their Beta-Glycoside Conjugates: Anti-tumor Isoflavones in Soy Bean Foods from American and Asian Diets"; *Journal of Agriculture and Food Chemistry* 41(11):1961-67, 1993.

"Foods That May Prevent Breast Cancer: Studies Are Investigating Soy Beans,

Whole Wheat, and Green Tea, Among Others"; *Primary Care and Cancer*; 14(2):10-11, 1994.

Fotsis, T., M. Pepper, H. Aldercreutz, et al.; "Genistein, a Dietary Derived Inhibitor of *In Vitro* Angiogenesis"; *Proceedings of the National Academy of Sciences USA* 90:2690-2694, 1993.

Franke, A. A., L. J. Custer, C. M. Cerna, and K. K. Narula; "Quantitation of Phytoestrogens in Legumes by HPLC"; *Journal of Agriculture and Food Chemistry* 42:1905-13, 1994.

Goodwin, Liza; "Soy to the World"; *Mirabella*, July-August 1997.

Getchell, K.; "The Role of Soy Products in Reducing Risk of Cancer"; *Journal of the National Cancer Institute* 83:8, 1991.

Herman, C., H. Aldercreutz, and B. R. Goldin; "Soy Bean Phytoestrogen Intake and Cancer Risk"; *Journal of Nutrition* 125:7575-7705, 1995.

Klatz, Ronald and Robert Goldman; "The Soybean Solution to Aging"; *Total Health* Vol. 19, No. 4, December 1997.

Lee, H. P., I. Gourley, S. W. Duffy, J. Esteve, J. Lee, and N. E. Duy; "Dietary Effects on Breast Cancer Risk in Singapore"; *The Lancet* 2:1197-1200, 1991.

Messina, M., and S. Barnes; "The Role of Soy Products in Reducing Risk of Cancer"; *Journal of the National Cancer Institute* 83:541-546, 1991.

Moltreni, A., L. Brizio-Moltreni, and V. Persky; *"In vitro* Hormonal Effects of Soy bean Isoflavones"; *Journal of Nutrition* 15:7515-7565, 1995.

Mulligan, Patti Tviet; "Experience the Powerful Benefits of Soy," *Health Counselor*, August-September 1997.

Thompson, L. U., and L. Zhang; "Physic Acid and Minerals: Effects on Early Markers of Risk for Mammary and Colon Carcinogenesis"; *Carcinogenesis* 12(11):1041, 1991.

Weed, Susun; *Breast Cancer? Breast Health! The Wise Woman Way*; Ashtree Publishing (Woodstock, NY), 1996.

Zara, David T.; *Nutrition and Cancer* 27:31-40, 1997.

New England Journal of Medicine 333(6):276-82, August 3, 1995.

Women's Health Advocate Newsletter, Vol. 3, No. 12, February 1997.

Chapter 8: Nutrient-Dense Green Vegetables Protective and Cleansing

Brody, Jane; "How to Feel Fitter, Eat Better, Live Longer"; *The New York Times Book of Health*, with reporters of the *New York Times; New York Times* Books, (NY), 1997.

Carper, Jean; *Food, Your Miracle Medicine*; Harper Perennial (New York), 1993.

Weed, Susun; *Breast Cancer? Breast Health! The Wise Woman Way*; Ashtree Publishing (Woodstock, NY), 1996.

Zhang, Yuesheng; "A Major Inducer of Anticarcinogenic Protective Enzymes From Broccoli: Isolation and Elucidation of Structure"; *Proceedings of the National Academy of Sciences USA* 89:2399-2403, 1992.

Chapter 9: The Hidden Power of Plant Foods

"Antitumor Effect by a Hot Water Extract of Chlorella vulgaris (CE) Resistance to Meth-A Tumor Growth Mediated CE-Induced Polymorphonuclear Leukocytes"; *Cancer, Immunology, Immunotherapy*; Department of Immunology, Kyoshu University, Japan, 1985.

"Astragalus Is Currently Under Investigation as an Adjunct for Cancer Therapy." *Women's Health Advocate*, December 1996.

"Augmentation of Antitumor Resistance by a Strain of Unicellular Green Algae, *Chlorella vulgariis*"; *Cancer, Immunology, Immunotherapy*; Department of Immunology, Kyoshu University, Japan, Spring 1984.

Brendstrup, Eva, and Laila Launso; "An Unconventional Cancer Treatment Model: A Research Project"; *Townsend Letter for Doctors and Patients*, July 1997.

Brenner et al.; "The Antiproliferative Effect of Vitamin D Analogs on MCF-Human Breast Cancer Cells; *Cancer Letter* 92(1):77-82, 1995.

Bresnick, G.; "Reduction in Mammary Tumorigenesis in the Rat by Cabbage and Cabbage Residue"; *Carcinogenesis* 11(7):1159-1163, 1990.

Byers, T., and C,. Perry; "Dietary Carotenes, Vitamin C, and Vitamin E as Protective Antioxidants in Human Cancers"; *Annual Review of Nutrition* 12:139-59, 1992.

Chasseaud, L. F; "The Role of GSH and GSH S-Transferases in the Metabolism of Chemical Carcinogens and Other Electrophotic Agents"; *Advances in Cancer Research*, Vol. 29, pp. 176-244, 1975.

"Co-Enzyme Q10 (CoQ10) as a Treatment for Breast Cancer;" *Alternative Medicine Review*, Vol. 2, No. 1, 1997.

Crayhon, Robert; "Chlorella"; Total Health Magazine, August 1996.

Cuskelly, G., et al.; "Effects of Increasing Dietary Folate on Red Cell Folate: Implications for Prevention of Neural Tube Defects"; *The Lancet* 347:657-9, 1996.

Dimitrov et al.; "Some Aspects of Vitamin E Related to Humans and Breast Cancer Prevention"; *Advances in Experimental Medicine and Biology* 364:119-27, 1994.

Diplock, Anthony T.; "Antioxidant Nutrients and Disease Prevention: An Overview"; *American Journal of Clinical Nutrition* Vol. 53 (Supplement), pp. 1895-1935, 1991.

"Food, Nutrition, and the Prevention of Cancer: A Global Perspective"; American Institute for Cancer Research and the World Cancer Research Fund, December 1997.

Forman, Henry, Jay Rui-MingLiu, and Michael Ming Shi; "Glutathione Synthesis in Oxidative Stress"; in *Biothiols in Health and Disease* (Lester Packer and Enrique Cadenas, eds.), Martin Decker, (New York), 1995.

Gregus, Z., et al.; "Effect of Lipoic Acid on Biliary Excretion of Glutathione and Metals"; *Toxicology and Applied Pharmacology*, Vol. 14, No. 1, pp. 88-96, May 1992.

Haynes, Joan; "Coenzyme Q10 and Breast Cancer"; *Townsend Letter for Doctors and Patients*, August-September 1997.

Hobbs, Christopher; *Foundations of Health: Healing with Herbs and Foods*; Botanica Press, (Santa Cruz, CA), 1992.

"Immunomodulation of a Unicellular Green Algae (Chlorella pyrenoidosa) in Tumor-Bearing Mice"; *Journal of Ethnopharmacology* 24:135-146, 1988.

Jain, M., et al.; "Premorbid Diet and the Prognosis of Women with Breast Cancer"; *Journal of the National Cancer Institute* 86(18)1390-97, 1994.

Katsouyanni, K., D. Trichopoulos, P. Boyle, et al.; "Diet and Breast Cancer. A Case-Control Study in Greece"; *International Journal of Cancer* 38:815-20, 1986.

Lockwood et al.; "Partial and Complete Regression of Breast Cancer in Patients in Relation to Dosage of Co-Enzyme Q10"; *Biochemistry Biophysics Research Communications* 199(3):1504-8, 1994.

Mangels, A. R., J. M. Holden, G. R. Beecher, M. R. Forman, and E. Lanza; "Carotenoid Content of Fruits and Vegetables: An Evaluation of Analytic Data"; *Journal of the American Dietary Association* 93:284-96, 1993.

Meister, Acton; "Strategies for Increasing Cellular Glutathione"; In: *Biothiols in Health and Disease* (Lester Packer and Enrique Cadenas, eds.); Martin Decker (New York City), 1995.

Michnovicz, Jon J., *How To Reduce Your Risk of Breast Cancer* (written with Diane S. Klein), Warner Books (New York), 1994.

"Oral Administration of *Chlorella vulgaris* Augments Concomitant Antitumor Immunity"; *Immunopharmacology and Immunotoxicology* 12(2):277-291, 1990

Passwater, Richard; *Lipoic Acid: The Metabolic Antioxidant*; Keats Publishing (New Canaan, CT), 1996.

Passwater, Richard; *Selenium as Food and Medicine*, Keats Publishing (New Canaan, CT), 1981.

Pressman, Alan H., and Sheila Buff; *The GSH Phenomenon: Nature's Most Powerful Antioxidant and Healing Agent*, St. Martin's Press (New York), 1997.

Raloff, J.; "Folate Supplements Needed But Allergenic"; and "Major Antioxidant Supplement Goes Bust"; *The National Council Against Health Fraud Newsletter*, Vol. 13, No. 1, January-February 1996.

"The Consumption of Seaweed as a Protective Factor in the Etiology of Breast Cancer"; *Medical Hypothesis*; 1981.

"The Effect of Dietary Seaweeds on 7,12-Dimethyl-Benz[a] Anthracene-Induced Mammary Tumorigenesis in Rats"; *Cancer Letters* 35:109-18, 1987.

Schardt, David; "Phytochernicals: Plants Against Cancer"; *Nutrition Action Healthletter*, pp. 1-4, April 1994.

Schwitters, Bert (in collaboration with Professor Jack Masquellier); *OPC's in Practice: The Hidden Story of Proanthocyanidins, Nature's Most Powerful and Patented Antioxidant*; published by Alpha Omega Editrice, Via San Damaso 23, 00165 Roma, Italy, 1995.

Sharoni, Y., et al.; "Effects of Lycopene Enriched Tomato Oleoresin on 7,12-dimethyl-benz(1)anthracene-Induced Rat Mammary Tumors"; *Cancer Detect. Prey* 21(2):118-123, 1997.

Sheck, Jack; "Nutrition and Health"; *Explore More!* No. 16, 1996.

Valenzula, A., M. Aspillaga, S. Vial, and R. Guerra; "Selectivity of Silymarin on the Increase of the Glutathione Content in Different Tissues of the Rat"; *Planta Med.* 55:420-2, 1989.

Whitaker, Julian; *Health and Healing Newsletter*; Phillips Publishing Inc., February 1997.

Wood, A. W., M. T. Huang, R.L. Chang et al.; "Inhibition of the Mutagenicity of Bay-Region Diol Epoxides of Polycyclic Hydrocarbons by Naturally Occuring Plant Phenols: Exceptional Activity of Ellagic Acid"; *Proceedings of the National Academy of Science USA* 79:5513, 1982.

Journal of Nutrition, Vol. 127, No. 3, p. 544-48(S), 1997.

Chapter 10: Herbs, Spices, and Mushrooms: Potent Enhancers of Flavor and Health

"Asian Spice May Help Fight Cancer"; *Energy Times*; February 1997.

Cichoke, A. J.; "Maitake: The King of Mushrooms"; *Townsend Letter for Doctors*, 432-433, May 1994.

Dolby, Victoria; "An Important Extract from Maitake Mushrooms Is an Important AntiCancer Agent"; *Better Nutrition*, March 1997.

Dorant, E., P. A. van der Brandt, R. A. Goldbohm, et al.; "Garlic and Its Significance for the Prevention of Cancer in Humans: A Critical View"; *British Journal of Cancer* 67:424-9, 1993.

Fortes, Cristina, and Francesco Forastiere; "Correspondence Re: Consumption of Olive Oil and Specific Food Groups in Relation to Breast Cancer Risk in Greece"; *Journal of the National Cancer Institute*, Vol. 87, No. 13, 1995.

Geng, Z. H. and B. H. S. Lav; *Phytotherapy Research* 11:54-6, 1997.

Hiroaki, Nanba; "Results of Non-Controlled Clinical Study for Various Cancer Patients Using Maitake D-Fraction"; *Explore!* (6)5, 1995.

Mukunden, M. A., M. C. Chacko, et al.; "Effect of Turmeric and Curcumin on BP-DNA Adducts"; *Carcinogenesis* 14:493–96, 1993.

"Mutagenesis"; *Journal of the American College of Nutrition* 13:7; 1992.

Wagner, V. H., A. Proksch, L. Riess-Maurer, et al.; "Immunostimulating Polysaccharides (Heteroglycans) of Higher Plants"; *Arzneim-Forsch* 35:1068-75, 1985.

Werbach, M. D., and N. D. Murray; "Curcuminoid Phenols in Turmeric May Protect Against Cancer"; *Journal of Ethnopharmacology*, Vol. 47, 1995, *Botanical Influences on Illness*.

Nutrition Science News, Vol. 2, No. 7, July 1997.

Chapter 11: Food, Hormones and Breast Cancer: What's the Connection?

"A Study Hints at Cancer Risk in Heart Drug"; *New York Times*, October 16, 1997.

Anderson-Parrado, Patricia; "Phytoestrogens Put up a Strong 'Fight' Against Menopause, Cancer"; *Better Nutrition*, October 1996.

Angier, Natalie; "New Respect for Estrogen's Influence"; *New York Times*, June 24, 1997.

Arditti and Schrieber; "The Environmental Connection," *Sojourner*, December 29, 1996.

Austin, Steve, and Cathy Hitchkock; *Breast Cancer: What You Should Know (But May Not Be Told) About Prevention, Diagnosis, and Treatment"*; Prima Publishing, (Rocklin, CA) 1994.

Beckham, N.; "Phytoestrogens and Compounds That Affect Estrogen Metabolism"; *Australian Journal of Medical Herbalism*, Vol. 7 (1), 1995.

"Breast Cancer: Environmental Factors," *The Lancet*, p. 904. October 10, 1992.

"Breast Cancer and Pesticides"; *Soil and Health*; January 1994.

Brody, Jane; "New Clues on Balancing Risks of Hormones After Menopause"; *New York Times*, June 11, 1997.

Cassidy, A., et al.; "Biological Effects of a Diet of Soy Protein Rich in Isoflavones on the Menopausal Cycle of Premenopausal Women"; *American Journal of Clinical Nutrition* 60: 333-340, 1990.

Cowan, L. D., et al.; "Breast Cancer Incidence in Women with a History of Progesterone Deficiency"; *American Journal of Epidemiology* 114:209, 217, 1981.

"Dietary Modification Can Reduce Estrogen Levels in the Body"; *Journal of the National Cancer Institute*, October 12, 1996.

"Early Puberty Onset Seems Prevalent," *New York Times*; April 9, 1997.

"EcoCancers"; *Science News*, July 3, 1993 (10013).

"Editorial: Postmenopausal Hormone Replacement Therapy—Time for a Reappraisal?"; *New England Journal of Medicine*; 336, June 19, 1997.

Ekborm, A., D. Trichopoulos, H. O. Adami, C. C. Hsieh, and S. J. Lan; "Evidence of Prenatal Influences on Breast Cancer Risk"; *The Lancet* 340:1015-1018, 1992.

Follingstad, Alvin H.; "Estriol, the Forgotten Estrogen?"; *Journal of the American Medical Association*, January 2, 1978.

Foltz-Gray, Dorothy; "The Miracle of the Loaves"; *Health Magazine*, October 1997.

Franceschi, Silvia, Adriano Favero, Adriano Decarlo, Eva Negri, Carlo La Vecchio, Monica Ferraroni, Antonio Russo, Simonetta Salvini, Dino Amadori, Ettore Conti, Maurizio Montella, and Attilio Giacosa; "Intake of Macronutrients and Risk of Breast Cancer"; *The Lancet*, Vol. 347(9012), p. 1351(6), May 18, 1996.

Gittleman, Ann Louise, M.S., C.N.S.; "Low-down on Fiber"; *Total Health Magazine*, Vol. 19, No. 5, January 1998.

Glasier, A., and A. S. McNeilly; "Physiology of Lactation"; *Bailliere's Clinical Endocrinology and Metabolism* 4:379-97, 1990.

Goldin, B. R. et al.; "The Relationship Between Estrogen Levels and Diets of Caucasian American and Oriental Immigrant Women"; *American Journal of Clinical Nutrition* 44:945-53, 1986.

Graham, Linda Carol; "Do You Have a Hormone Shortage?"; *Redbook*, February 1989.

Griffiths, J.; "New Osteoporosis Treatment: Progesterone Reported to Increase Bone Density 10% in Six Months"; *Medical Tribune*, p. 1, November 29, 1990.

Grodstein, Francine, Meier J. Stampfer, Graham A. Colditz, et al.; "Postmenopausal Hormone Therapy and Mortality"; *New England Journal of Medicine* 336:1769-1775, June 19, 1997.

Hargrove, Joel; *Infertility and Reproductive Medicine Clinics of North America*, October 1995, Vol. 6, No. 4.

Jordan, V. C., M. H. Jeng, et al.; "The Estrogenic Activity of Synthetic Progestins Used in Oral Contraceptives"; *Cancer* 71: 1501-1505, 1993.

Key, T. K. A. and M. C. Pike; "The Role of Oestrogens and Progestogens in the Epidemiology and Prevention of Breast Cancer"; *European Journal of Cancer and Clinical Oncology*, 24(1): 29-43, 1988.

"Kids Eat More Calories and Exercise Less"; *USA Today*, March 7, 1997.

Kirschmann, Gayla J. and John D. Kirschmann; *Nutrition Almanac*, Fourth Edition, McGraw-Hill (New York), 1996.

Kolata, Gina; "Study Discounts DDT Role in Breast Cancer"; *New York Times*, October 30, 1997.

Lee, John R.; "Is Natural Progesterone the Missing Link in Osteoporosis Prevention and Treatment?" *Medical Hypothesis* 35:316-318, 1991.

Lee, John R.; *Natural Progesterone, The Multiple Roles of a Remarkable Hormone*; BLL Publishing (Sebastapol, CA), 1993.

Lee, John R.; "Osteoperosis Reversal: The Role of Progesterone"; *International Clinical Review* 3:384-91 1990.

McCully, Kilmer; *The Homocysteine Revolution*, Keats Publishing (New Canaan, CT), 1997.

Marchant, D. J.; "Supplemental Estrogen Replacement"; *Cancer* 75:512-17; 1994.

Mauvis-Jarvis, et al.; "Antiestrogen Action of Progesterone in Breast Tissue"; *Hormone Res.*, 28:212-218, 1987.

Merzenich, H., H. Boeing, and J. Wahrendorf; "Dietary Fat and Sports Activity as Determinants for Age at Menarche"; *American Journal of Epidemiology* 138:217-24, 1993.

Michnovicz, J. J., and H. L. Bradlow; "Altered Estrogen Metabolism and Excretion in Humans Following Consumption of Indole-3-Carbinol"; *Nutritional Cancer* 16:59-66, 1991.

Mohr, P. E., et al.; "Serum Progesterone and Prognosis in Operable Breast Cancer"; *British Journal of Cancer*, 1996.

Murase, Y., and Lishma, H.; "Clinical Studies of Oral Administration of Gamma-ory-zanol on Climacteric Complaints and Its Syndrome"; *Ostetrics and Gynecology Proceedings* 12(5):147-9, 1963.

Northrup, Christiane, M.D.; *Health Wisdom for Women* newsletter, January 1998.

Northrup, Christiane; "Is Progesterone Good for Your Breasts?"; *Health Wisdom for Women Newsletter*. Vol. 4, No. 12, December 1997.

"Oral Contraceptive Use and Breast Cancer Risk in Young Women"; *The Lancet*; pp. 973–982, 1989).

Paulsen, Monte; "Women with Breast Cancer Have Been Found to Have High Levels of DDT, Dioxin, PCB, DDE and Other Pesticides in Their Fatty Tissue in Numerous Studies"; as reported by the *Detroit Press*, May 1993 .

Peat, Raymond,; *Progesterone in Orthomolecular Medicine*, Kenogen (P.O. Box 5764, Eugene, Oregon 97405, 503-345-9855).

Pelton, Ross, Taffy Clarke Pelton, and Vinton C. Vint; *How to Prevent Breast*

Cancer: A Lifestyle Guide for the Prevention of Breast Cancer and Its Recurrence with an Investigation of the Critical Risk Factors; Fireside Publishing (New York), 1995.

Pitchford, Paul; *Healing with Whole Foods Oriental Traditions and Modern Nutrition* North Atlantic Books, (Berkeley, CA), Chap. 10, p. 142, 1993.

Reaney, Patricia; "Research Shows HRT Increases Breast Cancer Risk"; Reuter News Service, October 10, 1997.

Sahelian, Ray; "Hormone Update: Melatonin Found to Inhibit Breast Cancer Growth"; *Health Counselor,* Vol. 9, No. 1.

Setchell, K. D. R., and H. Adlercreutz; "Mammalian Lignans and Phytoestrogens: Recent Studies on Their Formation, Metabolism, and Biological Role in Health and Disease." In *Role of Gut Flora in Toxicology and Cancer,* I. R. Rowland (ed.), *Academic Press,* London, pp. 315-343, 1988.

Stanford, J. L., and D. B. Thomas; "Exogenous Progestins and Breast Cancer"; *Epidemiologic Reviews* 15:98-107, 1993.

Tavani, A., et al., "Margarine Intake and Risk of Nonfatal Acute Myocardial Infarction in Italian Women"; *European Journal of Clinical Nutrition* 51:30-2, 1997.

Thompson, L. U., et al.; "Mammalian Lignan Production from Various Foods"; *Nutrition and Cancer* 16:43-52, 1991.

Tretli, S.; "Height and Weight in Relation to Breast Cancer Morbidity and Mortality: A Prospective Study of 570,000 Women in Norway"; *International Journal of Cancer* 44:23-30, 1989.

Trichopoulos, D.; "Hypothesis: Does Breast Cancer Originate In Utero?"; *The Lancet* 335:939-940, 1990.

Ullman, Dana, M. P. H.; *The Consumer's Guide to Homeopathy,* J. P. Tarcher, 1996.

Walker, A.; "Osteoporosis and Calcium Deficiency"; *American Journal of Clinical Nutrition* 16:327, 1965.

Wang, X., B. Guyer, and D. M. Paige; "Differences in Gestational Age-Specific Birthweight Among Chinese, Japanese, and White Americans"; *International Journal of Epidemiology* 23:119-128, 1994.

Werbach, Melryn R.; *Foundations of Natural Medicine: A Source Book of Clinical Research* Third Line Press, 1997.

Widhalm, K., J. Leibertseder, and M. Bavernfried; "Over- and Undernutrition in Europe"; Presentation by the Austrian Nutrition Society at the Seventh European Nutrition Conference, May 1995.

Wolf, B. M.; "Potential Role of Raising Dietary Protein Intake for Reducing Risk of Atherosclerosis"; *Canadian Journal of Cardiology* 11 (Supplement G): l27G-131G, 1995.

Yoo, K. Y., K. Tajima, et al.; "Independent Protective Effect of Lactation Against Breast Cancer—A Case-Control Study"; *American Journal of Epidemiology* 135:726-33, 1992.

Australian Journal of Medical Herbalism 7:1, 11-16, 1995.

European Journal of Cancer 28A(4/5):784-8, 1992

Gallagher Report, January 28, 1985.

Journal of the National Cancer Institute 83:541-6, 1991.

Life Sciences 18(54):1299-1303, 1994.

Time Magazine, May 26, 1997, from a study in the *New England Journal of Medicine*.
Townsend Letter for Doctors and Patients, August/September 1997.
Tufts Univ. Health and Nutr. Letter, April 17, 1997.
Science, June 7, 1996.
Science News 144:266-7, April 25, 1992.
Self Magazine, January 1997.
Women's Health Advocate, January 1996.
Your Health Magazine, May 27, 1997.

Chapter 12: Preventing Carbohydrate Overload: A New Equation for Health

"Benefits Found in Asian Fish Diet"; *New York Times*, July 4, 1997.

"Benzo(a)pyrene and Other Polynuclear Hydrocarbons in Charcoal-Broiled Meat"; *Science*, Vol. 145, July 1964.

Carper, Jean; *Food, Your Miracle Medicine*; Harper Perennial (New York), 1993.

"Clinical Debate: Should a Low-Fat, High-Carbohydrate Diet Be Recommended for Everyone?"; *New England Journal of Medicine*, August 21, 1997.

Cobias, L., et al.; "Lipid Lipoprotein and Hemostatic Effects of Fish vs. Fish Oil W-3 Fatty Acids in Mildly Hyperlipidemic Males"; *American Journal of Clinical Nutrition* 53:1210-16, 1991.

Crayhon, Robert; *Nutrition Made Simple*. Evans (New York), 1994.

Foltz-Gray, Dorothy; "The Miracle of the Loaves"; *Health*, October 1997.

Franceschi, Silvia, Adriano Favero, Adriano DeCarlo, Eva Negri, Carlo La Vecchia, Monica Ferraroni, Antonio Russo, Simonetta Salvini, Dino Amadori, Ettore Conti, Maurizio Montella, and Attilio Giacosa; "Intake of Macronutrients and Risk of Breast Cancer"; *The Lancet*, Vol. 347(9012), p. 1351(6), May 18, 1996.

Gittleman, Ann Louise; "The 40/30/30 Plan: Super Nutrition for the Next Millennium"; *Total Health*, Vol. 19, No. 3, pp. 55-57, 1997.

Hardman et al, "A High Fish Oil Diet Supplemented with Ferric Citrate. Safely Inhibits Primary and Metastatic Human Breast Carcinoma Growth in Nude Mice"; *Proceedings of the Annual Meeting, American Association of Cancer Research*; 36:679, 1993.

Hill, Michael J., ed.; *Epidemiology of Diet and Cancer*, Ellis Horwood Publishers, 1994.

Jeppesen, J., et al.; "Effects of Low-Fat, High Carbohydrate Diets on Risk Factors for Ischemic Heart Disease in Postmenopausal Women"; *American Journal of Clinical Nutrition* 65:1027-33, 1997.

Kaizer, et al.; "Fish Consumption and Breast Cancer Risk"; *Nutrition and Cancer* 12:6166, 1989.

Karmali, R. A.; "Omega-3 Fatty Acids and Cancer"; *Journal of Internal Medicine* 225 (Suppl. 1, 1989):197-200.

Kirschmann, Gayla J., and John D. Kirschmann; *Nutrition Almanac (Fourth Edition)*, McGraw-Hill (New York), 1996.

La Vecchia, C., E. Negri, A. DeCarlo, B. D'Avanzo, and S. Franceschi; "A Case Control Study of Diet and Gastric Cancer in Northern Italy"; *International Journal of Cancer*, 40:484-489, 1992.

Lee, H. P.; "Dietary Effects on Breast Cancer Risk in Singapore"; *The Lancet* 337:1197-1200, 1991.

Reaven, G. M.; "Role of Insulin Resistance in Human Disease"; *Diabetes* 37:1595-1607, 1988.

Wu, D., S. N. Meydani, M. Meydani, M. G. Hayek, P. Huth, and R. J. Nicolosi; "Immunologic Effects of Marine- and Plant-Derived N-3 Polyunsaturated Fatty Acids in Nonhuman Primates"; *American Journal of Clinical Nutrition* 63:273-280, 1996.

American Journal of Clinical Nutrition 62:621-32, 1995.

Gallagher Report, January 28, 1985.

Nutrition Review 54(4):5-169-75, 1996.

Nutrition, Diet and Cancer '82, National Academy of Sciences (Washington, D.C.), 1982.

Chapter 13: Rejuvenating Your Immune and Lymphatic Systems: What You Can Do Now

"Antitrans-forming Activity of Chlorophyllin Against Selected Carcinogens and Complex Mixtures"; *Teratogenesis, Carcinogenesis, and Mutagenesis* 14:75-81, 1994.

Bardychev et al.; "Acupuncture in Edema of the Extremeties Following Radiation or Combination Therapy of Cancer of the Breast and Uterus"; *Vopr. Onkol.* 34, No. 3:319-22, 1988.

Cayce, Edgar, and B. Ernest Frejer; *The Edgar Cayce Companion*, A. R. E. Press, (Virginia Beach, VA), 1995.

"Chemoprotective Properties of Chlorophyllin Against Vinyl Carbamate P-Nitrophenyl Vinyl Ether and Their Electrophilic Epoxides" ; *Cancer Letters* 94:33-40, 1995.

"Detoxification of Chlorodecone Poisoned Rats with Chlorella and Chlorella Derived Sporopollenin"; *Drug and Chemical Toxicology* 7(1):57-71, 1984.

"Dietary Chlorophyllin Is a Potent Inhibitor of Aflatoxin B1 Hepatocarcinogenesis in Rainbow Trout"; *Oregon Technical Paper* #10,505, Department of Food Science and Technology (V.B.J.H.D.A.G.B.) and Statistics (C.P.), Oregon Agriculture Experiment Station, Oregon State University, Corvallis, OR 97331, November 1, 1994.

Dwivedi, C., et al.; "Effect of Calcium Glucarate on B-gluuronidase Activity and Glucarate content of Certain Vegetables and Fruits"; *Biochem. Med. Metabol. Biol.* 1940:43-83, 1992.

Foster, Steven; "Milk Thistle: We Need This Weed!"; *Better Nutrition*, October 1997.

"Herbs to Keep Your Breasts Healthy"; *Vegetarian Times*, July 1997.

Hobbs, Christopher; *Foundations of Health: Healing with Herbs and Foods*, Botanica Press (Santa Cruz, CA), 1992.

"Inhibition of 2-Amino-3-Methylimidazo (4,5-F) Quinoline (Q)-DNA Finding in

Rats Given Chlorophyllin: Dose Response and Time Course Studies in the Liver and Colon"; *Carcinogenesis*, Vol. 13, No. 4, pp. 763-766, 1994.

Moore, M.; *Medicinal Plants of the Mountain West*, Museum of New Mexico Press (Santa Fe), 1979.

Pressman, Alan H., with Sheila Buff; *The GSH Phenomenon: Nature's Most Powerful Antioxidant and Healing Agent*, St. Martin's Press (New York), 1997.

Roloff, Janet; "Additional Source of Dietary Estrogens"; *Science News*, June 3, 1995.

Roloff, Janet; "Eco Cancers"; *Science News*, October 1993.

Salmi, H. and S. Sarna; "Effect of Silymarin on Chemical, Functional, and Morphological Alterations of the Liver"; *Scandinavian Journal of Gastroenterology* 17:517-21.

Schacter, Michael (of the Schacter Center for Complementary Medicine, Suffern, New York); "The Prevention and Complementary Treatment of Breast Cancer"; lecture presented at the American College for the Advancement in Medicine Meeting, Hyatt Regency Tampa Hotel, Tampa, Florida, April 24, 1997.

Singer, Sydney Ross, and Soma Grismaijer; *Dressed to Kill: The Link Between Bras and Breast Cancer*, Avery Publishing Group (Wayne, NJ), 1995.

Valenzuela, A., M. Aspillaga, S. Vial, R. Guerra; "Selectivity of Silymarin on the Increase of the Glutathione Content in Different Tissues of the Rat"; *Planta Med* 55:420-22, 1985.

Chapter 14: The French Mediterranean Diet: Natural Food at Its Best

Ainsleigh, H. G.; "Beneficial Effects of Sun Exposure on Cancer Mortality"; *Prev. Med.* 22:132-40, 1993.

Aviram, M., and K. Eigs; "Dietary Olive Oil Reduces Low-Density Lipoprotein Uptake by Macrophages and Decreases the Susceptibility of the Lipoprotein to Undergo Lipid Peroxidation"; *Annals of Nutrition and Metabolism* 37:75-89, 1995.

Brody, Jane; "Personal Health, The Nutrient That Reddens Tomatoes Appears to Have Health Benefits"; *New York Times*, March 12, 1997.

Burton, A. C., F. Cornhill; "Correlation of Cancer Death Rates with Altitude and with the Quality of Water Supply of 100 Largest Cities in the U.S."; *Journal Toxicology and Environmental Health* 3:465-478, 1977.

Caranee, W. K. and R. L. White; "The Genetic Basis of Cancer"; *Scientific American*, March 1995, 72-79.

Colston, K. W., et al.; "Possible Role for Vitamin D in Controlling Breast Cancer Cell Proliferation"; *Cancer* 1:188-91, 1989.

Conney Alan; "Designer Foods II"; paper on antioxidants presented at Rutgers Continuing Professional Education in Food Science Course, Piscataway, NJ, March 16–17, 1993.

Fox, Martin; *Healthy Water*; 1990 booklet. (*See* Resource Guide; available from Multipure Corp.)

Franceschi, Silvia, Adriano Favero, Adriano DeCarlo, Eva Negri, Carlo La Vecchia,

Monica Ferraroni, Antonio Russo, Simonetta Salvini, Dino Amadori, Ettore Conti, Maurizio Montella, and Attilio Giacosa; "Intake of Macronutrients and Risk of Breast Cancer"; *The Lancet*, Vol. 347(9012), p. 1351(6), May 18, 1996.

Gopnik, Adam; "Is There a Crisis in French Cooking?"; *The New Yorker*, April 1997.

Grady, Denise; "Study Favors Monounsaturated Fat: Lower Risks Cited for Breast Cancer and Heart Disease"; *New York Times*, January 13, 1998.

Harwood, Skippy; "Author Extols Foods as Preventive Medicine,"; *Palm Beach Post*, April 1997.

Helser, M. A., J. H. Hotchkiss, and D. A. Roe; "Influence of Fruit and Vegetable Juices on the Endogenous Formation of Nitrosoproline and N-nitrosothiazo-lidine4-carboxylic Acid in Humans on Controlled Diets"; *Carcinogenesisis* No. 12, 2277-80, December 1992.

Jenkins, Steve; *Cheese Primer*, Workman Press (New York), 1996.

Karmal, R. A.; "Omega-3 Fatty Acids and Cancer"; *Journal of Internal Medicine* 225 (Suppl. 1, 1989):197-200.

La Vecchia, Carlo, Eva Negri, Silvia Franceschi, Adriano DeCarlo, Attilio Giacosa, and Upworth; "Olive Oil and Breast Cancer Risk in Italy"; *Nutrition Research Newsletter*, Vol. 15, No. 2, p.12(1), February 1996.

Leak, A.; "Cardiovascular Effects of Omega-3 Fatty Acids"; *New England Journal of Medicine* 318:549-557; 1988.

Masquelier, Jack; "Why Wine Keeps the French from Heart Atttacks"; *Townsend Letter for Doctors and Patients*, December 1996.

O'Neill, Molly; "Living Dangerously"; *New York Times Magazine*, May 11, 1997.

Passwater, Richard A.; *Lipoic Acid: The Metabolic Antioxidant*; Good Health Guide, Keats (New Canaan, CT), 1996.

"Queen-Making Substance"; *Science News* December 15, 1962.

"Rutin Helps Repair Genes, Prevent Early Stages of Cancer"; *The Nutrition Reporter*, Vol, 8. No 3, 1997.

Richardson, S., and M. Gerber; "Nutritional Factors and Breast Cancer. A Case-Control Study in a French Mediterranean Region." In: *Epidemiology of Diet and Cancer* (M. J., Hill, A. Giacosa, P. J., Caygill, eds.), Ellis Horwood,(Chichester, UK), pp. 353-377 1994.

Richardson, S., M. Gerber, et al.; "The Role of Fat, Animal Protein, and Some Vitamin Consumption in Breast Cancer: A Case Control Study in Southern France"; *International Journal of Cancer* 48:1-9, 1991.

Salaman, Maureen, and James F. Scherr; *Foods That Heal*; MKS Publications, Menlo Park, Calif. 1989.

Sauer, H. A., "Relationship of Water to Risk of Dying." In: D. X. Manners (ed.) *International Water Quality Symposium: Water, Its Effects on Life, Quality*; Water Quality Research Council, (Washington, D.C.), pp. 76-79, 1974.

Save, W., et al.; "Dietary Omega 3 Polyunsaturated Fats and Breast Cancer"; *Supplement to Nutrition* 12:1, 1996.

"Study Hints at Cancer Peril in Chlorination"; *New York Times*, June 18, 1997.

"The Fat With the Power to Heal"; *Your Health*, January 1997.

"The Fat You Don't Know About."; Nutrition Update, *American Health*, March 1997.

Trichopoulou, Antonia, Klea Katsoyanni, Sherri Stuver, Lia Tzala, Charalambox Gnardellis, Eric Rimm, Dimitrios Trichopoulos; "Consumption of Olive Oil and Specific Food Groups in Relation to Breast Cancer Risk in Greece"; *Journal of the National Cancer Institute*, Vol. 87, No. 2, January 18, 1995.

Trichopoulou, Antonia; "Editorial: Olive Oil and Breast Cancer"; *Cancer Causes and Control*, Vol. 6, p. 475, 1995.

"Up Your Fish Intake for PMS Relief"; *The Natural Way*, January– February 1997.

"Up Your Intake of Oil-Rich Fish to Prevent Depression"; *Living Fit*, January-February 1997.

Winter, Ruth; *A Consumer's Guide to Medicine in Food*; Crown (New York), p. 59, 1995.

American Heart Association Report, Summer 1997. Leading scientific authorities call into question population-wide limits on egg consumption.

American Journal of Clinical Nutrition 61:549-554, 1995.

Wolk, Alicia et al.; "A Prospective Study of Association of Monounsaturated Fat and Other Fat with Risk of Breast Cancer"; *Archives of Internal Medicine*, January 12, 1998.

Women's Health Advocate; June 1996; on fish oil, heart disease and arthritis.

Chapter 15: Alcohol, Coffee, and Sugar

Boyle, C. A., G. S. Berkowitz, V. S. LiVolsi, et al.; "Caffeine Consumption and Fibrocystic Breast Disease: A Case Control Epidemiologic Study;" *Journal of the National Cancer Institute* 72:1015-1019, 1984.

Bernstein, J., S. Alpert, K. Nauss, and R. Suskind, "Depression of Lymphocyte Transformation Following Oral Glucose Ingestion"; *AM/CLN Nutrition* 30:613, 1977.

Carper, Jean; *Food, Your Miracle Medicine*; Harper Perennial (New York), 1 993.

Carroll; "Dietary Factors in Hormone-Dependent Cancers" *Current Concepts in Nutrition*, Vol. 6 of *Nutrition and Cancer*, Wiley and Sons (New York), 1992.

Crayhon, Robert; "Maximizing Bone Health"; *Total Health Magazine*, Vol. 19, No. 4, 1997.

Ferratoni, M., A. DeCarli, W. C. Willett, et al.; "Alcohol and Breast Cancer Risk: A Case-Control Study from Northern Italy"; *International Journal of Epidemiol.* 20.859-864, 1991.

Franceschi, Silvia, Adriano Favero, Adriano DeCarlo, Eva Negri, Carlo La Vecchia, Monica Ferraroni, Antonio Russo, Simonetta Salvini, Dino Amadori, Ettore Conti, Maurizio Montella, and Attilio Giacosa; "Intake of Macronutrients and Risk of Breast Cancer"; *The Lancet*, Vol. 347(9012), p. 1351(6), May 18, 1996.

Graham, S.; "Editorial: Alcohol and Breast Cancer"; *New England Journal of Medicine* 316(19):1211-13, 1987.

Lee, Laura; Interviews with Nancy Appleton; *Townsend Letter for Doctors and Patients*; May 1997.

Levi, et al.; "Dietary Factors and Breast Cancer Risk in Vaud, Switzerland"; *Nutrition and Cancer* 19(3):327-35, 1993.

Lowenfels, A. B.; "Alcohol and Breast Cancer (Correspondence)"; *The Lancet* 335:1216, 1990.

Lubin, F.; "Consumption of Methylxanthine-Containing Beverages and the Risk of Breast Cancer"; *Cancer Letter* 53 (2-3):81-90.

Minton, J. P., H. Abou-Issa, N. Reiches, and J. M. Roseman; "Clinical and Biochemical Studies on Methylxanthine-Related Fibrocystic Breast Disease;" *Surgery*, 90:299-304, 1981.

Northrup, Christiane; *Health Wisdom for Women*, Vol. 4, No. 11, November 1997.

Richardon, S., I. DeVincenzi, H. Pujol et al.; "Alcohol Consumption in a Case-Control Study of Breast Cancer in Southern France"; *International Journal of Cancer* 44:84-89, 1989.

Roberts, H.J., M.D., FACP, FCCP; "Aspartame and Hyperthyroidism: A Presidential Affliction Reconsidered"; *Townsend Letter for Doctors and Patients*, May 1997.

Roberts, H.J.; "Complications Associated With Aspartame (NutraSweet) in Diabetics"; *Clinical Research* 36:349A, 1988.

Rosenberg, L., L..S. Metzger, and J.R. Palmer; "Alcohol Consumption and Risk of Breast Cancer: A Review of the Epidemiologic Evidence"; *Epidemiology Review* 15:133-144, 1993.

Seely, S. and D F. Horrobin; "Diet and Breast Cancer: The Possible Connection With Sugar Consumption"; *Medical Hypothesis* 11(3):319-27, 1983.

Stacey, Michelle; "The Fall and Rise of Kilmer McCully"; *The New York Times Sunday Magazine*, August 10, 1997.

Tufts University Diet and Nutrition Letter, December 1996

Tufts University Health and Nutrition Letter, March 1997; "Research Update: Hip Way to Brew Coffee Not so Cool."

Welsch, C. W. et al.; "Caffeine (1,3,n-trimethylxanthine), a Temperature Promoter of DMBA-Induced Rat Mammary Gland Carcinogenesis"; *International Journal of Cancer* 32:479-84, October 1983.

Williams, P.; "Coffee Intake of Elevated Cholesterol and Apolepoprotein B Levels in Women"; *Journal of the American Chemical Society* 253:1407, 1985.

Winick, M., Editor; *Current Concepts in Nutrition, Volume 6: Nutrition and Cancer*; "Dietary Factors in Hormone-Dependent Cancers"; John Wiley & Sons (New York City), pp. 25-40, 1977.

Department of Health and Human Services; "Summary of Adverse Reactions Attributed to Aspartame"; April 20, 1995.

Food Network Website (http://www.foodtv.com/infood.htm). *In Food Today*; December 5, 1996; "New Estrogen Warning: Study Links Alcohol with Hormone Levels."

Journal of the American Dietetic Association 85:1, 127-132; "The Carcinogenicity of Caffeine and Coffee: A Review"; 1985.

Chapter 16: Power Teas

Austin, F.G.; "Schistosoma Mansoni Chemoprophylaxis With Dietary Lapachol"; *American Journal of Tropical Medicine and Hygiene* 23:412-419, 1979.

Bachun, N.R., S.L. Gordon, M.V. Gee, and H. Kon; "NADPH Cytochrome P-450 Reductase Activation of Quinone Anticancer Agents to Free Radicals"; *Proceedings of the National Academy of Science USA* 76:954-957, 1979.

Hardwell, J.I.; "Plants Used Against Cancer. A Survey"; in *The Book of Tea Okakura*, Shambala Publishing, by M.A. Lawrence, 1982.

Komori et al.; "Anticarcinogenic Activity of Green Tea Polyphenols"; *Japanese Journal of Clinical Oncology* 23(3):186-90, 1993.

McCarty, Meredith; *Fresh From a Vegetarian Kitchen*, Turning Point Publications, 1989.

Weed, Susun; *Breast Cancer? Breast Health! The Wise Woman Way*; Ash Tree Publishing (Woodstock, NY), 1996.

Let's Live, February 1985.

Vegetarian Time, July 1985.

Chapter 17: Mammography
Foods and Supplements That Offer Protection

Abrams, Martin B. et al.; "Early Detection and Monitoring of Cancer with the Anti-malignin Antibody Test"; *Cancer Detection and Prevention* 18(1):65-78, 1994.

"AMAS Review Published by the National Cancer Institute"; *Journal of Cell Biochemistry* 19:172-185, 1994.

Akizuki, Shinichiro; *Physical Constitution and Food*; pamphlet published by Dr. Akizuki and St. Francis Hospital (Hongen Machi 2-535, Nagasaki, Japan).

Ben-Amotz, A. et al.; *Radiation and Environmental Biophysics* 35:385-88, 1996.

Immen,Wallace; "Timing of Breast X-Rays Stressed: Accuracy Linked to Menstrual Cycle"; *The Globe and Mail*, Friday, August 15, 1997.

Kamen, Betty, Ph.D.; "Radiation, Detoxification, Immunity, and Chlorella: The One-Celled Wonder"; *Natural Food and Farming*, Vol. 33, No. 6, February 1987.

Keville, Kathi and Mindy Green; *Aromatherapy: A Complete Guide to the Healing Art*, The Crossing Press, 1995, pg.68.

Kushi, Aveline with Wendy Esko; *Macrobiotic Cancer Prevention Cookbook*; Avery Publishing,1988, p. 17.

Lucas, Richard; *Eleuthero (Siberian Ginseng), Health Herb of Russia*; R&M Books, 1973, pgs. 30-33.

Pelton, Ross, Pelton, Taffy Clarke, and Vinton C. Vint; *How To Prevent Breast Cancer: A Lifestyle Guide for the Prevention of Breast Cancer and Its Recurrence—With an Investigation of the Critical Risk Factors*, Fireside (New York City), 1995.

Pitchford, Paul; *Healing With Whole Foods: Oriental Traditions and Modern Nutrition*, North Atlantic Books, 1993, p. 73.

Scientific Proceedings for the 87th Annual Meeting of the American Association for Cancer Research, Washington, D.C., April 1996.

Sminia, P. et al.; "Hyperthermia, Radiation Carcinogenesis, and the Protective Potential of Vitamin A and N-Acetylcysteine"; *Journal of Cancer Research and Clinical Oncology* 122:343-350, 1996.

St. Clair, W.H., P.C. Billings, and A.R. Kennedy; "The Effects of the Bowman-Birk Protease Inhibitor on *c-myc* Expression and Cell Proliferation in the Unirradiated and Irradiated Mouse"; *Colon Cancer Letter* 52:145-152, 1990.

Weed, Susun; *Breast Cancer? Breast Health! The Wise Woman Way*; Ash Tree Publishing (Woodstock, NY), 1996.

Chapter 18: Secrets of a Healthy Kitchen

Bilger, Berkhard; "Guide to Fats"; *Health*, September1997.

Bittman, Mark; "Tangy Ways With Sea Scallops, Nature's Original Fast Food"; *New York Times*, September 24, 1997.

Bland, Jeffrey S., Ph.D.; "Cancer Fighting Foods: Natural Healing"; *Delicious!*, September 1997.

Brody, Jane E.; "Preventing Breast Cancer"; *New York Times*, May 7, 1997.

Brody, Jane E.; "Transfatty Acids Tied to Risk of Breast Cancer"; *New York Times*, October 14, 1997.

Brody, Jane; "What Is a Woman To Do To Avoid Breast Cancer? Plenty, New Studies Suggest"; *New York Times*, June 30, 1997.

Carper, Jean; *Food, Your Miracle Medicine*; Harper Perennial (New York City), 1993.

Epstein, Samuel S.; "Unlabelled Milk From Cows Treated With Biosynthetic Growth Hormones: A Case of Regulatory Abdication"; *International Journal of Health Services*, Vol. 26, No. 1, pp. 173-185, 1996.

Epstein, Samuel, M.D.; report for FDA Commissioner David Kessler, M.D; "Bovine Growth Hormone (BGH) May Increase the Risk of Breast Cancer"; 1994.

Fremerman, Sarah; "Goat Milk"; *Natural Health*, December 1997.

Halpern, G.M.; "Influence of Long-Term Yogurt Consumption in Young Adults"; *International Journal of Immunotherapy* VII(4):105-l0, 1991.

Harris, et al.; *New England Journal of Medicine* 7:473-480, 1992.

Kirschmann, Gayla J. and John. D. Kirschmann; *Nutrition Almanac, 4th Edition*; McGraw Hill (New York City), 1996.

Kolata, Gina; "Scientists Ease Up on Fears of Eggs"; *New York Times*, September 24, 1997.

Muse, Vance, *Self* magazine, September 1997.

Peterson, Cass; "The Jerusalem Artichoke"; *New York Times*, September 21, 1997.

Raloff, J.; "This Fat May Fight Cancer in Several Ways"; *Science News* 145(12):182-83, March :19, 1994.

Reddy, G.V.; "Antitumor Activity of Yogurt Compounds"; *Journal of Food Products* 46:8-11, 1983.

Sharoni, Y. et al.; "Effects of Lycopene Enriched Tomato Oleoresin on 7,12-dimethylbenz(l)anthracene-Induced Rat Mammary Tumors"; *Cancer Detect. Prev* 21(2):118-123, 1997.

Schoeneck, Annelies; *Making Sauerkraut and Pickled Vegetables at Home: The Original Lactic Acid Fermentation Method,* Alive Books (Vancouver),

Stevens, Richard G. et al.; "Dietary Effects on Breast Cancer"; *The Lancet* 338:186-87, July 20, 1991.

Stewart, J.C.; *Drinking Water Hazards,* Vol. 10; Ohio Envirographics, 1990.

Trichopoulou, Antonia; "Olive Oil and Breast Cancer"; *Cancer Causes and Control,* Vol. 6, 1995 (Harvard School of Public Health).

Van't Veer et al.; "Dietary Fiber, Beta-Carotene, and Breast Cancer. Results from a Case-Control Study"; *International Journal of Cancer* 45(5):82-88, 1990.

Weed, Susun; *Breast Cancer? Breast Health! The Wise Woman Way;* Ashtree Publishing (Woodstock, NY), 1996.

Yuan et al.; "Diet and Breast Cancer in Shanghai and Tianjin China"; *British Journal of Cancer* 71:1352-58, 1995.

Zara, David T.; *Nutrition and Cancer* 27:31-40, 1997.

Advances in Experimental Medicine and Biology, Vol. 401, 1996.

AICR; "Feast on Fruits and Vegetables"; 1995.

American Institute for Cancer Research; "Fruits and Vegetables Better Than Pills, Researchers Say"; Press Release, July 22, 1996.

American Journal of Public Health, Vol. 87, 1997.

International Journal of Health Services, January 1996.

Natural Health, January-February 1997.

New England Journal of Medicine 333(5):276-282, August 3, 1995.

PR Newswire; "Dana Farber Researchers Credit Processed Tomato Products With Reduced Cancer Risk"; March 12, 1997.

Science, Vol. 275, 1997.

Spectrum, March/April 1997.

Townsend Letter for Doctors and Patients; "Stop Breast Cancer in Its Tracks: Can Calcium D-Glucarate Reduce the Risk of Breast Cancer or Even Treat the Disease?"; May 1997.

Vogue, November 1997.

Xux, et al.; "Bioavailability of Soybean Isoflavones Depends Upon Gut Microflora in Women"; *Journal of Nutrition* 125:2307-15, 1995.

Chapter 19: Summary

Burros, Marian; "Folic Acid: Pop a Pill, or Eat the Food?"; *New York Times,* September 24, 1997.

Kohlmeier, Lenore et al.; "Adipose Tissue Transfatty Acids and Breast Cancer in the European Community Multicenter Study on Antioxidants, Myocardial Infarction, and Breast Cancer"; *Cancer Epidemiology, Biomarkers, and Prevention,* September 1997.

McCully, Kilmer S.; *The Homocysteine Revolution: Medicine for the New Millenium*, Keats Publishing(New Canaan, CT), May 1997.

Phillips, Roland C.; "Role of Lifestyle and Dietary Habits on Cancer Among 7th Day Adventists"; *Cancer Research* 35:3513-22, November 1975.

Stacey, Michelle; "The Fall and Rise of Kilmer McCully"; *New York Times*, August l0, 1997.

Zara, David T.; *Nutrition and Cancer* 27:31-40, 1997.

Chapter 20: Personal Care Guide

Ainsleigh, H.G.; "Beneficial Effects of Sun Exposure on Cancer Mortality"; *Prev. Med.* 22:132-40, 1993.

Belieu, Renee M., MD, FACOG; "Mastodynia"; *Obstetrics and Gynecology Clinics of North America* Vol. 21, No. 3, September 1994.

Bluchbauer, G. et al.; "Aromatherapy: Evidence for Sedative Effects of the Essential Oil of Lavender After Inhalation"; *Journal of Biosciences* Vol.46(11-120):1067-1072, 1991.

Boyle, W. and A. Saine; *Lectures in Naturopathic Hydrotherapy*, Buckeye Naturopathic Press (East Palestine, Ohio), 1988.

Brody, Jane; "What Is a Woman To Do To Avoid Breast Cancer? Plenty, New Studies Suggest"; *New York Times*, June 30, 1997.

Brody, Jane; "In Vitamin Mania, Millions Take Gamble on Health"; *New York Times*, October 26, 1997.

Brody, Jane; "How to Feel Fitter, Eat Better, Live Longer"; *The New York Times Book of Health*, 1997.

Colston, K.W. et al.; "Possible Role for Vitamin D in Controlling Breast Cancer Cell Proliferation"; *Cancer* 1:188-91, 1989.

Garland, F.C. et al.; "Geographic Variation in Breast Cancer Mortality in the United States: A Hypothesis Involving Exposure to Solar Radiation"; *Prev. Med.* 19:614-22, 1990.

Gateley, F.R.C.S., M. Miers, (Msc, RGN), R.E. Mansei (MS, FRCS), L.E. Hughes (D.S., FRCS); "Drug Treatments for Mastalgia: 17 Years' Experience in the Cardiff Mastalgia Clinic"; *Journal of the Royal Society of Medicine* ,Vol. 85, January 1992 (University of Wales College of Medicine, Heath Park, Cardiff, CF4 4XN).

Glucek, et al.; "Amelioration of Severe Migraine with Omega 3 Fatty Acids: A Double-blind Placebo-controlled Clinical Trial"; *American Journal of Clinical Nutrition* 43:710, 1986.

Gorham, E.D. et al.; "Sunlight and Breast Cancer Incidence in the U.S.S.R."; *International Journal of Epidemiology* 19820-24, 1990.

Hölzl, J.; "Constituents and Mechanism of Action of St. John's Wort", *Zeitschr. Phytocher* 14:255-65, 1993.

Itil, T.M., E. Eralp, E. Tsambis et al.; "Central Nervous System Effects of Ginko Biloba, a Plant Extract"; *American Journal of Therapeutics* 3:63-73, 1996.

Kolata, Gina; "Study Bolsters Idea That Exercise Cuts Breast Cancer Risk"; *New York Times*, May 1, 1997.

Kurfield, D.M., C.B. Welch, L.M. Lloyd et al.; "Inhibition of DMBA-Induced Mammary Tumorigenesis by Caloric Restriction in Rats Fed High-Fat Diet"; *International Journal of Cancer* 43:922-925, 1989.

Mayell, Mark; "25 Power Herbs"; *Natural Health Magazine*, October 1997.

Melchart, D., K. Linde, F. Worku et al.; "Immunomodulation With Echinacea— A Systematic Review of Controlled Clinical Trials"; *Phytomed* 1:245-54, 1994.

Simard, A. et al.; "Vitamin D Deficiency and Cancer of the Breast: An Unprovocative Ecological Hypothesis"; *Canadian Journal of Public Health* 82:300-303, 1991.

Thune, Inger, M.D., et al.; "Physical Activity and the Risk of Breast Cancer"; *New England Journal of Medicine* 336(18): 1269-1312, May 1997.

Weindruch, R., R.L. Walford, S. Fligiel, and D. Guthrie; "The Retardation of Aging in Mice by Dietary Restriction: Longevity, Cancer, Immunity, and Lifetime Energy Intake"; *Journal of Nutrition* 116:641-654, 1986.

Widhalm, K., J. Leibetseder, and M. Bavernfried; "Over- and Undernutrition in Europe"; *Proceedings of the Seventh European Nutrition Conference*, Austrian Nutrition Society, Vienna, May 1995.

AICR Special Release; "Fruits and Vegetables Better Than Pills, Researchers Say"; July 1996.

Advocate; "Researcher: Vitamin D May Help To Prevent Breast Cancer"; November 2, 1997.

Alternative Medicine Review, Vol. 2, No. 1, 1997.

Cancer Prevention News, Fall 1995; "Implants Pose Cancer Risk."

Chronic Pain Letter, Vol. XIII, No. 2, 1996; "Atypical Chest Pain Syndrome Associated With Breast Implants"; Box 1303, Old Chelsea Station, New York, NY 10011.

Diabetologia 40:344-47; "Vitamin D., Glucose Tolerance, and Insulinemia in Ederly Men"; 1997.

Health and Healing, Julian Whitaker, M.D.'s newsletter, July 1997, "Decrease Your Risk With Exercise."

Health Wisdom for Women Newsletter, Vol. 4, No. 6; "Reap the Benefits of Sunlight: Use Sun to Heal Your Body," June 1997.

Natural Health; "Ask the Experts," November/December 1997.

New York Times; "Study Finds Big Weight Gain Raises Risk of Breast Cancer"; November 5, 1997.

Southern Medical Journal 89:97-100, 1996. Correspondence: UCLA group, and Lousiana State University School of Medicine (New Orleans) group.

Townsend Letter for Doctors and Patients; "Breast Implants," April 1997.

INDEX

METRIC CONVERSION TABLE

1 teaspoon = 4.93 milliliters
1 tablespoon = 14.8 milliliters
1 fluid ounce = 29.6 milliliters
1 cup = .237 liter
1 pint = .48 liter
1 quart = 0.946 liter
1 gallon = 3.8 liters

Robin Keuneke has been a natural foods cook and counselor focusing on women's health for more than a decade. She is a frequent guest on holistic talk radio, both regionally and nationally, including the Dr. Robert Atkins and Gary Null shows. Keuneke is the Food Editor for *Total Health* magazine and has conducted workshops on women's health and food preparation at the National Gourmet Institute and Gullivers Macrobiotic Center in New York City, at the University of Connecticut, and at Danbury and Stanford Hospitals (in Connecticut).

Extensive travels bring a rich, multi-cultural perspective to Keuneke's recipes. She is also a fine artist whose work is in the permanent collection of the New York City Public Library, and her love of natural foods is expressed with an artist's touch.

Keuneke is a member of Chef's Collaborative 2000, a group of food writers and restaurant owners dedicated to personal health and the health of the planet. The members of Chef's Collaborative 2000 believe that vegetables, fruits, grains, beans, and breads are the foundations of both diet and health. The group is also dedicated to educating children about the relationships among food, health, and the environment. Chef's Collaborative 2000 is an education initiative of Oldways Preservation and Exchange Trust, in Cambridge, Massachusetts. The purpose of Oldways is to acknowledge the healthfulness of traditional diets (like the Asian and Mediterranean diets), and to educate people about their health benefits.

Keuneke's work is profiled in Gary Null's *Encyclopedia of Alternative Health* (Kensington Publishing). She lives in Connecticut with her husband Thomas.